# Free to Fly

## a journey toward wellness

*by*

### Judit Rajhathy

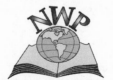

**New World Publishing**
P.O. Box 36075
Halifax, Nova Scotia
Canada B3J 3S9

The suggestions outlined in this book are recommendations, not prescriptions and are not intended as medical advice. Persons who are ill or on medications who wish to change their diet would be advised to contact a healthcare professional who understands the effects of diet on health. This book is meant to teach, not treat. The publishers regret that under no circumstances can they refer readers seeking medical advice to any of the medical practitioners or specialists mentioned in this book.

Although all sources have been thoroughly researched to ensure the accuracy and completeness of the information contained in this book, we assume no responsibility for errors, inaccuracies, omissions, or any inconsistency herein. Any slights of people or organizations are unintentional. All the characters in this book are fictitious. Any resemblance to actual persons, living or dead, is purely coincidental.

**Published by:**

New World Publishing, P. O. Box 36075, Halifax, N.S., Canada B3J 3S9

**Copyright** © 1999 New World Publishing ( Updated version )
© 1996 New World Publishing

Managing Editor: Francis G. Mitchell

Editors: Helen Lofgren, Michelle Paon, Peter A. Ackerman

Graphic Design/Illustration: Gizelle Erdei; 'toxic border' by Sandra Staple

Cover concept: Gizelle Erdei, Martha Kelder, Francis G. Mitchell, Judit Rajhathy

Layout & Typography: Francis G. Mitchell, R. Frederick Daugherty

Backcover photo: Florian Kuchurean, Photo 67, Halifax, N.S.

**Canadian Cataloguing-in-Publication Data**

Rajhathy, Judit
Free to Fly: a journey toward wellness

Includes bibliographical references and resource lists
ISBN 1-895814-04-9

1. Environmentally induced diseases -- Popular works. 2. Environmental
   health -- Popular works. 3. Self-care, Health. 4. Nutrition
   5. Chemicals-health aspects. 6. Sick building syndrome.

I. Title.    RA565.R34 1996                 613'.1                 C96-950027-0

Printed and bound in Canada on recycled paper  by *The Printer*, Halifax, N.S.
Printings: 1st - March, 1996);  2nd - October,1996;  3rd - November,1998 (updated version)

*For my children*
# Rachael and Jordan

*May this work contribute toward your
understanding of self-responsibility.*

*To you and your generation . . .
I pass the torch.*

*and to*

*each and every one of you who have struggled
for so long to find answers to your health problems
and who were told 'it's all in your head'!*

*In memory of my father, Dr. Tibor Rajhathy; my grandmother, ErzsébetRajhathy;
also young Aaron Dickson; Regine Stowe; and Arlene Zatzman*

## This book would not be complete without

# Special Thanks to:

My parents for their contribution to who I am today - my mother with her humor and my father with his insatiable thirst for knowledge.

My grandmother Erzsi Mami for showing me love and hope. My grandfather, Dr. Antal Weninger, for being an example of a truly holistic healer.

Janice Oliver, my dear friend, without whom I may not have survived. If it weren't for you, Janice, I might never have embarked on my own journey. Your ongoing support and encouragement have brought me through some difficult times. My thanks comes from the bottom of my heart!

Dr. William Crook for writing *The Yeast Connection*, the book that Janice pressed into my hands ten years ago - the same book that has helped thousands of others who never understood why they were so ill. Also, thank you for being the caring, loving person that you are.

Dr. Len Levine who started me on the road to recovery. Thank you for 'daring' to treat me through long distance phone calls and the postal system. You were instrumental in my first breakthrough.

Dr. Gerald Ross who actually listened, believed, and understood when I described my multiple symptoms on that memorable morning in New Minas, Nova Scotia. Since then, you have paved the way toward the understanding and acceptance of this condition and, along the way, have touched the lives of many.

Anna Protheroe, a fellow traveller, who gave so much of her time, patience and support when I took my first steps on my own path toward wellness.

Dr. David Rowland, publisher of *Health Naturally*, for teaching me that each of us must take responsibility for our own health. Thank you for providing me with the necessary tools and information so that I could share this knowledge with others. Thank you for providing unbiased, truthful nutritional information to the public. You are truly a great Canadian hero.

John Edmonds of Edmonds Environmental Services, Halifax, N.S., who heightened my awareness about the hazards of incinerators and chemical pesticides. Keep shining that organic light!

Jeff Schelew for planting the seed. Your idea of writing this book as a narrative was brilliant!

Dr. Doris Rapp for taking the time out of her busy schedule to write the foreword. Your work in helping children live fuller lives by identifying their sensitivities and encouraging them to adopt healthier lifestyles is invaluable. Thank you!

Dr. Carolyn Dean, for recognizing the value of *Free to Fly* and for writing the preface. You have brought the candida connection to the consciousness of many who would have otherwise fallen by the wayside. You are a true warrior in the relentless pursuit of truth. We need more physicians like you!

Drs. Theron Randolph, Albert Rowe, Herbert Rinkel, Marshall Mandell, William Rea, Orion Truss, John Maclennan, Jozef Krop, Marion Zazula, William LaValley, David Baker, Ross Mickelson, Jonathan Brostoff, George Lewith, Julian Kenyon, Ronald Greenberg, George Barber, Stuart Berger, Dean Ornish, Leo Galland, James Braly, Steven Gislason, Linus Pauling, Lendon Smith, Abram Hoffer, Richard Mackarness, Jean Munro, David Collison, Zoltan Rona, Carolyn DeMarco, Roy Fox, Patricia Beresford, Bruce Elliott, John Heisler and many others, who, like medical detectives, search for the underlying causes of ill health.

Dr. Carolee Bateson-Koch, for writing *Allergies: Disease In Disguise*, which offers one of the more comprehensive overviews of many of the underlying causes of chronic illness, and for showing me how it all fits together. Your formula has helped change many lives. Thank you again.

Dr. Elisabeth Gold, my personal physician. You continue to learn and grow by being open and listening to your patients. It truly is a gift. Thank you.

My many clients over the years who served as my true teachers, and who allowed me to participate in their own journeys toward wellness. You have taught me so much. Thank you.

Kathleen Helene Enders, author of *The Canary*, the poem that inspired the cover of this book. It was first published in *Esprit*, the magazine of the Evangelical Lutheran Women of Canada. Your words will resonate deep in the hearts of many for years to come.

Colleen MacLeod in Port Hood, Cape Breton, for her relentless search for better health for all those around her. You are a prime example of self-responsibility!

My dear friends Kiara Andrews, Bonnie Shubaly, Linda Goldwater and Karen Schlick for supporting my growth over the years; Helen Anne Bassani for her continual encouragement; and Margot Schelew, whose intelligence, honesty and directness I shall always treasure.

David Chilton, author of *The Wealthy Barber*, for taking time from his hectic life to talk to me about his experience in publishing. Your book inspired me to 'get down and do it'!

Groups such as Citizens for Choice in Health Care; My Health, My Rights; the Allergy and Environmental Health Association; Back to Basics; American Pie; Northwest Coalition for Alternatives to Pesticides; and other groups providing the public with information on complementary practices. A special thank you to Maggie Burston, founder and director of *Candida Research and Information Service*, for endlessly researching the role of fungus and parasites in human health and passing on the information to so many others.

All the health food stores and holistic health publications worldwide who offer us alternatives and encourage us to take responsibility for our own health.

Jackie Hart, Elizabeth Wuerr, Sheila Cole, Mary-Celine Ronayne, Gail Sardin, Kim Harper-Given and Lois Hare, for reviewing and critiquing various sections of the book. Your comments were very helpful.

Helen Lofgren, Peter Ackerman, and Michelle Paon who spent countless hours editing, commenting, and proofing - often under very tight timelines. Your skills, suggestions and positive energy kept the juices flowing! Helen, your enthusiasm and knowledge in the area of environmental health was invaluable! Michelle, your eye for the smallest detail and your support, especially given the pressures and constraints of time, was truly appreciated.

Jordan Schelew, my junior editor, age ten! Thank you for your interest in your Mom's work and your ability to see and hear words when they're misplaced.

To Rachael Schelew and her friends Jaime, Hilary, Cindy and Amy for their patience in listening to me read some of the earlier drafts.

Dr. Virginia Salares at Canada Mortgage and Housing Corporation, and Mr. Robin Barrett, president of Healthy Homes Consulting, for reviewing the chapters *Sleeping with the Enemy* and *For Whom the Bell Tolls*. Also, Melanie Briand and the Ecology Action Centre for providing valuable information for *Garden of Eden, Revisited*.

Martha Kelder, an art therapist, who helped elicit the background image for the cover; Sandra Staple, a young artist and high school student who created the 'toxic border' that surrounds the quote by Rachel Carson at the end; and a special thanks to Gizelle Erdei, an excellent artist and graphic designer whose ideas and skillfulness helped make the cover better than I had ever imagined it could be. It was fun working with you on the graphics. Thank you so much!

Fred Daugherty for his editorial suggestions as well as his technical expertise in formatting and overall book production; Max Moulton for scanning some of the illustrations for the book and video editing; Philip Durant for his patience, advice and help with the production of the manuscript, often on very short notice.

And last, but not least Francis Mitchell, co-publisher, project manager, chief editor, taskmaster, and dear friend, without whom this book may never have been brought to fruition - certainly not as quickly! You stood by me through thick and thin, and believed in this project from beginning to end. Your enthusiasm, original ideas, wise advice and general all around support and passionate commitment parallels none other! Thank you.

I am forever grateful.

# Preface

I first met Judit Rajhathy at health seminars I gave in Halifax, Nova Scotia during the late eighties.

That first year, she was performing detective work on her own health and that of her children. The following year she was studying nutrition; and the next time I saw her, she had a cable television show called 'It's Your Health', and I was one of her guests. And now, Judit has invented Jillian in *Free to Fly*, successfully transferring all that she learned over the past decade into an extremely readable and useful book.

*Free to Fly* is ten books rolled into one, which in itself is a very wise investment. It leaves no stone unturned. Often, a chronically ill person has to go on a very long journey to find the cause of their illness. With this book as a guide, the journey is shortened considerably. Most causes of modern day chemical sensitivities, allergies, as well as physical and even mental imbalances, are detailed and dissected, along with solutions and suggested therapies. All bases are covered - nothing is missed.

What I find appalling is that ninety-five percent of the information in *Free to Fly* was not available to me in medical school. As far as I can tell, it is still not available and may, indeed be frowned upon by the conventional medical community. In spite of the fact that our environment is now inundated by such an overwhelming array of additives, pesticides, herbicides, cleaning products, and so on, few doctors make the connection between these chemicals and our poor health. And since medicine is a monopoly, frustrated patients must depend on books such as *Free to Fly* in order to improve their lives.

Conditions such as candidiasis, a yeast overgrowth commonly brought on by the overuse of antibiotics, the birth control pill, or a highly refined sugar and white flour diet are also going unrecognized and under-diagnosed. It is important to realize that repeated vaginal yeast infections in women are symptomatic of a much deeper imbalance. This kind of inner ecological imbalance can produce symptoms from head to toe. For example, there are seventy-nine different toxins that yeast can produce in its life cycle. One is aldehyde which can damage the liver and cause mood swings. Another is alcohol, high enough to be detected by a Breathalyzer. Still other toxins include pseudo-hormones that can either block or enhance estrogen. And as if that weren't enough, some of these toxins can even mimic neurotransmitters that affect the brain. Symptoms from the growth of this yeast in the gut range from diarrhea to constipation. If your tongue has a white coating, your entire intestinal tract may be similarly affected. Malnutrition and chronic arthritis are only two examples out of hundreds of what a yeast overgrowth can do to your digestion, absorption and assimilation.

Chronic parasitic infections are now endemic in our 'civilized' world. In New York City, where I live, the water supply is known to be infested with several types of parasites. Everyone is potentially exposed! Parasites are even more dangerous than candidiasis. These organisms can migrate to vital organs and can cause ongoing damage. They even produce toxins that can paralyse or stimulate the gut. And when one has parasites, worms are often not far behind. We are seeing more and more cases of worm infestation today. These creatures migrate to the lungs and liver as well. Now, if the body were in balance - if it weren't already compromised by drugs and chemicals - it would stand a chance of combating these organisms. However, it is precisely that imbalanced state that favors their growth.

When asked why more physicians aren't like Dr. Rowland in the book, I am ashamed to say that conventional medical boards, run entirely by conventional medical doctors, investigate other doctors who practice this type of medicine and either scare them into reverting back to conventional approaches, or threaten to remove their licenses. Any young doctor who wants to keep his or her license, is warned not to dabble in unconventional practices. What would you do? It takes a 'saint' to fight this type of monopoly. And these 'saints' need your active help and support - because *you* already know the consequences. It takes medicine twenty to twenty-five years to recognize a new condition. We don't have that long! We are suffering the effects of ecological imbalance *right now*.

*We Are The Experiment* is the title of a book I thought I might write one day. But I think Judit has done it - done it better than I could. Since she has lived this experience, she is especially capable of sounding the alarm and offering solutions. She has recognized not only the impact of bad diets and chemicals on our children, but also how quickly the situation can be reversed so that healing can take place. However, you have to recognize the problem before you can find a cure.

Read this book thoroughly, seek out a sympathetic practitioner, follow what is advised. Then, when you feel stronger and more energetic, do what Judit did. Turn your attention to the underlying problems in a society that is poisoning us and demand changes before it is too late.

*Carolyn Dean, BSc., M.D.*

Dr. Carolyn Dean, a graduate of the School of Medicine at Dalhousie University in Halifax, Nova Scotia, practiced complementary medicine in Toronto, Canada for twelve years and now lives in New York where she does clinical research in homeopathic acupuncture. She is the author of *When You Can't Reach the Doctor, Complementary Natural Prescriptions for Common Ailments, Homeopathic Remedies for Children's Common Ailments,* and *Menopause Naturally.*

# Foreword

The trials and tribulations of Jillian Stowe, the main character in *Free to Fly*, accurately reflect the frustrations that face an ever-increasing number of environmentally ill adults and children in our society today.

Even though physicians might not have answers to these problems, this book can provide you with practical suggestions and direction. After some initial physical improvement, psychologists or counsellors may, at times, be needed to cope with the secondary effects often noted in individuals who have been chronically ill and misunderstood for years. The basic challenge, however, is to find out *why* you are ill, and this is exactly what *Free to Fly* helps you to do.

Many families are too ill to seek the help they need. Often parents, and even children believe that their illness is their fault - that if they were only "better" in some way, they would not be ill. It is not a question of bad parents or bad children - many simply have a health problem that has not been recognized. And the answers are not more expensive drugs, or another trip to the medicine cabinet. The ultimate answer is to study, read and pray that you will find, or be directed to, the right health information and provider.

*Free to Fly* clearly and realistically shows you that you can find viable alternatives - better ways to help yourself. You may have to crawl slowly at first, but in time, you'll be able to run freely and feel truly well, perhaps for the first time in years. Remember, no one knows you or your children as well as you do. Find a physician or other qualified health care professional who is familiar with your type of medical complaint and one who has guided others along the paths that this book discusses.

*Free to Fly* will help you recognize the cause of your ill health. Then, try an elimination diet, alter your home environment, improve your nutrition, avoid chemicals, and find someone who knows some of the newer, more precise ways of testing and treatment. These changes will make a difference in your health - in your life.

The information in this book will help not only your immediate family, but also your circle of friends and acquaintances who are faced with the same patterns of illness and the same skeptical opposition from colleagues, health professionals and educators. Knowing that you may face these kinds of attitudes will help prepare you for what's ahead. Just as Jillian Stowe experiences symptoms of withdrawal in this book, it's important to keep in mind that certain therapies, such as a change in diet, can initially make you feel worse. You must understand that this response is only temporary and will ultimately lead you to a much better level of health. With patience and knowledge, many have overcome both serious health challenges and opposition from those around them.

It is not uncommon for individuals who have Environmental Illness, or food and chemical sensitivities, to go through a process of denial or anger, and even to refuse to accept what they've been told. This may be true for you or someone close to you. However, following a period of increased awareness, it is possible to relax, enjoy and give thanks for the changes in your life. Most people merely need some practical direction and advice.

*Free to Fly* will take you on a journey that will open the door to better health and provide the answers that you wish you had known many years ago.

*Doris Rapp, M.D., F.A.A.A., F.A.A.P.*

Dr. Doris Rapp is a board-certified Pediatric Allergist and one of North America's leading specialists in Environmental Medicine. Dr. Rapp has appeared on numerous national television and radio shows and has lectured to physicians at national and international medical conferences, furthering the significance of the role that environment has on health, learning and behavior. Dr. Rapp is well-known, especially throughout school systems, for her books and videos on environmental health.

# Table of Contents

# Table of Contents

# Introduction

Like the canaries of long ago that were taken deep beneath the earth to warn miners of noxious fumes, a new generation of human canaries is now sounding an alarm for the rest of society - warning of the environmental hazards that we've created.

This I know only too well. Ten years ago, I joined the ranks of the human canaries.

After the birth of my second child, I became chronically ill, developing one infection after another. My doctors had one solution - medication, medication, and more medication. After endless rounds of oral and intravenous antibiotics, I became fatigued, experienced mood swings, headaches and yeast infections that never cleared up and was diagnosed with an irritable bowel. Like Jillian in *Free to Fly*, I was plagued with a new symptom every few days - yet all my tests were negative. In fact, medically, I was declared the picture of health. Sound familiar?

While all this was going on with me, my three year old was becoming increasingly ill-tempered, demanding and stubborn. On some days she seemed fine, yet on others it was one tantrum after another. The unpredictability was puzzling and frustrating. As she was my first-born, I thought it was normal, a 'phase' she would soon outgrow. On top of this, I felt an ongoing concern over my newborn son's chronic congestion and ear infections. Many days, I was reduced to a crumpled, sobbing heap. The diagnosis - post-partum blues and stress. Wrong.

*Free to Fly* is a culmination of my own study, research and experiences over the past ten years. Ill health is *not* a natural state of being and in most cases, can be reversed simply by identifying and eliminating the underlying causes - and not by merely suppressing symptoms through drug therapy.

*Free to Fly* is also a result of the journeys of many others, including my family, friends and clients - comprised largely of parents and children with chronic health problems - who have allowed me to walk beside them and listen to their stories. *Free to Fly* is also influenced by my many years of giving educational seminars on environmental health. The more anecdotes I added to my presentations, the more connections my audiences made. Only then did I fully realize how starved the public was for such information. Twenty-four months ago, I decided to put these thoughts and feelings on paper so you, too, could make these connections.

*Free to Fly* is first and foremost a teaching book - a primer on environmental health and nutrition. In choosing to write this book I felt the narrative style would make the subject more personal, more enjoyable - more easily understood. Through her story, I invite you to become involved in Jillian's journey - to learn as she learns. Each chapter probes a little deeper into the reasons for her symptoms - symptoms you, or those close to you, may have in common. It is also my hope that your children will be helped. The beauty of the approach I've outlined in *Free to Fly* is that results are experienced quickly - often within weeks, sometimes within only days!

I wrote *Free to Fly* not as a nutritionist, doctor, scientist or toxicologist. I am first and foremost a mother, sister, friend and neighbor who is deeply concerned about what we, the caretakers of this earth, have created and the legacy we will leave for our children. For it is they who must ultimately bear the brunt of our negligence. The reality is that we live in a toxic world. And in our denial, we assume that environmental deterioration is something in the distant future. What we don't realize is that the future is *now*. We *are* being affected now.

Medicated as never before, our children suffer from chronic conditions in epidemic proportions. Thirty years ago, allergies, asthma, ear infections and behavior problems were the exception; today, they're household words. Food and chemical sensitivities are growing in frequency, as are chronic fatigue and systemic yeast overgrowth. Even 'sick building syndrome' has become an all-too-familiar phrase.

Despite this alarming state of affairs, too many health professionals continue to operate in denial. Rather than find the root cause of illness, patients are encouraged to use prescription drugs to allay their symptoms, often making situations far worse. And when modern medicine has no answer, you may recognize this reply: "There's nothing more we can do for you" or "It's all in your head" - and off we're shipped to the nearest psychiatrist or child psychologist!

As a society, we've become conditioned to entrust our health to the experts - to government and the healthcare community - believing that they ultimately must know what's best for us. *Free to Fly* explodes this myth and many others perpetuated by our over-medicated society in an increasingly contaminated world. It seems that the more I learn, the more frightened I become. But we *need* to be frightened. We *need* to pay attention. We mustn't wait until we are all too sick to make changes, to make a difference. The time is now - *your* time is now.

And there *are* answers. The growing field of environmental medicine has identified many of the factors that contribute to our general ill health. Along with complementary practices, such as diet therapy, orthomolecular nutrition and a wide variety of other modalities, many are finding their way to wellness.

You, too, can begin your journey - right now, and *Free to Fly* can serve as your guide. It will take you on a learning curve from the conventional allopathic approach to medicine to a new and intriguing world of empowering alternatives. For those of you who wish to pursue the subject further, I've included a comprehensive reading and resource list. It is my hope that *Free to Fly* will be the book that changes the way that you, and your health caregivers, view sickness and health. Ask questions, listen, read, research . . . don't take no for an answer. If you're not being heard, move on. Find a health practitioner who will listen. But more important, listen to yourself, your intuition. Trust your instincts. They are usually right. Taking ownership of your health is a quantum leap - from wanting to be fixed to fixing yourself. It requires education to make intelligent choices and, ultimately, to take full responsibility for your own health.

So, I challenge each and every one of you to walk the path with Jillian, and I honor you for having the courage to do so. Any journey begins with a first step, and once you've taken yours, you'll never look back.

*Judit*

*Wellness*

*is a*

*Journey . . .*

*not a*

*Destination*

# The Canary

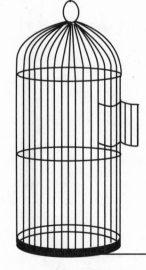

Born to fly
freely, soaring in the open breezes
with the light of the sun on its wings,
gliding in the updrafts of warm air
or sailing back to earth.  In joy
the canary sings.

Imprisoned, caged,
deep in the darkness of the mines,
a sentinel of danger in the stifling air,
drooping from the heat, feathers ruffled,
choking on poisoned air.  Miners warned,
the canary dies.

Born to live
freely, experiencing life's wholeness,
my spirit, soaring in the majesty
of mountains and skies, finds peace
in Earth's beauty, God's presence.  Rejoicing,
my soul sings.

Sickened, hemmed in
by walls invisible to unseeing eyes,
a sentinel of danger in our polluted world,
choking on the products of technology's
good life.  Take heed, be warned,
I am a canary.

**Kathleen Helene Enders**

First published in *Esprit*, May-June, 1990

*You are ultimately responsible*
*for your own health.*
*Your body has an incredible,*
*inborn ability*
*to*
*heal itself*
*-if given the conditions*
*it needs to do so . . .*

*There are many ways*
*to restore health,*
*and the more you know about them,*
*the more informed choices*
*you can make.*

David Rowland, Ph.D., Publisher
Health Naturally

# 1

# Devastation

*Modern medicine saved my life but couldn't make me well.*
**Wally Hersey, transplant recipient**

*I*'m sorry Jillian, there's nothing more I can do for you," sighed Dr. Klamer, avoiding eye contact as she closed my file. "We've done everything medically possible and all your tests have come back negative. Aside from sending you for a psychiatric consultation, I have nothing else to offer."

I felt like the floor had just dropped from under me.

A lump formed in my throat. "But . . . my problem is my *body* . . . not my mind," I stammered. "How's a psychiatrist going to help me?"

Dr. Klamer was my third family doctor in the last three years. At this point it was apparent I was no further ahead with her than I'd been with the previous two, not to mention the countless specialists I'd seen.

Since my youngest child Max was born, every morning began with pain. My joints hurt, my head ached, my sinuses were constantly infected, my stomach was always full of gas and bloated. I was freezing all the time and my hair had even started to fall out! Before Max's birth, I'd never had a weight problem. Now I was a good thirty-five pounds overweight, and diets just weren't working. Perfumes I once loved now smelled repulsive. Just the odor of fabric softener from a neighbor's dryer vent was enough to sicken me as I walked down the street.

I was falling apart and no one could help me.

Worst were the mood swings, chronic depression, and a total inability to focus on even the simplest tasks. It felt like my very being was deteriorating. I knew I was in real trouble when I couldn't grasp what I'd just read in my daughter's third grade reader. At times, I felt so spaced out that I blanked completely when asked for simple information over the phone, like my address or telephone number. Other times I'd drive down a street and wonder where I was. Was I going senile?

Most frightening were the panic attacks, overpowering waves of anxiety. My heart would race so fast I could feel it in my throat. Out of the blue, I'd be petrified of just about anything that crossed my mind. Even the thought of making the next meal was too much. I felt overwhelmed. There were times when I couldn't bear to leave the house. The thought of running into someone - anyone - and having to deal with them was more than I could handle.

God! What was happening to me? Maybe I was going insane.

When I did bump into someone I knew, it usually turned into a disaster. They smelled of cigarette smoke, perfume or some other scent I couldn't tolerate. I was tired of making excuses for my quick exits, and then later, apologizing.

"Jillian, I don't doubt that something is wrong, but over the past year you've been seen by so many different specialists. You've been to a neurologist for your migraines, not one but two gynecologists for recurrent yeast infections and pelvic pain, a urologist for bladder infections and a gastroenterologist for your bowels. We've checked your blood repeatedly and nothing shows. You've had two surgeries over the past five years for your sinuses . . ."

Yeah, I thought to myself. Two operations later, after having been assured that the problem would be resolved, I was still suffering. At least I got a new nose out of the last deal!

" . . . and after numerous tests and hospitalizations, you've been given a clean bill of health. Maybe you have that Epstein-Barr virus or some kind of Chronic Fatigue Syndrome. There's not much more I can do for you other than to advise lots of rest and possibly more medication to keep your symptoms under control."

Dr. Klamer folded her hands on the desk, looked at me and continued, "What more can I do? Do *you* have any other suggestions?"

Deep down, I was sure I had some dreadful disease - a tumor growing somewhere that was causing all these bizarre symptoms. I'd heard horror stories about people whose cancer had been repeatedly misdiagnosed until it was too late.

I had no obvious reason to be depressed, irritable or to have panic attacks. Michael, my partner of thirteen years, was a good husband and a great father to our three children. We had no financial worries. I was lucky to be able to take a leave from nursing to stay home with the kids. Aside from my sickness and the typical stresses that accompany family life, our lives were as 'normal' as the next.

"Look, I'm desperate! I can't go on this way anymore." The floodgates opened. "This isn't a life . . ." I sobbed. "There are times I can't even remember my own name! Do you have any idea what it's like to go to the grocery store and not remember why you're there? As if that's not enough, then I get violently ill just from being in the place. There are days my body hurts so much I don't know how I'll survive from one hour to the next. How would you like to be so sick you don't know if you'll make it out of bed? It's like a living death! Dr. Klamer, can't you see why I'm so upset?" My body heaved with sobs. "I can't stand it - not a minute longer! I've got to get well! My kids need a mother! And I don't care what you think, I *know* I'm not crazy!"

Dr. Klamer's expression softened. Her voice was quiet. "What I'm suggesting is that you at least give this last route a chance. Who knows, maybe it'll provide us with some answers."

"You think I've flipped - that I've lost it!" I cried, through my tears.

"Jillian, I don't think that's the issue. Dr. Hendrikson doesn't just do ordinary psychiatric work. He specializes in patients with chronic conditions. At this point we can't afford to dismiss the stress factor. I'd feel better, and for your own peace of mind, let's give it a try."

I felt defeated. Wiping my eyes with a Kleenex, I gathered my things to leave. It was a good thing I had worn a pair of sunglasses. No one would notice my swollen eyes.

As I walked toward the door, Dr. Klamer looked up and said, "Meredith will call you with an appointment. I'll try to get you in as soon as possible." I nodded in resignation and left, walking very slowly and feeling very depressed.

Something awful was happening to me.

When I was at my worst, I felt like a candidate for the mental hospital. I tried my best to hide it from Michael and the kids. They never knew the depth of my pain and despair. I knew deep down, though, that whatever was making me so sick was *physical*. I was sure - call it gut instinct or female intuition - that my *body* was betraying me, not my mind.

The thought of seeing another doctor was overwhelming. I'd have to go over my history yet again and my file was already as thick as a Russian novel. Reading it was a doctor's nightmare and a hypochondriac's delight. It contained just about every symptom imaginable.

I'd become reluctant to discuss my health with family and friends. My complaints were a standing joke - the 'oh no, here she goes again' routine. They were so tired of hearing about my aches and pains that they would often change the subject or even leave the room. As bad as it was not knowing what was wrong with me, the isolation was much worse. I was devastated that no one believed I was so sick.

On the outside I looked quite healthy. On the inside, I felt like the walking dead. My brother, the worst offender, would say things like, "Jilly, you're always complaining. Why don't you just get on with life? Live it fully and forget about every little ache and pain. You're too intense. Enjoy!"

I felt so alone.

To make matters worse, it seemed that lately no one close to me could do anything right. I was so irritable and impatient with Michael and the kids that they avoided me at all cost. Their faces were so solemn, as if waiting for the next round of criticism. I just couldn't seem to help my erratic behavior. The unpredictability was frightening - for everyone. I knew things were rapidly deteriorating the day Michael ducked as I moved a cleaver from one counter to the other.

I was desperate for help.

The more medication I took for my aches and pains, the sicker I became. It was a vicious cycle - I would get an infection, take an antibiotic, become weaker, start a new infection, take yet another antibiotic and feel even worse. It never ended. I was given pain killers for my headaches, laxatives and anti-inflammatory drugs for my bowels, antihistamines, decongestants, and steroid nasal sprays for my sinuses. Our bathroom looked like a drug store. Little Max was on a similar treadmill. He suffered from constant ear infections and spent a good part of his first two years on antibiotics, looking paler and sicker by the week. Many of our days were spent in doctors' offices trying to figure out why we were always ill. We both caught every virus that was on the go and all too often spent our evenings in the emergency department of our local hospital.

I don't know why I had agreed to see a psychiatrist. I knew there was nothing wrong with my mind. I really was *physically* sick. Just because no one knew what I had, did not mean it didn't exist. As I drove home, I rehearsed for the upcoming session by inventing reasons for my depression just so I'd have something to talk about. How absurd! And all this just to please my doctor.

I decided not to tell Michael about the appointment with Dr. Hendrickson. Quite frankly, I felt humiliated and embarrassed.

Tomorrow was September 3rd. After being able to sleep in all summer, I prayed for enough energy to be able to get up with the kids every morning. School started awfully early.

What was going to become of me?

*I am a great believer in
freedom of choice
in health care.
To have this freedom,
you must have information.*

*I also believe
that responsibility for health
does not belong to doctors,
other health care practitioners,
insurance companies, lawyers
or the government.*

*It belongs to the individual.*

Zoltan P. Rona, M.D., M.Sc.
Return to the Joy of Health

# 2

# The Meeting

*When the student is ready, the teacher will appear.*
anonymous

$\mathcal{D}$aybreak came only too soon. Typical morning sounds filtered into my consciousness - the shower on full blast, Michael belting out yet another Elvis song. At least someone over the age of ten was bright and energetic! There were times I felt jealous that Michael seemed so damned healthy. At the same time, I thanked God we both weren't sick. Other than a few digestive problems and the occasional headache, he really didn't seem to be plagued with anything out of the ordinary.

Slowly, I dragged myself out of bed, washed, dressed, and made my way into the kitchen. Although in pain, I tried my best to be cheerful - at least for the children's sake.

Excited about their first day back at school, the usual 'you're looking at me the wrong way' fights were forgotten. Nathaniel was guzzling down his regular two glasses of milk, while trying to wash an apple for recess.

Emma, between bites of toast, asked, "Mommy, are you walking us to school?"

"Of course, sweetheart. I wouldn't miss your first day back at school for the world!" It was the least I could do, considering my inability to be a full-time parent this past summer.

"Thkool! Thkool!" shrieked Max from his booster seat, blueberries dripping out of his cherubic little mouth. He was as excited as the other two.

"Has anybody seen the camera?" I asked. Every September, I'd made it a tradition to photograph all three kids in the same pose on our front verandah. It was our version of a growth chart.

As I took their picture, I couldn't believe how it seemed like only yesterday that Nathaniel had started kindergarten. Now here he was, tall and lanky, wearing a baseball cap and a big, black pair of Doc Martens. Where did the time go?

"All right, everybody, let's go!" I shouted, wiping faces and putting Max in his stroller. We headed off to the school, a few blocks away.

Nathaniel ran off with his friends as soon as we rounded the corner. Emma gave me some last minute hugs and kisses at the sound of the first bell. "See you at lunchtime, Mom," she shouted as she skipped to the line with her little friends. My eyes brimmed with tears as I watched her class go into the building. How many summers would I miss due to this horrible illness that no one believed I had?

After the doors closed, I wandered over to the playground so Max could play on the swings and slide. Feeling tired, fat and bloated, I settled in the shade of a tree while I let Max run loose. His favorite pastime was chasing butterflies.

I had just started to daydream when I heard "Whee! Up to the sky! Let's go higher and higher!" accompanied by screeches and giggles. I turned my head and saw a young woman swing high up, almost to the treetops! She had long auburn hair and held a little girl not much older than Max. The two of them were having such fun! The young woman looked so alive, vital, healthy. In comparison, I felt like a beached whale.

I watched her as she jumped off the swing, hoisted the child onto her shoulders, and began walking in my direction. She sat down next to me.

"Isn't it a great day?"

"I guess." I must have sounded flat.

She tried again. "I'm Jane. And this is Abby." She squinted from the glare of the morning sun, shielding her eyes with one hand. "Say hello, Abby."

"Hew-wo." Her reply was accompanied by a wide grin.

I couldn't help but smile back at her. She was a petite child with beautiful dark curls and large deep-set brown eyes. Her skin was as flawless as her mother's. She ran over to where Max was playing.

"She's so sweet . . . I'm Jillian and that's my son, Max. How old is Abby?"

"She's three and a bit. And your son?"

"Max just turned three, although he thinks he's ten!"

Jane threw her head back and laughed heartily, "They do want to grow up quickly, don't they?"

I nodded. "Imagine, in just a couple of years, their freedom will be history."

"That's right. Twelve years of noses to the grindstone! Structure, discipline, here we come!"

"There's a bit of sadness in that, don't you think?" I had an image of a bird with its wings clipped.

She nodded in agreement, smiling at Max and Abby playing together in the sandbox. "Just look at them . . . I think Abby's found a new friend." For a few moments, no one spoke. We just watched the kids.

Jane broke the silence. Her voice was subdued. "They're right where they need to be - in the moment - spontaneous, fresh."

"Yeah," I sighed wistfully. "They have no agenda - they just *are* ! We should be so lucky."

Jane smiled. "We *can* be like that - even as adults - if we choose to be. *Everything in life is a choice.* It's something I learned from one of my teachers years ago that has remained with me ever since."

"And you must be all of twenty-nine!" I exclaimed.

"Are you kidding? I'm probably older than you. I had my kids later in life. So late, in fact, that my husband tells everyone Abby was conceived by osmosis! I have a daughter in her first year of high school."

"I hope you don't mind me asking, but how old *are* you?"

"I'm forty-three . . ."

"I find that hard to believe! You don't look a day over thirty!"

"Why, thank you," smiled Jane.

"And where do you get all your energy? I'm lucky if I can make it through the day."

"I've never felt better in my entire life. Actually, I feel more alive in my forties than I ever did in my teens and twenties."

"What's your secret?" I really wanted to know the answer. Had she discovered the fountain of youth? "How do you do it? I can barely keep up with life, let alone the kids. I feel like everything's passing me by - like an old movie - and I'm missing it all." I felt a wave of sadness wash over me. I choked back my tears, looking down at the ground. "Have you ever felt like that?"

Jane stared off into the distance. It was as if she had gone back to a time that obviously wasn't filled with the vitality and joy she now exuded. Had she not always felt this vibrant?

"Ah, yes," she said softly. "I call it the 'black hole', the time in my life I choose to forget . . ." Her voice trailed off. She glanced at her watch.

"Oh, gosh! I've gotta run. But, before I do, let me write down the name of the doctor who helped me change my life. I should tell you, he lives near Springvale, in this nothing little place, but I can assure you it may well be the most important trip you'll ever take. You'll never look back." She scribbled a name and number on the back of a grocery receipt and passed it to me.

Quickly she cleaned off Abby's hands and feet. "It was great meeting you. Maybe I'll see you again. Good luck!" I watched her literally skip down the street, swinging little Abby's hand, her hair shimmering in the bright sunlight.

"God!" I thought to myself. "Give me even a third of that woman's energy and I'd have it made!"

I put the crumpled piece of paper in my pocket, gathered up Max and began our walk home.

That night, I told Michael about Jane. He rolled his eyes and muttered, "Not another miracle worker! And way out near Springvale, besides. How come we haven't heard of this doctor if he's as good as she claims? And why would someone so great be practicing out in the boonies?"

In the end, he simply said, "Look, if you feel this guy can help, go for it. You don't know till you try. But don't get your hopes up. We've been through this too many times for it to happen again. I just don't want you to be disappointed."

What did I have to lose? I must admit, I dreaded the thought of handing my file over to yet another doctor. But something told me this time might be different.

The next morning, I picked up the phone and, with some hesitation, dialled the number. A pleasant voice answered, "Bridgeport Wellness Clinic. How may I help you?"

"Hello. I'd like to make an appointment with Dr. Rowland."

"Have you seen Dr. Rowland before?"

"No, this will be my first time."

"Hmm. Just hold one moment please." I could hear pages rustling. Then she said, "How about Friday, December 3rd at 1:30?"

I nearly fainted. "December 3rd!" I exclaimed. "Why such a long wait? I thought Dr. Rowland was a G.P., not a specialist."

"He is, but Dr. Rowland is one of the few holistic physicians in the area and a three month waiting list is really not that unusual."

I sighed. "Well, I guess I'll just have to wait." I felt disappointed but determined. "Book me in."

"You'll take the December 3rd appointment?"

"Yes."

I gave her my name, address and telephone number. This time, I could actually remember them.

She continued. "The appointment with Dr. Rowland will take an hour. Then, after a half-hour break, you'll be seen by our nutritional consultant who will advise you in-depth about your diet. Count on a minimum of two and a half hours at the clinic. We'll send some forms and a fee schedule to you today. Do you have some paper and a pen handy?"

"Yes. Just a moment." I wondered where I would find these sacred tools in a house with three kids who love to borrow. I dug them out of the junk drawer. "Okay, I'm ready to roll!"

"This questionnaire should be completed and mailed back to us at least two weeks before your appointment. The first section requires a detailed history of your health, from infancy. The second part asks for a family health history, including your mother, father, grandparents, siblings, nephews, nieces, and your children, if you have any. Third, we need you to describe the environment in which you currently live and work; and the last part asks for a detailed dietary description for any three day period between now and your appointment. Also, list all your symptoms in order of severity. The more information you can provide, the better."

"Believe me, I've gathered enough data about myself to fill a book!" I exclaimed, thinking of the enormous health file I'd accumulated over the past few years.

"And we ask that you not wear perfumes or any scented personal care products whatsoever. Many of our patients are very sensitive and cannot tolerate odors of any kind."

"Like perfume?"

"Yes . . ."

"I don't wear it anymore, so that's not a problem . . ."

"I also mean scented hairspray, deodorant, fabric softener . . . that sort of thing . . . anything that has a smell."

"I understand.  No problem."

"And oh, yes, Ms. Stowe, along with the questionnaire and fee schedule, I'll enclose directions to the clinic.  We're rather hard to find."

"That's great.  Thank you.  See you December 3rd."

How would I ever wait three months?   But at least now I could look forward to something.  I figured this Dr. Rowland must be pretty good if he was so booked up.  With my luck there'd be a snow storm and I'd have to wait another three months!

I decided then and there to cancel my appointment with the psychiatrist.

I marked the date on my calendar, dragged myself into the kitchen and started making lunch.

*Usually one cannot become a healer
without first passing through
sickness to health.
In our culture,
one cannot become a psychoanalyst
without being analyzed,
but one can become a medical mechanic
without ever experiencing
the need for a repair.*

*The denial of empathy benefits no one.*

*As mechanics, we doctors
always fail in the long run,
but as counselors,
teachers,
healers and caregivers
we can always contribute . . .*

**Bernie Siegel, M.D.
Love, Medicine & Miracles**

# 3

# Believed at Last!

*Holistic medicine's philosophical approach emphasizes the individual as opposed to the individual's disease. The holistic approach encourages personal responsibility for one's health.*
**Zoltan P. Rona, M.D., M.Sc.**

*F*inally! My day with Dr. Gabriel Rowland had arrived. I awoke earlier than usual. I was excited and nervous at the same time. Would he really be as Jane described him? I just wanted someone to save me, to fix me, like Humpty Dumpty, and put me back together again.

The weather couldn't have been better. Perhaps it was a good omen - maybe this trip was meant to be.

I packed a few snacks. As I kissed the children goodbye, I reminded Michael about their lunches in the fridge and Nathaniel's hockey practice after school. It was a good thing I had written everything down. Otherwise, I'd never have remembered.

The trip to Bridgeport was a welcome relief from city driving. Although the leaves were gone, an early morning frost made everything shimmer. When I pulled up to 58 Cedar Grove Lane, what I saw surprised me. I had expected a boxy, commercial building. Instead, here was a contemporary house with natural wood siding, full of windows and skylights. Outside was a carved sign that read:

> *The doctor of the future*
> *will give no medicine,*
> *but will interest his patient*
> *in the care of the human frame,*
> *in diet and in the*
> *cause and prevention of disease.*
> *Thomas A. Edison*

Just inside the front door, next to a 'no smoking' sign, was a colorful poster:

> *No scents please. Many of our patients have*
> *environmental sensitivities and cannot tolerate*
> *perfume, scented hairspray, deodorant and*
> *aftershave, cologne or other scented products.*
> *Thank you.*

The waiting area was filled with patients, chatting as if they'd known each other for years. I caught little bits of conversation here and there, most of which revolved around a variety of health issues. After checking in and filling out some forms, I settled in a corner and picked up a couple of magazines I'd never heard of - *Health Naturally* and *Alive*. Most of the articles focused on healthy eating habits and natural remedies for every ailment imaginable. I was intrigued.

Occasionally looking up, I caught glimpses of a wiry man in his mid-forties with an energetic stride going in and out of several different rooms.

"Excuse me, but is that Dr. Rowland?" I asked an older woman next to me.

"Sure is. That's the man who saved my life . . ."

"And mine," interjected a gentleman sitting next to her. He appeared to be in his late fifties and looked quite fit. "I wasn't sick a day until they decided to carpet the office where I worked. I've never been the same since. None of the doctors knew what was wrong - until Dr. Rowland. Who knows where I would have ended up!"

"You know, people come to him from all over," added the woman. "He's a godsend." Her tone became reflective. "I don't know where I'd be without him. I was slowly dying from asthma, you know. Couldn't get air. There's nothing worse than not being able to breathe."

"I can imagine how awful that must be," I said, thinking of the many times I'd held Emma as she gasped for air. "I find it unbearable to watch my little girl during her worst attacks."

"Oh, and how old is she, dear?"

"She's only eight, and I'm really worried about all the medication she's on . . ."

She barely acknowledged my reply. "For years I lived on steroids, inhalers - all sorts of medications. I'm finally free and clear, except for the occasional flare-up once or twice a year."

"Hmm, interesting. What kind of treatment does Dr. Rowland use?" I asked. I would have done just about anything to help Emma.

"Well, he uses different approaches for each person. He had me working on my diet, and with vitamins, minerals, herbs, homeopathy - even a bit of acupuncture!" She grinned, sensing I knew nothing about any of this.

"Diet?" I asked naively. "What did your *diet* have to do with your asthma?"

"Just about everything! I had to stop eating dairy products, yeasty foods and all kinds of goodies, like sugar and . . ."

"Ms. Stowe, Dr. Rowland's ready to see you now," said the receptionist. She ushered me into an office to our right and invited me to sit down.

I was so nervous, afraid that one more doctor would think my ill health was all in my head. As I looked around, I realized that this room was very different from the sterile, impersonal atmosphere of other doctors' offices I'd frequented. One entire wall was all window and overlooked a wooded area. Its effect was soothing. Another wall was covered with health-related books, enclosed in glass. There were hardwood floors and bright, simple, cotton-covered furniture.

In one corner of the room was a lecture board displaying a figure captioned *Is This You?* (fig. 1). On one side were *Physical Symptoms*, and on the other, *Psychological Symptoms*. I'd just begun to examine the physical ones when Dr. Rowland walked in, extended his hand and said, "Well, do you recognize yourself? Most of the people I see have almost every symptom on the chart." His informal, outgoing manner immediately put me at ease. I could feel my anxiety begin to subside.

I shook his hand and gestured toward the chart. "Boy! I'm down to the arthritic pains and irritable bowel and I can't believe it. It's *me*!"

"And all your tests are negative, right?" he grinned, as he put my file on the desk in front of him.

"Right! Nothing significant ever shows up, and I'll tell you, I've had every 'iscopy' and 'oscopy' imaginable. I cringe when I think of all the tests I've been through and all the doctors I've seen."

"Well, as invasive and costly as those tests are, they really are important because they can rule out some very serious diseases. In fact, before you leave here today, we'll order some new bloodwork and a few other tests so we'll have a baseline for future reference. He handed me several books. "Glance through these while I review the material you sent us. It appears that you've been ill for quite some time."

"It feels like forever," I sighed. "I can't remember when my life was normal, if such a thing ever existed."

Dr. Rowland nodded. "If you don't mind, I'll tape our session. Most of my patients have some memory impairment when they first arrive at our clinic and . . ."

"I can relate to that! I feel like I have premature Alzheimer's."

He chuckled. "We're going to cover a lot of territory in our hour together. Taping it will enable you to have the information right at your fingertips."

I glanced at the books on my lap: *An Alternative Approach to Allergies* by Dr. Theron Randolph and Ralph Moss, *Tired or Toxic* by Sherry Rogers, M.D., and *The Yeast Connection* by Dr. William Crook.

He peered over the top of his reading glasses. "These books are a must read and can be signed out from our lending library. Self-education is of utmost importance. Your recovery will be based upon *you* taking responsibility for your own health. All I provide is the map. It will be entirely up to you to follow it."

I was still intrigued by the chart and went back to studying it. Once I got through the physical symptoms, I began reading the psychological

# Is This You?
## (fig. 1)

**"PSYCHOLOGICAL" SYMPTOMS**

**PHYSICAL SYMPTOMS**

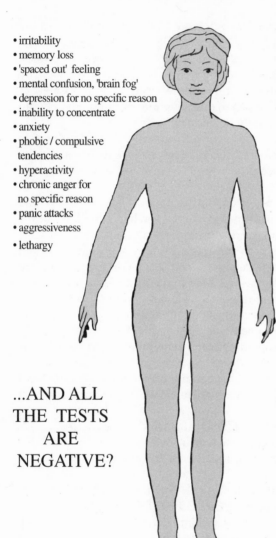

- irritability
- memory loss
- 'spaced out' feeling
- mental confusion, 'brain fog'
- depression for no specific reason
- inability to concentrate
- anxiety
- phobic / compulsive tendencies
- hyperactivity
- chronic anger for no specific reason
- panic attacks
- aggressiveness
- lethargy

- extreme fatigue
- headaches
- ear problem
- nasal congestion (sinusitis, rhinitis)
- tonsillitis or recurrent 'strep' throat
- chronic bad breath
- coated tongue
- itchy, watery or 'dry' eyes
- acne
- skin flushing
- asthma
- recurrent bronchitis
- heartburn
- eczema, hives, dermatitis
- chronic indigestion/living on antacids
- cold all the time especially in extremities
- P.M.S., pelvic pain
- recurrent vaginitis, prostatitis, jock itch
- spastic colon or irritable bowel
- abdominal gas and bloating
- constipation, diarrhea
- loss of sexual drive
- cystitis, repeated bladder infections
- eating disorders (i.e., binge eating)
- arthritic pain (worse on damp days)
- fluid retention
- weight gain - weight loss
- increasing food and chemical sensitivities (e.g., to perfumes)

...AND ALL
THE TESTS
ARE
NEGATIVE?

It may <u>not</u> be 'all in your head' !!!

ones - irritability, memory loss, 'spaced out' feeling, depression for no apparent reason, inability to concentrate - the list went on and on. All my symptoms were there. It was incredible!

After a few minutes reviewing my file, Dr. Rowland turned to me and said, "You know the 'psychological' symptoms you've experienced over the past few years? I have every confidence that they're *physiologically* based. From your health and environmental history, it's quite clear that you're *not* mentally ill."

Tears of relief rolled down my cheeks. Someone finally believed me! At the same time, I was angry - angry with all those who had doubted me over the years.

Dr. Rowland leaned over and gently touched my shoulder. "I know," he said, "it's such a relief to have someone believe you. To finally have acknowledged what you've known all along - that your *body* is sick, not your mind. Our focus in recent years has been more on how the mind influences the body. Although one very much affects the other, we tend to ignore the fact that physical illness can produce psychological symptoms."

"I've known that all along, but no one would believe me," I said, choking back the next flood of tears. I was embarrassed by my display of emotion. "I've been accused of everything - from being lazy, having housewife blues, to being a hypochondriac."

"Ms. Stowe - may I call you Jillian?"

I nodded.

"In all my years of practice, I've met only two people I would consider hypochondriacs. Everyone else's problems were *physiologically* based."

He continued in a quiet manner. "You know, the tears you shed today signify the beginning of your journey. Anne Frahm, an incredible woman who beat breast cancer and subsequently wrote a book about it, says that anger is like a cancer of the mind - devouring the emotional energies of a person. Your healing process will be quicker if you allow those feelings to come out. Your energy can then be focused on getting well. Would you like a Kleenex?"

Wiping my tears, I sniffled, "Why didn't those other doctors believe me? It's bad enough they couldn't find out what was wrong with me, but worse, they denied my experience."

"Do you mean that if it didn't fit with their sense of reality or the standard medical model, it doesn't exist?"

I nodded while blowing my nose. "And now, here you are, being totally sympathetic. Why? What makes you so different?"

"I learned early on in my practice to be an active listener. My patients serve as my best teachers. They're also their own best teachers. After all, who knows the body better than its owner? I listen carefully to their stories. The more we talk, the more pertinent information I get. In many cases, they can actually diagnose themselves. *They* are the real doctors. In fact, a patient's story often provides far more information than any tests. However, my real learning came as a result of my own illness."

"You were sick?"

"I sure was. When I recovered and felt well for the first time ever, having found answers to my own problems, I began to listen . . . with great care. At last, not only could I understand what my patients were going through, but I could actually help them find answers to their own health problems. Illness can be a great teacher."

"I can't imagine my illness teaching me anything!" I blurted. "It's ruining my life!" I choked back more tears.

"You'll soon discover that your symptoms, unpleasant as they are, can be positive signs . . ."

"What do you mean?"

"Well, your body is signalling you that something is very wrong. It's an opportunity to change habits, to begin to heal. Just think, many people never get any signs that something is wrong."

"Should I consider myself fortunate?" I asked, a touch of sarcasm in my voice.

"I know you can't possibly see the whole picture from where you are at this moment. There are many people who seem healthy all their lives who suddenly become critically ill or drop dead without warning."

"So what you're saying is that my symptoms are a warning before things really get out of hand?"

"Absolutely. Illness is the body's way of providing information - it's the language our body uses to tell us that it's upset, that we need to listen. You'll soon find out that there's so much to learn, not only about your body, but also about the environment in which you live, and how you interact with that environment."

"I just want to get well! I'm so tired of feeling this way. I'm sick of repeating my history over and over again to doctors who look at my body like it's an old cadaver with special interest parts - and then can't find anything wrong."

"It must be very frustrating . . ."

"It's humiliating! I'm looked at like a bladder, a bowel, or an adenoid- as if these parts were unrelated to the rest of me. It's so damned impersonal! It leaves me feeling totally insignificant . . . fragmented."

"You've just made a very important point. Modern medicine, like so much of our society, has become increasingly specialized. You see, doctors are taught to be mechanics, technicians. In medical school we're taught about disease, but learn nothing about what it means to the person who's experiencing it. In his book, *Peace, Love & Healing*, Dr. Bernie Siegel sums up the problem pretty well: *While I don't think most physicians are villains, I do think the training process of physicians is villainous.*"

We both laughed. It couldn't have been better said! There was something very genuine about him. In just a short time, he had shown me more compassion and understanding than I'd had since becoming ill.

He continued. "I feel very strongly that we must backtrack, and once again view the human being as a *whole*, encompassing the spiritual, mental, emotional and physical aspects, as this illustrates." He pointed to a poster on the wall entitled *Wholeness* (fig. 2). The words 'Mind, Body, Spirit' encircled a human figure. "Treating the individual, not the disease, is the

# Wholeness
### (fig. 2)

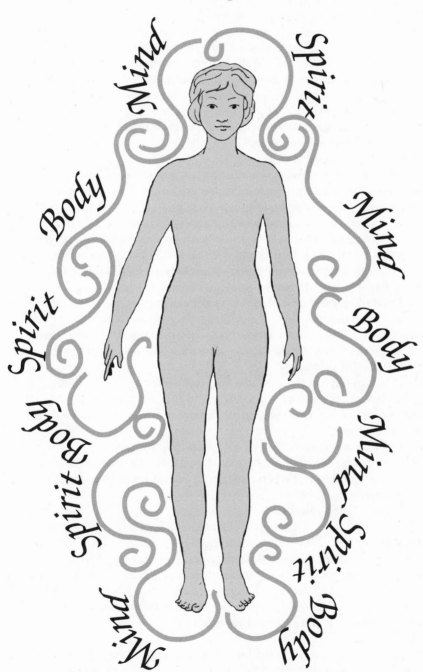

most effective course of action. Every part of your body is always very intricately connected to every other part. Ideally, it should be the family doctor's detective work that identifies the impact of the environment on a patient's health . . ."

"The environment?"

"Yes. Unfortunately, there's an enormous lack of information and education about the impact of the environment on our health." Dr. Rowland leaned closer to me. "What does the word environment mean to you?"

I thought for a moment. "Well, I think of things like acid rain, the destruction of the rain forest, baby seals, air pollution - that sort of thing."

"Most people think of the environment in that way, but rarely do we connect ourselves directly to it in an intimate, personal way. I see us as vital, pulsating organisms intricately connected to all three levels of environment: exterior, interior and internal."

"I'm not sure I understand."

"Well, your *exterior* environment is the environment outside," he said, pointing out the window, "and includes pollutants like auto exhaust, pesticides, and incinerator emissions. Your *interior* environment is the indoor environment - at home, work or school. It can include cleaning compounds commonly found under your kitchen sink, building materials, carpeting, personal care products and even air ventilation systems. Finally, your *internal* environment is the body - *your* body - which is influenced by what you eat, drink, and breathe on a daily basis."

Dr. Rowland picked up a book, opened it to a marked page and quoted from a Dr. David Reubin: *"People of America, the greatest threat to the survival of you and your children is not some terrible nuclear weapon. It is what you are going to eat from your dinner plate tonite.* You may well ask, what has this to do with my health problems?"

I nodded, assuming there would be a connection.

"The crux of the matter is - and I'll repeat this many times during our sessions together - what you eat, drink and breathe every day has a direct effect on your well-being."

"It reminds me of that old saying, *you are what you eat* ."

"But it's much more than that." He paused for a moment, walked over to his bookcase, and said, "When a fish in an aquarium displays psychotic behavior, do you call a fish psychiatrist?"

I laughed. "Who said that?"

He held up a book. "Dr. Stephen Gislason, in *Core Diet for Kids* - another good resource for you. Getting back for a moment to psychotic behavior, you wouldn't assume the fish was crazy and just leave it at that. You'd check the oxygen concentration, temperature, and pH of the water. You'd probably clean the tank or try changing its diet. So, I ask, why should humans be any different? You change the *physical environment* first because it's the most tangible, the easiest to work with."

It made sense.

"I know I must sound like a broken record, but the most important message I can give is that you must change what you're eating, drinking and breathing. You can go to therapy for years - not to say that therapy isn't useful - it is - but the therapy won't be nearly as effective if the body isn't balanced."

This way of thinking was totally new to me, but it made more sense than anything I'd heard yet.

"Every doctor I've seen has been quick to prescribe medication or write me off as a nut case. *You're* not doing that. Does this have anything to do with your own experience of being sick?"

"It certainly does. Because I want you to fully understand the connection we've just discussed, I'll share my story with you. But before I do, I'd like to examine you." Pointing to a door on our right, he said, "Why don't you go in there and slip on the robe that's draped over the table. I know you've had your share of physicals, but I'd like to make sure nothing's been missed. We can continue our discussion during the exam."

I could hardly wait to hear his story. In a few moments, there was a gentle knock on the door.

He began to check my blood pressure.

"You were just about to tell me about your illness . . ." I prodded.

"Oh yes. Throughout my childhood, I was quite a sickly kid. I caught everything that was on the go. By the time I got to medical school, I felt lousy and was a good fifty pounds overweight. I had weekly migraines that would last two to three days at a time, suffered from a variety of bowel problems, and had great difficulty concentrating . . ."

"That's how I feel!" I exclaimed, immediately identifying with his story.

"And believe me, you're not alone. But let me continue so you'll identify even more. Many mornings I felt like I couldn't breathe - my sinuses were so congested. I was exhausted most of the time, and my moods were up, down, and all over the place, making me very difficult to live with. I'm amazed I still have friends!"

I chuckled, thinking of my own mood swings and how everyone around me always walked on eggshells. I was starting to get the picture - he was once exactly where I was now.

"Now, keep still for just a moment so I can listen to your heart and lungs. Take a deep breath and exhale very slowly."

Despite his efforts to warm the stethoscope in his hands, it was still cold.

"Breathe in again. Out. Inhale. Exhale . . . and one more time. Good. So . . . back to my story. I was eating the standard diet that's touted as being so healthy, but was getting sicker and sicker. No wonder the abbreviated version of the standard American diet is S.A.D. - it's sad indeed, because this diet doesn't work for an increasing number of people. The truth is, there's no such thing as one diet that's appropriate for everyone. We're each biochemically unique, especially in North America, where there are so many different races and ethnic groups. Putting it quite simply, one man's food is another man's poison."

Dr. Rowland laid down his stethoscope. "Then one day I met an elderly physician who had been working in the field of environmental medicine. I owe much of my recovery and the way I choose to conduct my practice to this wonderful man. I've never looked back."

"But what was the actual *cause* of your illness?"

"The cause of my illness? My inner ecology was out of whack, as was the environment around me. So I guess I could say it was environmentally triggered."

"Environmentally triggered?" I was confused.

"Yes, I had become sensitive to almost everything I was eating, drinking, and breathing."

"What did you do to get better?"

"First, I stopped eating foods to which I was sensitive - common foods like sugar, wheat and dairy products."

"Regular foods caused all those problems?" I asked, with the same skepticism I had displayed in the waiting room. All of a sudden, it dawned on me, "Do you mean foods like bread, pasta, milk and cheese? Desserts?"

"Exactly. Everyday foods were killing me, slowly but surely . . ."

"But what's left to eat if you can't have milk and bread? Bread is the staff of life!" I was beginning to wonder about this Dr. Rowland.

He chuckled. "Typical response! I think I'll keep you in suspense until our nutritional consultant sees you in a little while. She'll be able to go into greater detail with you. I promise we won't keep you hanging!" he teased.

"Thank goodness for that!"

He continued the examination. "So far, everything seems fine."

"It always does." It was hard to contain my cynicism.

"Well, let's at least be thankful all the obvious things are normal. I'll meet you back in the other room."

Feeling somewhat reassured, I dressed and ran my fingers through my hair, stealing a glance in the mirror by the examining table. It was as if a stranger were looking back at me. I looked awful. My face was puffy and pasty. I had bags under my eyes and my hair was dull, dry and lifeless. I hurriedly dabbed on some lipstick and went back to the outer office.

Dr. Rowland, starting the tape again, motioned for me to sit down. "Now, getting back to my story. Foods were only part of the problem. Vitamin and mineral deficiencies and yeasts also played an important role. Other environmental factors such as everyday chemicals, cleaning agents used at the hospital, and even airborne irritants like dust and mold were also making me sick."

"Chemicals? What kind of chemicals?"

"Many toxic chemicals found right under our noses. Did you know that the average home can contain well over a hundred potentially dangerous chemicals, ranging from pesticides to bathroom cleaners? My home was no exception. Fumes from these products, combined with working extremely long hours in a hospital - subsequently found to be a sick building - and eating foods to which I was sensitive were slowly destroying my health. My memory was shot. I couldn't focus on anything important . . ."

"I know what that feels like!" I commiserated.

"My worst experience was going to deliver a baby and not knowing what to do. I'd delivered hundreds of babies - to the point where I could have done it blindfolded. But I was so mentally fogged, I couldn't remember even the most basic things."

It struck a responsive chord. I'd been there many times. "It must have been awful!"

"It was. I had to stop practicing. I took a long-term leave. I felt as if I had the flu all the time, but was, in fact, reacting to all those irritants."

"Boy, it's difficult for me to imagine you sick and overweight. You're so trim and seem to have all kinds of energy."

"Well, with a lot of intensive re-education and major lifestyle changes, I must say I'm healthier than I've ever been. And in just a few short weeks, you too, will begin to feel much better."

"If only I could believe that."

"I know, it's hard to see light at the end of the tunnel when you're standing in the dark. I hate to repeat myself, but if there's one thing to be learned from this session and any others we may have in the future, it's that there's an intricate connection between . . . between what?" he smiled.

"Between my health and what I'm eating, drinking and breathing on a daily basis - right?" I asked, eager to get it right.

"You've got it! You learn quickly!"

Dr. Rowland checked his watch. "Wow! We're already at half-time and we still haven't gotten into specifics - *your* problems." He stood up to change the tape, opened the windows a little wider and said, "Let's take a few deep breaths, stretch a bit and continue, shall we?"

I nodded in anticipation, ready for part two of our session. It wasn't completely clear just how all of this related to my own health. I had serious reservations, but having heard his story, I knew that Dr. Rowland had lived my nightmare. Maybe there *was* something to all this environmental stuff. His words began to resonate deep within.

Was truth staring me in the face?

*The alternative physician,*

*with the zeal of a medical detective,*

*seeks to find the cause*

*of your problem*

*rather than*

*merely treating symptoms*

*with a battery of drugs.*

**Jane Heimlich**
**What Your Doctor Won't Tell You**

# 4

# The Diagnosis

*All disease is biochemical.*
*The trick is to find the biochemical key that fits the lock.*
**Derrick Lonsdale, M.D.**

*J*illian, I'd like to elaborate on what we discussed a few minutes ago because it's fundamental to the principle of complementary, or as we often call it, wellness medicine. Do you remember what I said about the role of symptoms?"

"The part where you said we should feel fortunate that we're not feeling well?"

"Well . . . kind of," he chuckled. "You see, symptoms are the language of the body - the only way it knows how to communicate with its owner. For example, a fever that accompanies the common cold or flu, gives us the message that something is wrong. It also helps the body defend itself against these invaders."

"Normal protocol would be to reduce the fever right away - often with medication."

"Yes. But unless it's very high, accompanied with a lot of discomfort, there's no good reason to do that. In fact, by doing so, we interfere with the body's natural defense mechanisms. You see, within the confines of standard medical practice, we're taught to silence or mask symptoms through drugs or surgery, both of which are often needless."

"What would be an example of needless surgery?"

"Tonsillectomies are one of the best examples. Most cases of tonsillitis are caused by undiagnosed sensitivities. The tonsils swell in self-defense - a great warning signal that the body has ingested something it shouldn't have. At least we're not performing nearly as many as we once were. As well, consider the thousands of needless hysterectomies performed for complaints such as 'non-specific pelvic pain'. I can't begin to tell you how many women I see who still suffer from the same problems - *after* their reproductive organs have been removed! The underlying cause or causes were never addressed."

"So are you saying that by just treating symptoms, we can make ourselves even sicker?"

"We sure can. And by treating symptoms alone, we encourage the sick to continue to indulge in lifestyle habits that make them unwell in the first place. It's a big cover-up." Dr. Rowland stood up and walked across the room. "The key is to find the root cause of illness."

"But if I have a headache, wouldn't it be in order to take something to relieve the pain?"

"Absolutely, by all means. But if you get headaches two or three times a week, it's critical to find out *why*. Or, if you have eczema and the itch is driving you around the bend, a tiny bit of cortisone cream goes a long way. These are situations where we can count our blessings that we have such medications. But the next logical step would be to take a close look at our lifestyle or nutritional deficiencies for the real solution."

"Can you give me an example?"

"Take for instance, dermatological disorders. Other than in cases of contact dermatitis, digestive disturbances are often underlying factors. Once digestion improves, usually the skin condition also clears up."

"Who would ever have guessed!"

"Exactly! No one looks beyond the immediate." He pulled a rather large, black soft-covered book from his collection. "We treat our cars better than we do our bodies. Let me read you this short excerpt from *The Medical Mafia*, written by a Canadian physician, Guylaine Lanctôt:

> . . . let us look at the car. As soon as we hear a strange noise, we rush to the garage and ask them to check it out. They will look for the cause in order to fix the real problem before the car breaks down and we are stuck somewhere . . .
>
> When it comes to ourselves, we rush to take an aspirin for a headache. An anti-acid tablet for heartburn. Or a Valium for nerves. All to get as far away from the pain as possible. It will come back and we start taking the pills again, until finally, the 'breakdown occurs'

I can't emphasize enough how important it is to look for the *cause* of illness. Also, if a mechanic does a poor job on our car, we generally shop around for another who can do the job properly. But do we shop around for a doctor?"

"Rarely. It's almost considered heresy to do that kind of thing."

"Exactly. We need to take back ownership and exert our power so we can become equal partners in health with our physicians."

"That's a quantum leap," I replied, "especially considering the current dynamic between doctors and patients."

"As patients discover their own answers to many of their health problems, you'll find that dynamic change." He put the book away and turned to face me. "Now . . . getting back to you. Let's take a look at this fragmented little guy." Dr. Rowland pointed to a picture entitled *The Puzzle of Chronic Illness* (fig. 3). It was a simple drawing of an androgenous figure divided up like a jigsaw puzzle.

"Each piece represents influences and stressors inflicted upon us on

# Puzzle of Chronic Illness
## (fig. 3)

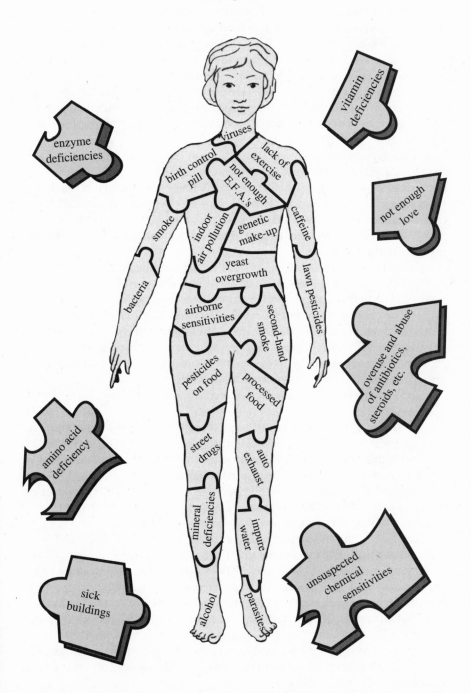

any given day. Some are physical, some are emotional, while others are spiritual. Our primary focus today will be on the physical."

As he explained the pieces of the puzzle, I couldn't help but notice how animated he was - his hands, his expression - everything. His whole being seemed integrated. I couldn't quite pinpoint what the quality was, but he had something that reminded me of the woman I had met at the playground in September - the one who had launched me on this journey. There was a sense of presence, focus, self-assurance - a balance about both of them. I'd never been around people who seemed so comfortable with themselves. Their energy was vibrant, yet calm.

"Let me show you in simple terms how these various stressors can affect your immune system. Take a look at this." He pointed to a chart showing a huge barrel with black, goopy-looking stuff flowing from the top (fig. 4).

"This represents the Total Load Theory  and is the most important concept you'll learn here today. It was developed by Dr. William Rea at the Environmental Health Center in Dallas, Texas and Dr. Richard Mackarness from England. The original model focused primarily on chemical overload. I've added some other common stressors that can be a daily burden for many,  such as vitamin and mineral deficiencies, drugs, improper diet and so on."

I gave him a sideways glance, "Life in the nineties, right?"

"That's right. Now, let's take a closer look. "This barrel is your immune system. The black liquid running out of it represents the symptoms you saw on the chart when you first walked in here. On any given day your immune system is bombarded by these stressors. Some of these include: improper diet, indoor and outdoor pollution and chemicals in food. The object here is to remove them one by one in order to bring your symptoms under control. Then the barrel won't overflow."

"Do you think I'm stressed?" I asked, worried about the implications of the word.

"Absolutely. But I'm focusing on physical stressors. It's much simpler to work with the body first. Once that's balanced, it's so much easier to work with the other aspects. In your case, I think physical stressors play a major role, causing many of your psychological symptoms."

I sighed with relief. It felt like a huge weight had lifted. My eyes began to tear again. "Do you know how good . . . how real  that sounds? To think I'd almost been convinced I was a mental case."

He added, "At the same time, we mustn't lose sight of the fact that you've been  unwell for a long time. That alone creates an enormous amount of emotional stress. It goes back to viewing the person as a whole. Mind, body, and spirit must work in harmony with one another - like instruments in an orchestra - in order to bring about balance and wellness."

"But all my weird symptoms . . . panic attacks, mood swings, irritability."

"From reading your history, I'm convinced those are physiologically induced." His words sounded so good - a confirmation of what I had known deep down all along.

# Total Load Theory
## (fig. 4)

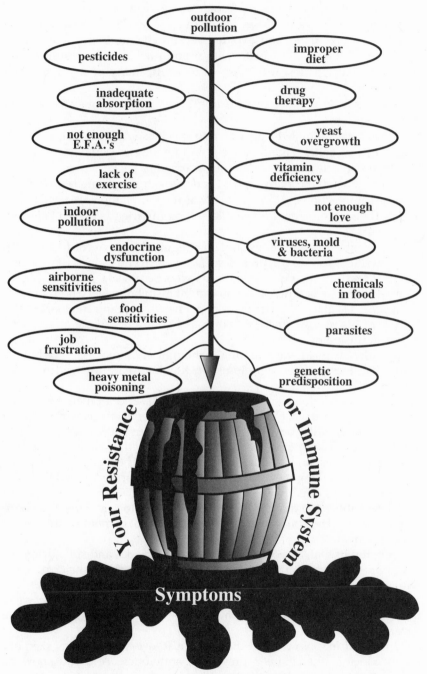

Adapted from an original concept by Drs. William Rea & Richard Mackarness.
Used with the permission of **William Rea, M.D., F.A.C.S.**, Environmental Health Center, Dallas, Texas.

"Now, getting back to the *Total Load Theory*. If you had only one or two stressors affecting you at any given time, chances are your immune system wouldn't be irritated, and your symptoms probably wouldn't have manifested in the first place. Symptoms develop when a person exceeds his or her tolerance of these stressors, or their total load."

"I feel a little stupid," I said. "Could you give me a concrete example?"

"Sure. I'll use my own story to illustrate. When I stopped eating foods that were problematic, and avoided certain chemicals in my everyday environment, I coped much better with airborne irritants like dust and mold. My total load was lessened and, as a result, many of my symptoms subsided."

"So what do you see overloading my barrel? What's stressing *my* immune system?"

"Good question. Let's get down to specifics. As an infant, your first symptom was colic. Then you went on to have excessive diaper rashes, chronic ear infections and bedwetting problems . . ."

I remembered the many nights I had awoken screaming from the pain of those ear infections. Added to that was the humiliation of waking up in a soaked bed. For years I lived a lie, telling my friends I wasn't allowed sleepovers.

". . . You were given antibiotics on a regular basis. According to what you've written, your next symptom surfaced when you were seven - chronic 'strep' throat. In the end, your tonsils were removed. In grade school, your resistance was down and you caught just about every bug that was on the go." He glanced up from the paper he was holding and looked over the top of his reading glasses "For many children, asthma and eczema kick in at this point . . ."

By now my head was spinning. I thought of Emma and Max, both of whom had many of the symptoms Dr. Rowland had just read from *my* childhood history.

"Then came adolescence - sugar, fast foods, and an increase in milk consumption, since most 'good' mothers insist their teenagers drink at least three glasses of milk a day. It's no coincidence your battle with acne began at this point. To counteract *that*, you were given Tetracyclene. As a result, your chronic yeast and bladder infections began. Then, adding fuel to the fire, you began taking the birth control pill which further altered the inner ecology of your body."

"I remember the day I started them. My doctor gave them to me to help my cycle. They only made me feel worse - not to mention the weight I packed on."

"On top of that," he continued, "more antibiotics and sulfa drugs for your bouts of cystitis and sinus infections and - voilà! - a major problem with your bowel. These drugs altered your intestinal flora and resulted in a diagnosis of irritable bowel, which, by the way, is a fancy label for 'we're not quite sure what's wrong with you.' Shortly thereafter, your fatigue began . . ."

I jumped in. "Now that I think about it, every time I was sick, our family doctor immediately prescribed antibiotics. And you know, he hardly ever took a swab of my throat!"

"Yes, that's a common oversight in our 'fix me fast' society. You know, Jillian, as health professionals, we're all thankful to have modern drugs because they do save lives - thank God. But let me tell you, they're grossly overused and abused in this society. A 1994 *Newsweek* article stated that various studies have concluded that fifty to sixty percent of all outpatient prescriptions are inappropriate."

"Dr. Rowland, I think you're right. When I worked in Emergency, nearly every child walked out with a prescription for an antibiotic - often to treat a virus. Doctors would justify it by telling parents it was a preventive measure."

He shook his head. "I read recently that seven out of ten Americans routinely take antibiotics as a treatment for the common cold, even though they're effective only against bacteria. We have a habit of prescribing antibiotics for anyone who looks sick. It's not unusual for me to see a child only twenty-four months old who's been on eighteen or twenty rounds of antibiotics. And, of course, there are times when it's the patient who demands them. As a nurse, I'm sure you're familiar with this scenario."

"I most certainly am. It's normal protocol, particularly for chronic ear infections. I used to see it all the time. But what else can you do when a child has a raging ear infection?" I thought again of my poor little Max, whose earaches had been chronic since he was six months old.

"If you're not familiar with diet therapy, homeopathy and other alternatives, you'd probably treat it with antibiotics - although studies from England and Scandinavian countries are showing they're not as effective as we once thought. One study that immediately comes to mind is from the University of Copenhagen in Denmark, where Drs. Marcus and Betil Diamant concluded that eighty-eight percent of patients never need antibiotics and that the frequency of recurrent ear infections in the untreated group was much lower than in the group that was treated. In fact, studies show that if children are given an antibiotic within the first day or two of the onset of symptoms, they're more likely to get another ear infection within the month . . ."

"So what's the solution?"

"Parents and physicians ought to wait at least a couple of days before they resort to antibiotics. It's been my experience that more often than not, mild analgesics, a bit of warm oil, heat and monitoring the situation is enough. Obviously, if the fever escalates and the pain doesn't let up, action must be taken."

"Funny you should bring this up . . . my little guy, Max, is on this same treadmill. In fact, on many occasions, our doctor would diagnose an ear infection during a routine checkup when there weren't any visible signs - no fever, no pain. Many of my friends have similar experiences, but the medical community puts the fear of God into you. We're made to feel so guilty, that eventually we just give in."

"I understand. It's obvious that many of my colleagues need to keep more up to date with the literature. But again, the bottom line is that after one or two bouts of ear infections, it would be only logical to try to find the *cause*."

"You mean what caused it in the first place?"

"Yes. You see, in those cases where there's a chronic pattern, *food sensitivities* - especially to dairy products - are often the culprits. And to make matters worse, what do we give kids after tonsillectomies and ear surgeries?"

"Ice cream!"

Dr. Rowland shook his head. "Isn't it amazing? And when the suspect food or foods are eliminated, more often than not, the problem resolves itself. No more colic, bladder or ear infections, or tonsillitis, and therefore no need for antibiotics. And even more amazing, behavioral issues can become a thing of the past." He noticed my puzzled expression and smiled. "I know it may seem too simple, but in most cases, it really *is* that simple!"

"But why are dairy products such a problem all of a sudden? People have been drinking milk and eating cheese for ages."

"And our society has been plagued with chronic disease for nearly as long. Some of my colleagues suggest that cow's milk is for calves, not humans, its purpose being to take a ninety pound calf and nourish it to nearly a ton within nine months. They argue that the milk of each animal is structured precisely to meet the needs of its young and not the young of other species. In fact, when you think about it, we're the only animal that drinks the milk of another. Have you ever seen an elephant nursing a horse? Or a dog being fed by a goat? And to make matters worse, we even drink it well beyond the weaning stage."

"I've heard that argument before, but thought it was because humans are intelligent enough to figure out an alternative food source . . ."

"Perhaps to our detriment. One study, reported in the *Archives of Disease in Childhood*, concluded that forty percent of children are sensitive to cow's milk. Dr. David Collison, in *Why Do I Feel So Awful?*, cites several research papers that describe the damaging effect of cow's milk on psychiatric patients - many of whom are afflicted for years with confusion, fatigue, even paranoia. In one of these studies, eighty percent of patients made significant, and sometimes complete, recoveries from these symptoms upon removal of cow's milk. In fact, any of my more holistically inclined colleagues will tell you that dairy products are one of the most common culprits underlying today's health problems."

"Unbelievable!"

"Maybe, but nevertheless, very real. John Robbins in *May All Be Fed* says he grew up believing in dairy products the way some people believe in the Bible - thanks to the milk marketing boards. I tell you, milk is the most political food in North America . . ."

"You mentioned symptoms. What kinds of symptoms?"

"The list of symptoms is as long as is the list of benefits obtained by sensitive individuals who remove dairy products from their diets. Dairy products can cause gas or bloating, cramps, hyperactivity, muscle pain, sinus congestion, asthma, depression, eczema, ear infections, enlarged tonsils and adenoids, irritability - you name it. And this relationship of symptoms to dairy products has been cited in prestigious publications such as the *Lancet, Advances in Pediatrics, Gastroenterology* and the *Journal of the Canadian Medical Association*."

"Other than lactose intolerance causing a bit of gas, bloating and maybe some diarrhea, I'd certainly never heard of these connections - and I'm a nurse!"

"Don't feel bad, most physicians don't make these connections either. But let's get back for a moment to the influence of the powerful milk marketing boards . . . I've had very young patients who lived year after year on antibiotics and heavy-duty steroids to combat the multi-faceted symptoms that dairy products provoked. Their parents were terrified to remove dairy from their diets, even though it would reduce and often resolve the symptoms. They felt more comfortable giving their children continual doses of medication to control their symptoms than removing milk from their diets!"

"Everywhere you look, from magazine and television ads to billboards, the message is loud and clear - milk is nature's perfect food."

"Hopefully, that image will change as more and more people, as well as physicians, begin to make these connections. Another reason to re-evaluate the benefits of cow's milk is that an overwhelming number of people - especially those who are not of Anglo-Celtic origin - are lactose intolerant, unable to digest the natural sugar found in milk. In fact, some of the literature suggests that many stop manufacturing lactase - the enzyme necessary to break down milk sugar - between early childhood and adolescence . . ."

"I wonder if Greeks fall into that category. Some of my mother's people are from the island of Crete."

"One study published in the *Medical Journal of Australia*, showed that among Greek children, 56 percent showed malabsorption. Asian children fared the worst, with a 93 percent deficiency in lactase . . . But I'd like to address your earlier question about why cow's milk seems to be even less tolerated today than ever before. The milk our ancestors drank was straight from the cow - raw, full of enzymes. Later, with the advent of large dairies, pasteurization and homogenization came on the scene. Milk became a processed food. Parallel to that development, we began to see a significant increase in chronic ailments such as those I listed a few moments ago."

"But why?"

"Because processing strips the milk of most of its essential enzymes, placing tremendous demands upon the digestive system. So for an increasing number of people, dairy products are not the best source of calcium. Raw, unpasteurized milk contains an enzyme which splits calcium from phosphorus, allowing calcium absorption to take place. However, when it's pasteurized, it actually loses some available calcium. According to recent studies, low fat or skim milk prohibits calcium absorption even further because it's missing the fat which is essential for the transportation and absorption of calcium. But it's been my experience that children who are already sensitized, can't seem to tolerate either form - skim milk even less, because it's higher in protein. If you cannot digest it, you certainly can't absorb its calcium. Then again, would we want to consume dairy products daily when they're often contaminated with antibiotic and hormone residues?"

"Well, no . . ."

"Dr. Charles Simone, a nationally renowned cancer specialist and author of *Cancer & Nutrition*, connects milk and cancer in several ways. One of these is the repetitive exposure to milk contaminants such as DES, or diethylstilbestrol, used as a growth promoter for cattle. He stresses that there needs to be more long-term research on continuous low-level exposure to DES and its link to cancer. And then there are other dairy contaminants such as pesticides, industrial residues, and heavy metals that could be detrimental to our health. These are concentrated in the cow as it consumes tainted, processed feed mixtures, and even some grasses."

"Things the average person doesn't even think about! Well, here goes another 'perfect food' myth out the window!"

"And who knows, maybe it was a perfect food - at one time - before it was tampered with. Suddenly Dr. Rowland broke into a grin. "I was just thinking of something I heard on the radio last night, sponsored by the Veterinarians' Association. They were urging cat owners not to feed their pets milk because it often causes gastrointestinal distress. In fact, one woman who called in told a story of her Doberman who had developed a severe skin condition. For two years, she had tried medication, lotions and shampoos - all to no avail. She discovered that the dog was sensitive to dairy products and that whey powder, a component of dairy, was in almost everything he was eating. So, these problems are not unique to humans."

"But if you don't drink milk, where do you get calcium?"

"There are many good alternative sources of calcium such as nuts and seeds - as well as milks and pastes made from them - soya products, salmon, dark green vegetables, especially the leafy ones, plus concentrated green drinks . . ."

"Green drinks?"

"Yes, you might want to discuss that in more detail with Eva. Many ethnic foods use these products. For example, middle eastern cuisine uses a lot of sesame seed paste - tahini - in their dishes. Oriental dishes often call for soya products. I often cook with seaweeds as well, which are full of trace minerals, including calcium. If you're worried, you can always take supplements, but make sure you don't take calcium without magnesium. Overall, one of the most significant things you can do, is to keep your dietary protein intake at a fairly low level. The latest in nutritional research clearly and consistently indicates that the typical North American high animal protein diet, rich in phosphorus, can create a calcium imbalance, regardless of how much calcium we take in. According to John Robbins, the few studies that didn't find this connection were all financially supported by the meat and dairy industries."

"So what about all those celebrity milk mustache ads in magazines and on T.V.? If what you're saying is true, they're awfully misleading."

"They certainly are. In fact, I read recently that the Physician's Committee for Responsible Medicine (PCRM) has lodged a complaint with the Federal Trade Commission in Washington, D.C. stating that this ad campaign is deceptive . . . "

"But what about osteoporosis?" I interrupted.

"Interestingly, North America has a high percentage of osteoporosis in spite of its high rate of dairy consumption. This is also true for Finland, Sweden, Israel and the United Kingdom - all countries where the intake of animal protein is very high. Compare this with China where the intake of calcium is half of what we ingest. They obtain their calcium primarily from vegetable sources. You see, loss of bone mass is typically caused by excessive calcium *loss*, rather than inadequate calcium intake. This is why the PCRM claims that these ads are misleading. In fact, in 1989, the *British Medical Journal* published a comprehensive review of the scientific literature on calcium intake and osteoporosis, suggesting the idea that increased calcium intake can offset bone loss is *clearly misleading and not supported by experimental observation*. Countries with high calcium diets even have higher fracture rates compared to those with a lower calcium intake. For example, while the average calcium intake in Singapore is less than half the recommended daily allowance (RDA), the fracture rate in Singapore is five times lower than in the U.S. where the intake is much higher. Again, it's our diet and sedentary lifestyle that encourage the loss of calcium."

"And leafy green vegetables still make up such a small percentage of our grocery stores . . ." I thought of all the aisles of processed, boxed junk.

"Absolutely, especially when compared to an Asian grocery store! And don't forget that caffeine consumption and the use of refined sugar and salt also contribute to calcium loss, all of which comprise a major part of the average North American diet. Then there's the role that dairy sensitivities play - if you can't digest it properly, you certainly can't absorb its nutrients. What puts this entire dairy issue into perspective is that a significant proportion of the world's population does not consume dairy products at all, and their teeth and bones are perfectly fine. John Robbins, in his book, *May All Be Fed*, goes into it quite extensively, citing many studies to support this view. It would be interesting to conduct bone density studies on children with a dairy sensitivity who drink milk and those who don't, but who get calcium from other sources."

He paused for a moment to gather his thoughts. "But let's get back to the basic issue we were discussing. The most frightening thing about unidentified food sensitivities is that the symptoms they create are often treated with broad-spectrum antibiotics. These drugs don't differentiate between the beneficial and the harmful bacteria in your body. They destroy the intestinal flora, or internal ecology, upsetting the natural balance in your system. As a result, a secondary problem can occur - a massive yeast overgrowth in the gut, because there's no longer adequate healthy bacteria left to keep it in check. Once that happens, the gut becomes permeable and multiple food sensitivities can occur. You know, Jillian, holistic health care providers have a saying: *More than one antibiotic per year equals hidden food sensitivities*."

Max! Every few weeks he'd wake up screaming with a terrible ear infection. This meant a round of antibiotics almost every month, each course lasting a minimum of ten days. One didn't need to be a genius in math to figure out that he was practically living on the stuff! And he was getting crankier and sicker by the week.

I was confused. "But going back to my own story, what do infantile colic and childhood ear infections have to do with one another? And how are bladder infections and irritable bowels related? Am I missing something?"

"There's a definite connection. Environmental medicine identifies these as target organs. It's well known that swelling of tissues is an effect of allergy or sensitivity. Just as the tiny eustachian tubes swell, so can the bladder, and in some cases, even the brain may be affected in this way. Where certain foods cause children to misbehave, we call it a cerebral or brain allergy. In other children, the lungs, bowel or bladder become the target organs, resulting in asthma, chronic bronchitis, irritable bowel or bedwetting. The same foods that caused the original problem can be responsible for many other symptoms down the line."

I was starting to see the pattern - and it was a little too close to home. "Am I hearing you correctly? Foods can actually cause disease?"

"Absolutely. At least twenty-five major disease states can be connected to common foods and chemicals we encounter daily."

"What kinds of disease?"

"Migraines, bladder and bowel problems, arthritis, some forms of obesity, a variety of manic-depressive disorders, schizophrenia, and many of the problems on the chart you looked at when you first came in here."

"They can actually be caused by *foods*?"

"Yes. In fact, a typical picture is the middle-aged woman who is advised to increase her milk intake to prevent osteoporosis. Within weeks or months, she develops an irritable bowel, chronic headaches, or sinusitis. This is also probably the same woman who had an intense dislike for milk most of her life, suffered from colic as an infant, and had ear infections as a child. And no one ever makes the connection! Then the endless rounds of medication begin. Many people unwisely assume that unless something they're ingesting causes an immediate reaction, they can eat, drink or breathe anything - that they're invincible. These same people often end up with arthritis, diabetes, heart disease or cancer and ask, 'why me'?" With his eyes downcast, and sadness in his voice, he said, "My own father was an example of this kind of thinking . . . and in cases where the disease is not directly caused by foods, certain foods can worsen the illness."

"And our quick fix is to medicate," I mumbled. "Almost everyone I know takes one thing or another. If it's not Tylenol for their headaches, or Tums for their upset stomachs, it's Claritin or Seldane for their sinuses, or Ex-lax for their bowels. Come to think of it, many of my friends' children are on antibiotics a good part of the year."

Dr. Rowland nodded in agreement. "The whole pattern is a medical nightmare, and what's worse, is that most orthodox medicine just doesn't see the connection. Almost daily I witness the end result of what I consider pharmaceutical abuse - children and adults plagued with chronic bowel dysbiosis, whether yeast or parasitic in nature. And these conditions often underlie multiple food sensitivities."

"Do you mean vaginal yeast?"

"No, I mean overgrowth of yeast in the bowel. You see, vaginal yeast is only one indicator of this problem . . ."

"I *live* on Monistat and Gyne-Lotrimin! I often joke with my friends and tell them that I, alone, keep these companies in business."

"As far back as the 1970's, a study was published in the *Journal of the American Medical Association*. The conclusion was that vaginal yeast is *always* accompanied by yeast in the stool. It further concluded that a *cure* for vaginitis would not be possible without prior eradication of yeast from the gut. Despite this and other studies, many of my colleagues refuse to acknowledge that such a condition even exists."

He paused for a moment as if deep in thought. "Of course, in addition to yeast, the other horrendous problem caused by the overuse of broad spectrum antibiotics is that the immune system becomes compromised and can't ward off the next little bug that comes along. You see, the body defences are now unable to fight without assistance."

"Maybe that's why we're sick all the time."

"That may be one of the reasons," said Dr. Rowland. "Almost all bacteria nowadays have strains that are resistant to at least one of modern medicine's array of antibiotics. The worst scenario - which is already becoming a reality - is that when you need an antibiotic for a serious bacterial infection, none will be effective. The rise in drug-resistant bacteria is frightening and will only worsen."

"So, are you saying the microorganisms are winning?" It sounded like an episode of Star Trek.

He nodded. "That may be one reason for the resurgence of diseases we thought had been eradicated."

"Do you think I have this yeast imbalance?" I asked, looking at *The Yeast Connection* on my lap.

"Judging from your history, I would say it's highly likely. But you also need to address your immediate environment, your surroundings."

"My surroundings?"

He carefully looked over a page in my file. "I see here that many of your symptoms got much worse after you started working on a newly renovated floor at the hospital . . ."

Oh my God! The new link. Now, it was all coming back to me . . . "That's right! I'd get sore throats, splitting headaches and catch everything that was going around. I always felt better on weekends and on my days off. But I always chalked it up to stress."

"We attribute most everything to that catch-all word, and in some cases, justifiably so. But let me continue. About a year ago, you renovated your home. Your fatigue and many of your 'psychological' symptoms increased significantly. You know, Jillian, the two most common stories I hear from environmentally sensitive women are that they were fine until the birth of their second or third child, or until they moved into their new home, or renovated an existing one."

"Well, I fit into both of those categories."

"You sure do. Add this to a toxic workplace, a history of undiagnosed sensitivities treated inappropriately with massive doses of antibiotics, and you've toppled your load - like this." He pointed to a chart entitled *Breaking Point* (fig. 5), depicting a human figure weighted down by a stack of bricks,

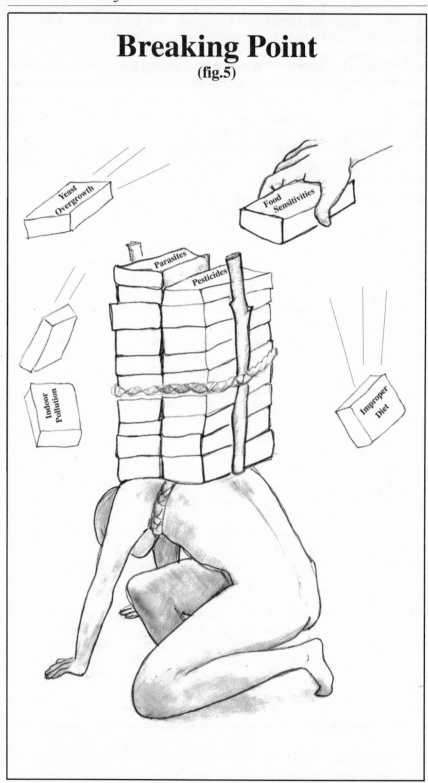

each brick representing an environmental assault. "To regain your health, you'll need to unload many of these bricks. It could take considerable time and patience, but you'll get there."

"I'm still confused. What exactly do you think I have?"

"You seem to be hypersensitive to a range of substances in your environment - to things you encounter every day. This condition is commonly known as Environmental Illness or E.I. but many prefer to call it Multiple Chemical Sensitivity or M.C.S. In reality, they're the same thing."

I now had a real disease. It had a name! I was so relieved to be taken seriously at last. As if reading my mind, Dr. Rowland gently explained. "Yes, there is actually such a condition as Environmental Illness. However, I prefer to use the term 'environmentally challenged'. It's a more positive approach. Jillian, there are thousands of people just like you, walking around with vague symptoms, but who never connect them to the actual causes."

"So I had a third baby and renovated my house," I debated. "Lots of people do both and feel just fine."

"Ah, but remember," he smiled, "your external environment is only part of the problem. Another part is the environment in here," he said, pointing to his body, "the internal environment."

"Where does yeast fit into this?"

"That's a story in itself and would take much longer to explain than we have right now. As a start I'd like you to read *The Yeast Connection*. We'll discuss it further during your next visit. The first step in removing some of these stressors will be to unmask your food sensitivities through re-education and elimination."

"It sounds as if I'm in for the long haul," I said, feeling somewhat defeated.

"But think of how long it took you to get this way. Disease is a gradual process. It develops as we prolong our exposure to low levels of toxins in the air, water and food supply. It doesn't just happen overnight. Nor does recovery. But I can guarantee you'll be surprised at the changes that will occur over the next few weeks."

"Aren't there any tests for all this?"

"There are, but they're expensive and painstaking. I always prefer to try the simple approach first - working with diet, reducing yeast, healing the gastrointestinal tract, and controlling the environment in which you spend most of your time. It puts you directly in the driver's seat - right where I like my patients to be. This way the responsibility for your health is back in your control."

"But how long do you think it will be before I see any visible changes?"

He noted my discouraged expression and reassured me with a smile. "Judging from your health history, you should see some pretty dramatic results within two weeks. If, after this period of time, there's no improvement, then we'll do more extensive tests. Fair?"

"Fair."

There was a gentle knock. The door opened a crack, and a woman's voice announced, "Dr. Rowland, your next patient is ready."

He looked at his watch. "Emily's right. Our time is up." He thanked her and said he'd be just a few more minutes.

"My role over the next while is to help you relate theory to what's actually happening to you. I'll also refer you to several experts in the field of environmental health. We'll start today with Eva Sandor, our nutritional consultant, who'll go over an elimination diet with you. She'll help you understand how masked food sensitivities and contaminants in our food play a major role in chronic illness, as well as explain the food-mood connection. I would say that in your case, foods are a major culprit right now."

"I've already seen several dieticians . . ."

He grinned. "And I'll bet they told you to eat a balanced diet based on the four food groups."

"Four? I thought there were five basic food groups now."

"Well, it depends upon where you are. The American Food Pyramid has five and Canada's Food Guide to Healthy Eating has four. The only difference is that the former separates vegetables and fruits into two categories while the latter groups them into one."

"So that's the difference. In any case, the more I followed it, the worse I felt."

"That's not uncommon. An increasing number of people are becoming sensitive to many common foods listed in these groups. Eva specializes in orthomolecular and environmental nutrition. It's a great combination since both work together in bringing about wellness."

"What's orthomo. . . whatever it was you just said?"

"Ortho means to straighten, so it quite literally means 'to straighten molecules'. The term was coined by two time Nobel Prize winner, Dr. Linus Pauling. The focus of Eva's approach is to bring about balance in the body through diet and food supplements. In other words, the body must receive adequate amounts of nutrients in order to heal itself or prevent sickness in the first place. However, when Eva talks about diet, she focuses on what are known as masked food sensitivities and the *quality* of the foods you eat, not just the basic food groups. You'll love her energy. She's a dynamo and is extremely knowledgeable to boot."

He closed my file. "We'll also need some routine blood, urine and stool samples. You can pick up requisitions for those from Emily at the front desk."

He smiled and looked directly at me. "How are you feeling?"

"Dr. Rowland, just being *believed* is a relief. Being told there's something I can do about all this is more than I had hoped for."

"There are many things you can do to heal yourself, and we're here to help you learn to do just that."

"All I want is to feel well. I'll do anything it takes!"

"It'll mean making some major lifestyle changes."

"I'm ready for whatever needs to be done. By the way, when do I see you again?"

"Normally, we'd have you back in two weeks, but due to the holidays, we'll have to wait about a month. Emily will book you on the same day as your follow-up with Eva. We usually coordinate our appointments. Don't forget to follow her instructions to the letter and be sure to read the books I recommended. Education is the key to understanding. Then comes first-hand experience - actually *doing* it. Remember, Jillian, no one else can give you good health - no one but yourself."

He walked over to the recorder and popped out the cassette. "Don't forget your tape." Extending his hand, he smiled and said with conviction, "I *know* you can do it! Have a wonderful holiday. See you in the new year."

Emily showed me out. I had half an hour to relax before my appointment with Ms. Sandor.

My head was spinning, but I had a gut feeling that finally, I was on the right track. All this information was very different from what I had been told over the past three years, but it felt right. More important, I was *believed*. I hadn't felt this optimistic in years.

And . . . I wasn't crazy after all.

*In 1940 about 20 percent of the food*

*consumed in this country*

*was processed.*

*Today it is close to 75 percent.*

*We consume the elements*

*of our own destruction,*

*with our excessive intake of sugar*

*. . . fats, loss of bulk or fiber,*

*elimination of vitamins and minerals,*

*and the pollution of food with chemicals*

*never demonstrated to be safe.*

**Abram Hoffer, Ph.D., M.D. & Morton Walker, D.P.M.**
**Orthomolecular Nutrition**

# 5

# Chemical Soup

*We are faced with the increasing use of substitute ingredients, sham foods that get much of their taste and appearance and nutrients not from nature, but from a chemical factory.*
**David R. Collison, M.D.**

*I*t was 3:15 by the time I saw Eva Sandor. I'd taken a short walk to refresh myself and called home to make sure everything was under control. Michael would be home by suppertime to take over from the sitter. Good thing I'd brought a snack with me - I was starved!

I was so glad my session with Dr. Rowland had been taped. I couldn't possibly have retained all the information we covered. During my walk, I tried to make sense of my life in terms of my health over the years, particularly the last three. It was also becoming clear that my kids had many of the same symptoms I'd had as a child. Could there be a connection?

Emily escorted me to Ms. Sandor's office on the top floor of the clinic. On the way we passed a well-equipped kitchen. She said they held regular cooking classes at the clinic and that people came from all over to learn how to prepare healthy meals. Next to the kitchen was a large room, empty except for mats and cushions along the outer wall.

"That's where we have meditation, yoga and t'ai chi classes," she said.

"And these offices?" I asked, pointing to several other doors as we made our way to the third floor.

"Oh, those are used by practitioners specializing in acupuncture, homeopathy, massage, psychotherapy and other complementary practices."

We walked past a tall window. Outside, two women wearing white cloth face masks were getting out of a car. Seeing my puzzled expression, Emily explained that their sensitivities were so severe they had to wear charcoal-filter masks for protection. I felt grateful I wasn't as sick as they were.

By the time we reached the waiting area outside Ms. Sandor's office, I felt like I'd just walked several miles instead of up three flights of stairs. I sat down, still huffing and puffing, closed my eyes, and tried taking some deep breaths as Dr. Rowland had suggested.

Suddenly, the door opened. A very attractive, slim young woman came toward me. Her hair was chin length with very short, spiked bangs. They accentuated her large, deep-set hazel eyes. Smiling, she said, "Hi! I'm Eva. You must be Jillian. Come in."

I noticed how light her step was, how her body seemed to flow as she walked - briskly, but with grace. I felt like an elephant next to her. Her hair glistened in the sunlight that streamed in the window above her desk.

She motioned towards a chair and said in a rather jovial manner, "Please, have a seat and welcome to Nutrition 101. Aha! Here it is. The very thick file of Jillian Stowe."

Glancing up at me, she asked, "How was your appointment with Dr. Rowland? Are you saturated yet?"

"Am I! I'm on information overload, but I'm ready for more. Taping the sessions was a great idea. I'd never be able to remember everything. But you know, Ms. Sandor . . ."

"Please, call me Eva."

"He's the first doctor in three years who not only believes that I'm really sick, but is sure he can help me."

"Jillian, you're in the best of hands. If it weren't for Dr. Rowland, I don't know where I, and many others, would have ended up. We owe our lives to that man."

"You were sick too?" I asked, curious to hear her story.

"I sure was. And, like you, I went to just about every specialist in the area. When I was at my worst, I even went to one of the largest medical centres in North America. No one knew what was wrong with me. Then, I met Dr. Rowland. Over the years, he's helped thousands of people just like us."

"I'd been to so many nutritionists, dieticians and doctors who just kept telling me to take my medications and eat the foods outlined in the Guide. The more I followed their advice the sicker I became!"

"That's because the Guide is meant to be just that - a very general guide for the public at large. What it doesn't take into account is the *quality* of the recommended foods. It doesn't address pesticide residues, nutrient content after transportation, or the fact that more and more people have developed sensitivities to foods. . ."

I quickly interjected. "Dr. Rowland said the same thing, but *why* are so many people developing sensitivities?"

"Food sensitivities have been around since recorded history. There are references as far back as the Old Testament. In this century, connections between food and mood were cited in the medical literature as early as 1908. Today, we're simply becoming more aware that sensitivities are at the root of many chronic illnesses."

"But is it not true that more people suffer from sensitivities today than ever before?" I asked.

"Absolutely. The frequency has increased dramatically, especially since the Industrial Revolution - and not just to foods."

"What price, progress!" I lamented.

"In 1987, I attended a National Academy of Sciences workshop. At that time, it was estimated that fifteen percent of the United States population were chemically sensitive."

"And that was quite a few years ago. I wonder if it's higher today."

"Well, Dr. Doris Rapp, a pediatric allergist and author of many books on this subject, suggests that seventy-five percent of the North American population suffers from some form of sensitivity to one thing or another."

"But *why* such a dramatic increase?"

"Today, people are exposed to concentrations of chemicals far higher than those experienced by any other generation in human history. Over 70,000 new chemicals have been added to our environment since the 1940's, with hundreds of new chemicals introduced every year. . ."

"That's incredible!"

". . . and the production of synthetics has increased from 1.3 billion pounds in 1940 to 320 billion pounds in 1980 - in only forty years."

"Those figures are staggering!"

"You're right about that! From the moment of conception until death, we're subjected to a host of dangerous chemicals. The combined effect of these on our health is, as yet, unknown - particularly when it comes to children. But the bottom line is that we're not meant to live the way we're living - sedentary, in an increasingly toxic world. Here at the clinic, we refer to these combinations as a chemical soup. . ."

"An eerie description!"

"You see, our environment, diet and way of life have changed so dramatically over the past century - especially the last forty-five years - that our bodies haven't been able to compensate for all these stresses."

"Do you mean the stresses that can overload the immune system?"

"Yes. First, let's look at what we eat. If we compare the food supply of the 1950's to today, it begins to make sense. One example is your corner grocery store. Two-thirds of the aisles are full of packaged, processed foods. They're loaded with harmful fats, additives and preservatives to prolong shelf life and are almost totally devoid of nutrients." As she spoke, Eva became more animated and passionate, reminding me of Dr. Rowland.

All of a sudden, she whirled around in her chair, opened a drawer and pulled out a box . . . of dog biscuits! With her other hand, she picked up some small, familiar-looking packages - treats I often gave to the kids for recess - including snacks like glazed fruit chews and chocolate-covered granola bars.

"Your *dog* eats better than you do! Just take a look. Read the list of ingredients on this box of dog biscuits. They're all natural and free of additives and preservatives. Now, take a look at *this*!" She held up the goodies in her other hand.

"I buy those for my kids," I said, sheepishly.

"Yes, you and any number of other parents who don't realize what's in them. They're full of hydrogenated fats, dangerous additives and preservatives, as well as loads of sugar. There's even *shellac* in this one!" She held up one of the more colorful packets.

"Shellac? Isn't that what we use to finish wood?"

"Quite correct. And although this is food-grade shellac, it's not much better for you."

"What was that hydrog . . . hydrogen . . . whatever it was that you just said?"

"Hydrogenated fat is an altered fat used to preserve shelf life. It's been strongly linked to heart disease and is a suspected carcinogen. Read a book called *Fats that Heal, Fats that Kill* by Udo Erasmus, an expert in this field. A friend of mine who specializes in nutritional medicine refers to these types of fats as 'liquid plastic'."

"It really is a buyer-beware society! But how do we know what to look for?"

"Education is the key. We really have to start reading labels. Take a look at this." She picked up a food wrapper. "We think that when we eat these, we're eating ice cream. Heck, I can't even pronounce the chemicals listed in here, can you?" She passed me the wrapper.

I stumbled over the words. "Polysorbate 80 and/or polysorbate 65, propy . . . propylene glycol algi . . . alginate, mono and/or digly . . . diglycerides . . . what are these things?"

"Exactly my point! Why eat what you can't pronounce? And these ingredients are always written in fine print and tucked away very neatly. Few people would ever notice them, not that most even know to look. But more important, many of these additives and colorings have potentially serious health consequences. Take carrageenan as an example - one I always assumed to be among the safest. It's used as a texture-modifying agent in many foods from ice cream to prepared meats and salad dressings. According to *Additive Alert*, prepared by one of Canada's leading public environmental interest groups, Pollution Probe, it's associated with ulcers, colitis, colon cancer, and decreased numbers of live births in pregnant animals."

"And we're allowed to eat it!"

"We're all but force-fed hundreds - no, thousands - of even far more harmful additives and preservatives. The most intelligent approach is to limit or eliminate your consumption of these substances."

"What are some of the others?" I asked, becoming more and more concerned.

"BHA, short for butylated hydroxyanisole and BHT, butylated hydroxytoluene, are both commonly used preservatives in dried breakfast cereals, salad dressings, margarines, meat by-products and even parboiled rice."

"What specific health risks would be associated with them?"

"Again, according to *Additive Alert*, these chemicals accumulate in body fat and are associated with symptoms such as vomiting, dizziness and stomach cramps. They can also cause allergies, kidney damage, behavioral changes, nerve and reproductive system damage, birth defects, and even cancer.

"Who would ever make the connection?"

"Very few. Many of those symptoms could easily be chalked up to stomach flu or food poisoning . . ."

We looked at each other and laughed. It was as if we could read each other's minds. It *was* food poisoning! A slow, chemical poisoning!

"Jillian, I can't begin to tell you about the many adverse effects of additives, preservatives and colorings on the children I see. Symptoms range from gastrointestinal disorders and behavior problems, to suicidal tendencies - to name only a few."

"Oh, how awful!" I was mortified.

She took out the ice cream sandwich wrapper again. "Propylene glycol is used in ice cream to prevent ice crystals from forming. According to Beatrice Trum Hunter in *Consumer Beware*, this chemical is used in germicides, antifreeze and paint remover. Some of my little patients can tolerate brands of chemical-free ice cream made from natural ingredients, similar to what our parents and grandparents ate, but they become totally hyperactive when given one of these." She waved the wrapper in the air.

I thought of all the foods I naively packed into my grocery cart every week that were probably full of horrible things.

"Included in the foods we consume every day, are virtually thousands of additives, synthetic flavors and dyes, many of which have been banned in Europe and in several Scandinavian countries. Obviously, they're health risks. Dr. Ross Hume Hall, a biochemist at McMaster University who regularly advises the Canadian federal government, suggests that we don't have the proper tools for measuring the health risk of low-level exposure over decades. The current method is to expose laboratory mice and rats to large amounts of a suspected toxic compound and to watch to see some evidence of cancer."

"So we don't know much about the hazards of exposure over the long haul."

"No. And not only do scientists not measure the effects from low-level chemical exposure over time, but they have virtually no way of measuring the toxicity *in combination* of everything to which we're exposed. It's the chemical soup we referred to earlier. It's a problem no one addresses. From cradle to grave we're victims of slow poisoning, and we're not even aware of it. What we do see is an increasing number of deaths from cancer and heart disease, and a population plagued with chronic, degenerative illnesses."

"And no one makes the connections?" I was aghast.

Eva nodded. "Sad, isn't it? Here's an anecdote from Ross Hume Hall's foreword to *Additive Alert*. It would be amusing if it weren't so frightening:

> Imagine sitting at the breakfast table and telling your five-year old, 'Go ahead, eat your Crunchies with their 100 deliberately added emulsifiers, acidulants, firmers, enhancers, humectants, sequestrants, stabilizers, texturizers, anti-caking agents, their 150 pesticide residues, their 2,000 petroleum- based residues rubbed off the packaging. Don't worry, because the government food regulations say all those additives are safe.' I think your child would be a bit sceptical.
>
> I'm sceptical. Like a five-year-old I keep asking 'how can you be sure?' How do you know that the great mix of additives buried in every spoonful of Crunchies is safe?

One book of many that makes well-documented connections between cancer and diet is *Cancer & Nutrition* by Dr. Charles Simone . . ."

"Oh yes, I think that's one that Dr. Rowland mentioned . . ."

"Well, Simone states that it's now estimated and generally accepted that diet and nutrition appear to be factors in 60 percent of cancers in women and 40 percent in men, as well as about 75 percent of cardiovascular diseases. He goes on to make a very important statement: *You have almost total control over the destiny of your health and the health of your family! Do something about it.* One person who comes to mind who *did* something about it is Dr. Lorraine Day, who was chief of orthopedic surgery at San Francisco General Hospital. She was diagnosed with breast cancer and subsequently healed herself - primarily through nutrition. I shuddered when I heard her state: *Cancer is found at the end of your fork.*"

"What an absolutely horrible thought!"

"It may well be, but from my experience over the years, it's very accurate. A clear example is the link between sodium nitrite and cancer. This additive is found in almost all processed meats . . ."

I thought of the sandwiches my kids ate every day and our wienie roasts in the summer.

". . . Nitrites combine in the stomach with amines - a natural substance produced in the human body - to form nitrosamines, which are potent poisons. Despite studies which clearly link this additive to cancer, nitrites are still being used and there is no indication that they will be outlawed. In fact, *The Lancet*, ever conservative, warned as far back as 1968 of 'the gravest concern' over this chemical."

"But if there's such concern, how do food processing companies get away with it?"

"Probably because of economic pressures. It's the cheapest preservative that protects against botulism. The argument put forth by the food industry is that people are better off avoiding immediate death from botulism than worrying over the longer term possibility of death from nitrosamine-caused esophageal or stomach cancer."

"What a choice! Pay now or pay later? Maybe we should avoid these meats altogether."

"Not a bad idea." She then returned to her explanation of why so many people suffer from sensitivities today. "The second reason is the phenomenal growth of the fast food industry. It, too, has contributed significantly to our ill health. Back in the fifties when most of our food was cooked at home, we knew what ingredients went into our stomachs. Today, who knows? Fats and sugars are only two of the evils. Again, additives, dyes and artificial flavors are in almost all fast foods - from 'homemade' soups made from a powder base, to burgers full of tenderizers and coloring agents. According to Simone, the number of fast-food outlets increased from 30,000 to 140,000 in just the ten year period from 1970 to 1980. He added that most disturbing of all, is that fast-food chains have expanded to elementary and secondary schools, colleges, military bases, and even hospitals."

"Like our local Children's Hospital," I interrupted.

"Can you imagine the message we give to our young people by encouraging junk food in a healing institution? They're already inundated from an early age with foods devoid of essential nutrients, high in fat and low in fiber, with excess sodium and questionable additives. This all contributes to the increase in chronic degenerative diseases, and along with that, a rise in healthcare costs. In fact, at a recent conference on adolescent nutrition, doctors reported that blockages of arteries, hypertension, and reductions in liver function can start even before the teen years."

"It appears to be a no-win situation."

"It is," she replied. "Even in Japan, where the traditional diet consisted of rice and fish, fatty foods have become a mainstay and the average child's cholesterol has risen to a level now exceeding that of the United States. Japan's average fat intake is eight times higher than it was in the 1960's, while the percentage of obese children has tripled, as has the average cholesterol count. Dr. Richard Deckelbaum, a nutritionist at Columbia University, correlates the rise in childhood obesity around the world to the increase in packaged, convenience foods."

"Which only goes to show that much of degenerative disease is due to lifestyle factors such as diet, rather than to genetics."

"Exactly my point. According to the scathing nutritional report card published in 1988, the *Surgeon General's Report on Diet and Health*, poor diet was blamed for increased incidence of coronary heart disease; high blood pressure; cancer; diabetes; obesity; skeletal, dental, kidney and gastroinestinal diseases; infections and lowered immunity; anemia; and neurological disorders. According to the report, the likelihood of developing any of these diseases can be reduced by *dietary modifications alone.* This report also stated that diet was the primary cause of the 2.1 million deaths in the U.S. in 1987."

"This only confirms what Drs. Simone and Day are suggesting . . ."

"The message is clear. The question is: Do we live to eat, or do we eat to live?"

Eva pulled a chart from her top drawer. "Bad enough that these foods are full of fats and sugars - take a look at this." She wheeled her chair closer. "These lists are extremely alarming and contain issues the Food Guide does *not* address. It's much the same in the U.S. Food Pyramid. For example, most people would think that ordering a fish fillet from one of these fast food joints might be a healthier alternative. But look at the *twenty-five* possible additives that are permitted in that one item alone! It really is awful. And what about a 'healthy' milkshake? Take a good look at this chart (fig. 6)."

I peered over her shoulder. I was horrified! Nearly *thirty* ingredients, names I couldn't possibly pronounce, jumped out at me. "No wonder everyone's sick. We just don't think about what we're putting into our bodies!"

"Exactly. And look here," continued Eva, "Even if you order a salad, this is what's in the dressing alone."

I looked at the list of chemicals. I was shocked. "God! At any one meal, you could be eating close to one hundred chemicals. What about government agencies? Aren't they supposed to protect us?"

# Additives in Fast Foods:
## a few examples
### (fig. 6)

**Additives in a fish fillet from a popular fast-food outlet:**

calcium silicate, monosodium glutamate (hydrolyzed plant protein, autolyzed yeast), sodium hexametaphosphate, sodium tripolyphosphate, modified corn starch.

The following are permitted food additives which may or may not be present in the flour of this product: acetone, amylase, ammonium persulphate, ammonium chloride, ascorbic acid, azodicarbonamide, benzoyl peroxide, bromelain, calcium carbonate, calcium sulphate, chlorine, chlorine dioxide, dicalcium phosphate, glucoamylase, lactase, lipoxidase, l-cysteine (hydrochloride), magnesium carbonate, potassium aluminum sulphate, potassium bromate, protease, sodium aluminum sulphate, tricalcium phosphate, monocalcium phosphate.

**Additives in a milkshake from a popular fast-food outlet:**

artificial flavor, calcium sulphate, carob bean gum, carboxymethyl cellulose, calcium chloride, carrageenan, citric acid, cellulose gum, color, disodium phosphate, guar gum, lactic acid, lecithin, lipase, locust bean gum, microbial enyzyme, mono- and diglycerides, polysorbate 80, pepsin, propylene glycol, potassium sorbate, rennet, sorbic acid, sodium citrate, sodium bicarbonate, sodium benzoate, xanthan gum.

**Additives in condiments such as salad dressings, dipping sauces, jam, peanut butter, gravy from a popular fast-food outlet:**

alum, artificial flavor, BHA, BHT, citric acid, color, cellulose gum, disodium guanylate, disodium inosinate, disodium EDTA, gum arabic, guar gum, mono- and diglycerides, microcrystalline cellulose, natural flavor, potassium sorbate, polysorbate 80, pectin, propylene glycol alginate, polysorbate 60, phosphoric acid, sodium acetate, sorbic acid, sodium benzoate, sodium citrate, xanthan gum.

Information from: **Additive Alert,** The Pollution Probe Foundation

"As long as there's no proof of harm, government policy allows a large array of chemicals into our food supply. Contrast that with Norway, where many food additives are not permitted. They're presumed guilty even if claimed to be harmless. All synthetic food colors have been banned there since 1979. Randee Holmes, author of *Additive Alert*, finds the Canadian government's attitude hard to swallow. For example, Citrus Red Dye No. 2, used to color Florida oranges, and BHA, an oil preservative, are both considered carcinogenic by health authorities in other countries, but are still permitted here . . . "

"That's outrageous!" I was becoming incensed.

"Outrageous perhaps, but true. In *Diet for A Poisoned Planet*, David Steinman points out, *We are told constantly that the level of a toxin in a certain food is 'absolutely safe'. But how many 'absolutely safe' doses does it take before it's not safe anymore?* Two good examples are DDT and Alar. DDT, for example, was used for thirty years before it was banned in the early seventies and it still continues to haunt us. High concentrations can *still* be found in those who were exposed to it, some of whom developed breast cancer. Even the foods that are supposed to be healthy for us - fruits and vegetables - are contaminated. There are more pesticides used on our food than ever before - more chemicals in general. These put very heavy stresses on our immune system. We're literally digging our graves with our teeth."

"And the cancer societies keep telling us to eat more of these foods! They never mention pesticides."

"That's right. This reminds me of last night's trip to the grocery store. Over the bags of carrots, there was a sign that read: *For every pound of carrots purchased, three cents will be donated to the cancer society.* Interestingly, when I went to the organic section to buy *my* carrots, I noticed there was no such sign. What irony!"

"Doesn't sound quite right, does it?"

"No. There's something very wrong with this picture. According to Simone, pesticide residues are commonly found in human tissue in most Americans, averaging six parts per million in fatty tissue. And I'm sure Canadians are not far behind. These residues have also been found in both human and cow's milk, and have even been known to cross the placental barrier, entering the human fetus. According to the National Academy of Sciences, pesticide residues on food crops cause 14,000 new cases of cancer each year out of 1.3 million total cases. That one percent may appear to be insignificant, unless, of course, you happen to be one of the 14,000 . . ."

"Or a friend, or family member!"

"Yes, of course. And what's not factored into statistics are the chronic illnesses that arise as a result of pesticide exposure - the walking wounded- those still alive, but chronically unwell. Few of us suspect that our daily apple or potato may be so contaminated with chemicals that it's the direct cause of the chronic fatigue, flu-like symptoms, arthritis, or headaches we've come to take for granted."

"Who'd ever believe it?" I couldn't believe what I was hearing. Yet, it all made perfect sense. How could we continue to deny that these exposures don't affect our health? I realized, of course, that I was part of that denial.

"We just buzz along, busy as bees, seldom giving any of this a second thought - until we're sick and are forced to take a closer look. For many, it's too late."

"I know just what you mean."

"A fourth reason for this rise in sensitivities, and perhaps one of the more significant, is the epidemic overuse and abuse of prescription drugs."

"Like antibiotics?" I asked, reflecting on my discussion with Dr. Rowland.

"Yes." She held up a sheet of paper. "This is just one article of many that talks about the perils of unnecessary antibiotic usage. It says that along with the 1.5 million pounds of tranquilizers and 800,000 pounds of barbiturates, Americans ingested *four million pounds* of penicillin last year. And according to a *New York Times* front page article, prescription drugs kill between 30,000 and 60,000 people each year. This doesn't even include the thousands who suffer permanent side effects or who develop new diseases caused by the drugs themselves. The owner of a pharmaceutical company once stated that the only safe drug is an ineffective one."

"It really is a shame that so many people practically live on all this stuff. And my family is certainly no exception . . . but we're given no alternatives."

"I'm not defending the medical establishment, but many of my colleagues and friends who are doctors tell me that their patients actually demand prescriptions."

"But don't you think it's because we're conditioned to think that way?" I asked, thinking of the massive numbers of medications my family alone had been given over a relatively short period of time.

"Yes. We're a quick-fix society wanting instant solutions for everything, including our health. As a result, we pay for it in the long run."

"We sure do. I'm a prime example. Look where it's gotten me," I moaned.

"You have a lot of company in that regard," said Eva, smiling. "Then, added to all the prescriptions routinely dished out, there are the drug residues in the animal products we eventually wind up eating. We get a double dose. No wonder we have serious health problems!"

"What kinds of drugs?" I asked.

"Hormones to enhance animal growth, and antibiotics that are given to livestock. Many of these have never been approved for humans, yet we inadvertently consume them when we eat meat products from these animals. We've seen numerous incidents of people reacting to these substances. Just yesterday, a woman came in with a badly swollen face. It happened every time she ate turkey. When tested for pure, drug-free turkey, she didn't react at all. She'd lived with this situation for years, being treated with one medication after another, which only compounded her problem."

"Think how many other symptoms we might experience which we never connect to the root cause," I remarked.

"According to a recent magazine article, there's been a fourfold increase in the sale of hormones used for livestock in the past ten years. Approximately ninety-five percent of all cattle are treated with them. And not only is meat contaminated with them, but so are some farmed fish. I often wonder about the connection between this and the rise in breast cancer over the past ten years."

"Or the fact that our daughters are developing breasts at such an early age!" I exclaimed, thinking of several young girls in our neighborhood who were maturing far too quickly.

"Actually, there have been human horror stories that substantiate the connection between contaminated meats and premature puberty. One that comes to mind is in *Diet For A Poisoned Planet*. Steinman refers to a situation in Puerto Rico in the early 1980's. Children under the age of eight began to menstruate, and developed breasts and pubic hair in epidemic proportions. Physicians studying the problem removed chicken and milk from the children's diets, and that alone significantly reduced the problem. Researchers found extremely high estrogen levels in some samples of pork and chicken as well as synthetic hormones circulating in the bloodstreams of the children."

"Oh, that's absolutely terrible!" As much as I didn't want to believe it, I knew intuitively that the connection was a very significant one. "What are some of these hormones?"

"Estradiol, progesterone, testosterone, zeranol and melegestrol acetate. The latter two are synthetically produced. Just the other day, Dr. Rowland mentioned the significant increase in what's called estrogen-dependent cancer among relatively young women. You see, Jillian, it's not just the fat that causes the problems; it's what's *in* the fat. Yet, this issue is never addressed by nutritionists or cancer societies."

"Are these hormones allowed to be used everywhere?"

"No. I understand they're not permitted in Sweden and in 1989, the European Economic Community (EEC) banned the use of hormones in all animals used for human consumption. As a result, North American meats and poultry can no longer be exported to any of the twelve countries belonging to the EEC. Some people say it was an economic move . . ."

"Who cares about the original motive. At least they're not eating contaminated meat! We have to do the same here. We have a *right* to know what's in the food we eat!"

"Yes, we do. When was the last time you saw artificial flavors, colors, pesticides, drugs or other additives listed on a package of ground beef or on a turkey? Meat and dairy producers are not required by law to label their products. A government report in the early eighties discovered that out of 150 drugs and pesticides contained in meat and poultry, forty-two were potential carcinogens, twenty were linked to birth defects, and six had adverse effects on fetuses. And how many more substances are there that we know nothing about?"

"They should be *forced* to list everything that's given to the animals, right from birth to the time they're slaughtered."

"I couldn't agree more, Jillian. And if you've ever tasted a free-range chicken, you'd never go back to the supermarket variety. The flavor is out of this world!"

"Where do you buy them? I'd like to try one."

"We have lists of where you can buy them at the front desk. The staff can help you . . . Grocery stores should be required by law to list all additives - not only what's in processed foods, but in all other foods as well. Anything added to our food should be itemized, right from chickens to grapes and potatoes. As you said, we, as consumers, have a *right* to know what we're eating - especially for our children's sake. These kids suffer not only from pesticide exposure if living in agricultural areas, but from the very food they eat. What pops into my mind is that National Academy of Sciences figure of 1.3 million total cases of cancer from pesticide residues."

"How can this be allowed to happen?"

"You tell me," replied Eva, shaking her head. "According to the General Accounting Office (GAO), the investigative arm of Congress, the Food and Drug Administration samples only one percent of domestically produced fruits and vegetables for pesticide residues. In 1985, the FDA devoted only 3.4 percent of its annual $397.5 million budget to monitoring pesticides."

"And I suppose some of the pesticides banned in the U.S. and Canada are still used in the countries from which we import our produce."

"That's quite correct. And are you aware that by the time a child reaches the age of six, cumulative exposure to just eight of the pesticides used on produce alone can reach toxic levels?"

I shook my head. This session was turning into a rude awakening!

"And this doesn't even include the contaminants found in dairy and meat products. Nor does it take into account the impact processed or fast foods, a high fat-diet, the overconsumption of sugar, and environmental contaminants have on a child's health. Pretty scary stuff."

I nodded in agreement. "And it all goes back to education, doesn't it?"

"It sure does. Education and freedom of information. We all need to have a Who's Who of pesticides on our kitchen table. As Rachel Carson said so eloquently in *Silent Spring* over thirty years ago: *If we are going to live so intimately with these chemicals - eating and drinking them, taking them into the very marrow of our bones - we had better know something about their nature and their power.* Imagine if produce departments were required by law to list all of the chemicals used on all fruits and vegetables: carbaryl, diazinon, dicolfol, ethion, malathion, methyl parathion, thiabendazole, phosalone . . ."

"No one would buy anything!" I cried.

"You bet. Or, they'd think twice about choosing foods that don't contain these chemicals. Each fruit and vegetable may have been treated with up to forty allowable pesticides. These may be used at any given time and in any combination. And they're all approved by government agencies. What comes to mind is a recent interview with Lorraine Day on a local radio phone-in show. . ."

"Is that the doctor who healed herself of breast cancer?"

"Yes. She said: *Imagine a mother serving her children a beautiful, luscious salad freshly picked from the garden. All of a sudden, she says, 'I'll be right back. I'm just going to get a bottle of pesticide and spray the salad.' How's that any different than the farmer spraying?"*

It wasn't any different. She was right. The only difference was that one was blatantly obvious, and the other, we ignored - perhaps because we were not properly informed in the first place.

She continued. "Think of even one typical meal - you could be eating over three hundred different pesticides, additives and colorings - and never even know it. And, do we know, for example, how the pesticides on tomatoes interact with the preservatives used in making spaghetti sauce?"

I was aghast at the thought. "Now I know what you mean by the term 'chemical soup'!"

"If everyone were aware of this, the demand for organically grown produce would escalate dramatically and prices would come down accordingly."

"What do you mean by organically grown?"

"Pesticide-free and grown without synthetic fertilizers . . . I must tell you a quick story. A friend of mine who's a biologist at one of the universities on the Canadian east coast, recently told me that they were doing a series of experiments with eight hundred grasshoppers. Their main food source was organic lettuce from a local producer. One day, due to a snowstorm, the organic lettuce couldn't be delivered. The technician went to the local supermarket and bought some regular lettuce - the kind that you and I, and everyone else out there eats. The next morning, all eight hundred insects were dead! Postmortem analyses revealed that the deaths were due to synthetic pesticides. You know that luscious-looking piece of broccoli sitting in the cooler of your neighborhood grocery store in the middle of January? It's probably been aerial-sprayed with who knows what and shipped thousands of miles to get here in time for dinner. Chances are the soil was deficient in most trace minerals - unless organically grown."

She looked up, eyebrows raised, "The real question remains: Which of the chemicals or drugs used today will be banned tomorrow, once their neurotoxic or carcinogenic effects are finally proven?"

"Like thalidomide, DES, and breast implants - all believed to be perfectly safe at one time?"

"Precisely. As were DDT and Alar as well. We've known for years that anything that's not free of pesticides just isn't safe - especially for children. Yet, we continue to use them. The National Academy of Sciences recently stated that by the time a child is five, he or she will have received up to *thirty-five percent* of his acceptable lifetime dose of carcinogenic pesticides."

"I guess the bottom line remains unchanged, if they kill pests, they can also kill us - slowly but surely." I couldn't ignore this awful thought. "Where can I get more information?"

"Reading Steinman's book would be a good beginning," replied Eva. "He lists all the drugs, pesticides and additives in everything you eat and drink, and categorizes them according to their level of safety. If everyone were to read this book, grocery stores carrying safe, pesticide-free foods would be popping up everywhere."

"As would more healthy cereal and snack food choices. Boy! There could be great business opportunities out there for anyone wanting to provide healthy alternatives. As it stands now, we're nothing more than guinea pigs for food industry experiments!"

"We certainly are."

"So what can I do right now - even before I read the book?"

"A first step would be to read labels. Remember the simple rule of thumb - avoid packaged foods that contain words you can't pronounce. I used to advise people to shop around the periphery of their grocery store and leave out the middle aisles entirely, where all the processed junk seems to be. But, as I said earlier, what's even more unfair is what we're *not* told about - all the drugs and pesticides in meats, dairy products, fruits and vegetables."

"It's more than unfair, it's criminal!" I felt angry and helpless at the same time. "What can I do about pesticides on my fresh produce?"

"If you can't buy organically grown produce, peel what you can, and soak the rest in a solution of vegetable-based soap and water. A good scrub brush will remove surface pesticides. Brand names for recommended soaps can be found in this book, *Clean & Green* by Annie Berthold-Bond." She held up a rather attractive book with a picture on the cover of a hand cleaning the earth. "But keep in mind, many residues cannot be scrubbed away - they're not only *on* the plant, but *in* it."

"So the reality is that residues will be eaten by the unwary consumer anyhow?"

"That's probably closer to the truth. And remember, we've only touched on the pesticides sprayed on our foods while they're still in the ground. What about the waxes, fungicides, and chemicals used to fumigate dried fruits or the gases used to artificially ripen tomatoes and bananas? But we haven't enough time to discuss this in detail. So . . . let's get back to your original question about the increase in sensitivities. Another reason is the introduction of the birth control pill, which has contributed significantly to changing the internal flora of women."

"And externally," I joked. "It not only made me feel sick and bitchy, but I gained weight like crazy!"

She smiled. "Yes, it's amazing how everyone thought the pill was the answer to all our prayers. Only now are we finding out the long-term problems associated with it. Apart from the sorts of effects you just mentioned, it can also create vitamin and mineral deficiencies which further predispose women to sensitivities. I don't know if you're aware of this, but it's estimated that seventy percent of those who are environmentally ill are women."

"I didn't know that. Come to think of it, though, it seems it's mainly my female friends who are chronically ill - rarely their husbands. Why is that?"

"There's nothing conclusive, but Dr. Rowland links it to four basic factors: women have more physical stressors such as childbirth, the pill, and hormonal fluctuations; we tend to frequent doctors' offices more often, and are therefore medicated more; women tend to spend longer periods in what is often a toxic home or office; and last, but not least, there's the superwoman syndrome. Being on call twenty-four hours a day as mother, wife, chauffeur and maid, combined with a career is exhausting."

"You're telling me! The best thing I ever did was take a leave of absence after my last child was born."

"I'll bet. Do you ever wonder how much worse you might have been had you kept on working?"

"I couldn't have survived," I said quietly, as I thought of the past three years, much of it a blur. "I barely had enough energy for myself - being so sick with two young children and a baby."

"Which brings me to yet another reason for the dramatic increase in sensitivities. Although it's changing, the trend over the past forty years has been to bottle-feed instead of breast-feed. The formula industry is a huge business that has created far too many health problems."

"I don't understand the connection . . ."

"Breast milk provides essential fats and enzymes that make it highly digestible and includes substances which enhance immunity. On the other hand, formulas lack many of these vital components. One example cited in the *British Medical Journal* demonstrated that out of 339 infants with gastroenteritis, 338 had been bottle-fed. Study after study consistently shows that bottle-feeding is associated with the development of a variety of chronic diseases in later life."

"I tried to breast-feed my youngest, Max, but my milk supply dwindled. I was afraid he'd starve. Then I followed the advice of the nursing staff and began supplementing him with formula. Eventually, I ran out of my own milk."

"You know, Jillian, the notion that mother's milk dries up is one of the biggest myths perpetuated by our society. And I hear it all the time. So many women are told the same story. The truth of the matter is that the breast is an incredible machine, functioning perfectly as it was intended, on the law of supply and demand. In order for milk to be produced, the baby must suckle . . ."

"But he did, and nothing happened."

"You mean, at first you had milk and then the supply dwindled, right?"

"Right."

"How long did you wait before supplementing him with formula?"

"Ten or twelve hours. That's when I was told to start."

"Sometimes it takes as long as twenty-four hours for more milk to be produced. Of course, if the baby is supplemented, he won't feel like sucking and then the milk supply will dwindle. It's a Catch-22 situation. The mother should be encouraged to keep suckling the baby until more milk comes in. It's simply letting nature take its course. By doing so, we could prevent many problems from developing later on."

"Are breast-fed babies free from sensitivities?"

"Not necessarily, but statistically they have a much better chance. And, if they do suffer from them, at least we can alter the mother's diet to alleviate the problem. If formula-fed, the choices are very limited."

"I can't believe how much I'm learning today!"

Her charisma was spellbinding. Eva's eyes danced, her body language was as articulate in conveying her message as were her words. She leaned forward, gently sweeping a strand of hair behind her ear.

"Well, I have even more information for you," she said, smiling. An additional reason for the rise in sensitivities was the seventies' energy crisis that gave birth to airtight homes and sealed buildings. This, in turn, led to the development of mechanical ventilation systems. They're often operated and maintained improperly, and consequently, wreak havoc on our health."

"Like the new wing of the hospital where I last worked! Not only was it a sealed unit, but the air exchange system was turned down on weekends to save money."

"In some office buildings, those systems are turned off completely on weekends, and turned on about an hour before people show up for work on Monday morning. This practice stirs up bacteria and molds which are then inhaled by the occupants. We see so many sick people as a result of such negligent habits. By the way, if these systems were properly maintained, bacteria and mold wouldn't be as much of a problem to begin with."

"Wow, if management only knew what it was costing them in terms of reduced productivity, sick leave and disability payments!"

"What's even worse is seeing sick children as a result of these practices in schools. It truly is a tragedy. We see the casualties here at this clinic."

I shook my head in disgust.

"Yet another factor for this increase in sensitivities is our habit of repetitive eating. This can create shortages in the body . . ."

I interrupted. "What do you mean?"

"Well, the habit of eating the same foods too often can short-change people with respect to some very essential nutrients. For the person predisposed to food sensitivities due to a permeable gut, it's a sure way of developing full-blown problems."

"But haven't people always eaten this way?"

"Not really. When you think about it, our grandparents ate seasonally. For example, apples were available in the fall and berries in summer. Their bodies had a break from different foods throughout the year."

"Why is that significant?"

"Repetitive eating, especially of cooked, denatured foods, tends to deplete the enzyme system because the same ones are called into action day in and day out. But you have to keep in mind, for many of our forebears, their total load was at a minimum. Their air, water and food were essentially free of chemical contaminants. I hate to sound repetitious, but the bottom line - the basic, hard-core truth - is that most allergies or sensitivities largely stem from the past few decades of over-medication, the increase of chemicals in our environment, and abusive eating habits."

"Abusive eating habits?" I felt like a parrot, echoing her every phrase.

"Yes, our society is brainwashed into eating foods that are overcooked, over-processed and devoid of essential nutrients. Did you know that the most frequently consumed foods in America are coffee, white bread, and sugar - in that order?"

"I didn't know it was that bad . . ."

"It's even worse - hot dogs were fourth. Let me tell you about Pottenger's famous cats. Back in the thirties, Dr. Pottenger conducted a series of studies with over nine hundred cats. One group of cats was put on a diet of raw foods, while the others were fed cooked foods. The first group had healthy offspring over several generations while the latter gave birth to kittens plagued with allergies. Each generation became substantially worse - some even stillborn. You see, raw foods contain all the essential enzymes, while cooked, processed foods don't. People are no different."

"So again, it goes back to diet."

"You've got it!"

I laughed. "Now you sound just like Dr. Rowland!"

"Thank you! That's quite a compliment," said Eva, smiling. "In any case, poor diet combined with the other things we discussed, can deplete the immune system to the point where the body is weakened and can't cope with common healthy foods that ordinarily wouldn't be a problem."

"Does that go back to the *Total Load Theory* - that it's really a combination of things that overloads the immune system?"

"Yes. The body weakens and can't handle even the simplest things - like dust and dust mites. But there *is* good news!"

"That's a relief. What is it?" I could handle a bit of good news right about now.

"As the body is strengthened through proper diet, yeast management, and appropriate supplements, some of these sensitivities can die down - especially the cumulative ones. In fact, successive generations can actually be strengthened, if care is taken."

"You mean you can actually reverse the situation?"

"To some degree, yes. For example, a colleague of Dr. Rowland had a highly sensitive daughter who was pregnant. Her underlying yeast condition was treated and she was given supplements for the nutrients she lacked. He supervised her diet throughout her pregnancy by eliminating problem foods and rotating all the rest. She ate lots of uncooked, organic, raw foods. The end result? She gave birth to a relatively healthy son - much healthier than she had been."

"It's a relief to know there's hope."

Eva smiled reassuringly. "It's important to know we can make positive changes in spite of the toxic world in which we live."

"What did you mean by supplements?"

"Vitamins, minerals, enzymes, essential fatty acids, herbs . . ."

"Far too many doctors laugh at the idea of taking vitamins. They say all it does is create expensive urine."

"Yes, sadly, that's a common attitude. But just between you and me, I know many who pop them like crazy and still won't advise their patients to take them. In fact, according to the 1992 *Medical Tribune*, eight out of ten doctors take antioxidants for long-term health."

I couldn't quite see Dr. Klamer doing that!

"It seems that the more information that comes out about antioxidants and their importance in our toxic world, the more seriously it's taken. I don't know if you've noticed, but over the past couple of years, the covers of magazines like *Time*, *Newsweek* and *MacLean's* have featured vitamins on several occasions."

"I have noticed. In fact, I took one of those magazines to my doctor, as well as to the dietician I was seeing."

"It's a sign of changing times. Basically, it indicates an increased awareness among the general population, which in itself is very significant. We'll go into detail about supplements during your follow-up visit. It's vital that we focus strictly on food elimination first, so we can learn how specific foods affect you."

"But why do we need supplements at all?"

"One good reason is the increased incidence of bowel disorders, which, in turn, result in impaired absorption. But we also need supplements because our food is low in essential nutrients - processing being the main culprit."

Eva got up, walked over to a cupboard by the door, and pulled out a loaf of sliced, white bread. "Here's a great example. We strip all the nutrients out of the whole grain in order to make it more appealing." She took out a few slices, squished them into a ball and tossed it to me. I caught it with my left hand. It felt like a lump of playdough!

"To produce this, the processor removes the better part of twenty-four nutrients from whole wheat, replaces *four* of them, and then has the nerve to call it enriched! Imagine what this does to your gut. There's almost no fiber left, and people wonder why they need laxatives. There are enough additives and preservatives in here to pickle a horse! What bugs me the most is how they indiscriminately throw a few of the vital nutrients back in, and call it enriched! It's dishonest."

Listening to Eva, I felt like I was in the midst of an ongoing drama. I never knew what she was going to say or do next. It was never dull!

She picked up a small book and opened it to a flagged page. "Listen to this:

> Food technologists . . . replace only a few of the multi-
> nutritional substances removed and label their product
> 'enriched'. This is the same as being held up at gunpoint
> on a dark street and ordered to strip naked. The thief takes
> clothes and valuables, notices your shivering embarrassment,
> then returns your underwear and fifty cents to take the bus
> home. Do you then feel enriched? "

I had to laugh. "That's great! What's it from?"

"It's from *Orthomolecular Nutrition* by Abram Hoffer, but he's actually quoting Roger Williams in *Nutrition Against Disease*. Can you see how ridiculous the term 'enriched' is?"

"I do now," I replied. "But the reality is that most people never stop long enough to think about it. I never did. I just accepted everything at face value."

"Then we end up in shock and disbelief when illness strikes, never thinking for a moment that our diet might be one of the underlying causes of our poor state of health. It seems that every time I pick up a newspaper, they've discovered a genetic link to just about every conceivable illness. I think it's a convenient way of removing responsibility from us and redirecting the blame to a 'mysterious illness' that just pops out of nowhere. And the magic solution? A yet-to-be discovered wonder drug! Or, one that's already been discovered - like Prozac, for instance. It's the nineties' cure-all. According to *Maclean's* magazine, there are over *eleven million* people on this drug. After all, it can 'cure' anything from depression to P.M.S.!"

"It must work if so many people use it."

"Once again, in a crisis situation, great - go for it. But then, once the condition is stabilized, the object would be to dig a little deeper and try to identify some underlying causes - whether physical or emotional in nature. If they're not identified, they'll only rear their ugly heads at a later date."

Eva put the bread away and sat down again. "Oh yes, another significant factor is that modern agricultural methods have robbed the soil of trace elements. Many of them are not necessary for the plant's growth, but are essential for human development. Unless you eat pesticide-free, locally grown food all year round as well as meat that's free of antibiotics and hormones, you can't expect to get all your nutrients from food."

"Why does it have to be locally grown?"

"Aha! I was hoping you'd ask, because that brings me to my next point. The shipping of foods alone, from one end of the continent to another, causes a loss in nutrient value. Just think about it. Our food - especially if you live in a more northern climate as we do - is shipped thousands of miles. How many nutrients could possibly remain by the time it finally reaches your dinner plate?"

"I'd never really thought about it. But it does make sense. But why is it that some people have sensitivities and others don't?"

"Good question. That's where heredity meets environment."

"Heredity meets the environment?" I asked, puzzled. It sounded like a bad science fiction film.

"This is where genetics can legitimately play a significant part. Some individuals are more predisposed than others. Statistics show that if one parent has sensitivities, there's a forty percent chance the offspring will have them too. If both parents have sensitivities, the percentage increases to seventy. Look over here . . ." Eva pointed to a chart entitled *Family Patterns of Hidden Sensitivities* (fig. 7).

My eyes jumped to the statement at the bottom: *Each generation's health is slightly more compromised than the previous one due to environmental deterioration.*

"Notwithstanding genetic factors, you can't escape the fact that the environment plays a significant role. Just look at the chronic illnesses on this chart. The first generation had their share of difficulties, but notice that problems increase substantially with each successive generation. The third one is plagued with all kinds of ailments, just like Pottenger's cats. But guess what?" Eva looked smug.

"What?" I replied, waiting for the punch line.

"The underlying causes of these ailments that are passed from generation to generation have never been addressed."

"What causes?" I asked dumbfounded.

"Sensitivities to foods, chemicals and airborne irritants."

# Family Patterns of Hidden Sensitivities
### (fig. 7)

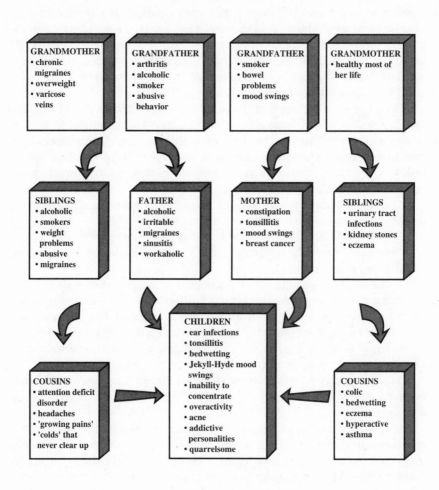

**GRANDMOTHER**
- chronic migraines
- overweight
- varicose veins

**GRANDFATHER**
- arthritis
- alcoholic
- smoker
- abusive behavior

**GRANDFATHER**
- smoker
- bowel problems
- mood swings

**GRANDMOTHER**
- healthy most of her life

**SIBLINGS**
- alcoholic
- smokers
- weight problems
- abusive
- migraines

**FATHER**
- alcoholic
- irritable
- migraines
- sinusitis
- workaholic

**MOTHER**
- constipation
- tonsillitis
- mood swings
- breast cancer

**SIBLINGS**
- urinary tract infections
- kidney stones
- eczema

**CHILDREN**
- ear infections
- tonsillitis
- bedwetting
- Jekyll-Hyde mood swings
- inability to concentrate
- overactivity
- acne
- addictive personalities
- quarrelsome

**COUSINS**
- attention deficit disorder
- headaches
- 'growing pains'
- 'colds' that never clear up

**COUSINS**
- colic
- bedwetting
- eczema
- hyperactive
- asthma

**Each generation's health is slightly more compromised than the previous one due to environmental deterioration**

At this point, I couldn't decide whether Dr. Rowland and Eva were bordering on the insane or were absolutely brilliant and as yet, undiscovered.

Eva continued. "Let me give you an example. I was told for years that my personality was wild, explosive and flamboyant because I'm Hungarian. My whole family's like that - crazy and off the wall."

"I was wondering what kind of name Eva Sandor was."

"Actually, my surname is pronounced 'Shandor' - the S is pronounced Sh. In any event, our house was the noisiest on the block. I bought into the story that we were all like that due to our expressive natures. Years later when I discovered I had food and chemical sensitivities, and decided to do something about them, I no longer behaved like the rest of my family."

"What kind of behavior do you mean? Give me an example."

"Lots of shouting, negativity - even abusive behavior."

"I have such a hard time imagining you in that kind of atmosphere." In fact, I couldn't see it at all.

She went on. "When I go home for a visit and indulge in my old comfort foods, not only do some of my old physical symptoms return, but I also start acting like the rest of my family - highly irritable and depressed. As a result, we all end up fighting with one another. If I stay on track with my diet, I can sit back, watch them all drive each other crazy, and remain quite sane. Like me, my dad had lots of digestive problems. He spent years going from one specialist to another trying to get help - without success. The tragedy is that he eventually ended up with bowel cancer."

"So are you and Dr. Rowland saying that these food sensitivities not only can cause chronic ill health and behavior problems, but can also result in more serious disease?"

"Yes. One of the best books I've read on the subject is by Dr. Chris Reading, an Australian physician. It's called *Your Family Tree Connection*. He links the constant stress on target organs with the eventual progression of disease in these same organs. It makes perfect sense, doesn't it? If there's continual wear and tear on a specific organ like the bowel, for example, does it not make sense that disease might occur there?"

I was skeptical. "If something as basic as *food* can cause all these illnesses, why don't dieticians and most doctors out there know about it?"

"Sometimes it can be as simple as not asking the right questions. And not only can foods cause illnesses, but so can underlying causes such as yeast infections and parasites." Eva stood up and walked over to the window. She looked as if she were about to deliver a lecture. "You see, Jillian, in our overly scientific world, anecdote or personal experience no longer seem to count. If a rat in a laboratory doesn't confirm what we suspect, the problem doesn't exist. We rely almost exclusively upon experimental evidence instead of listening to patients and their experiences. If the tests don't show it, they don't have it!"

"That's what's happened to me. My tests are always negative, yet I'm as sick as a dog!"

Eva chuckled, "Maybe it's because you're eating people food instead of dog food!"

I laughed with her. "But seriously, getting back to my earlier question, why don't most of the other doctors know this stuff?"

"As I said, anecdote is not accepted in medical literature. As you'll soon discover, doctors who value this type of evidence, and who have a grasp of how the environment influences human health, tend to publish books for the public. For example, William Crook wrote *The Yeast Connection*, Doris Rapp, *The Impossible Child*, Stephen Gislason, *Core Diet For Kids*, and so on. The most positive aspect of writing for the layperson rather than for medical journals, is that it puts the responsibility for people's health back into their own hands, a concept long overdue. Then, of course, there are the politics . . ."

"Politics?" I asked, wondering how politics, nutrition, and environmental health were linked.

"Well, who's going to make money by helping people get well? You can bet it won't be pharmaceutical companies or the processed food industry. They all want to keep the cogs of their big multinational corporations turning. In fact, by finding out the cause of disease, they stand to lose billions of dollars every year. Even the dairy and meat marketing boards are primarily focused on making money, often to our detriment."

"I feel like I'm just waking up from a deep sleep," I said. "I still find it mind-boggling that we're all so unaware of what's really going on. We mechanically perform our day-to-day functions with a complete lack of understanding of the bigger picture."

"Unfortunately, that's exactly how many of us live our lives. We entrust our health to everyone but ourselves. In the spring of 1991, a major press conference was held in Washington, D.C. by a group called Physicians Committee for Responsible Medicine . . ."

"Oh yes, the group opposed to the milk-mustache commercials . . ."

"Yes, no wonder . . . Well, this same group announced a plan to establish four entirely new food groups - whole grains, legumes, vegetables and fruits. The meat industry immediately called its own press conference and attempted to dismiss the PCRM as having no scientific merit. This sort of thing happens all the time. The question is, who decides what we eat?"

"Industry?" I was getting the picture.

"Right. I have to read this bit from *May All Be Fed*. It quotes Marion Nestle, who was managing editor of the Surgeon General's landmark report on Nutrition and Health in 1988. Obviously, she wasn't impressed with the food groups created by the USDA, which, by the way, are not significantly different from those in Canada. She says:

> The standard . . . food groups are based on American
> agricultural lobbies. Why do we have a milk group? Because
> we have a National Dairy Council. Why do we have a meat
> group? Because we have an extremely powerful meat lobby."

"So we're constantly dictated to by powerful lobby groups."

"All the time." Eva paused for a moment. "And then there are some non-profit organizations that raise funds year after year for scientific research . . ."

"You mean health societies and foundations?"

"Yes. Dr. Rowland and I, as well as many of our colleagues, have volunteered to conduct workshops for groups like these. We include topics which deal with chronic degenerative disease and childhood hyperactivity - especially Attention Deficit Hyperactive Disorder, better known as A.D.H.D. We explain our approach - altering lifestyle habits - but they're not the least bit interested."

I thought of Nathaniel. His teacher had recently suggested that he be tested for A.D.D. "You mean to tell me that A.D.D. is also linked to environmental factors?"

"Often, it can be - especially to foods and chemicals. It can also be due to a nutritional imbalance. There are many studies that show that dietary factors play a major role in this condition. Some can even be found in conventional medical journals."

"So if that's the case, why wouldn't these groups be interested in learning about other options?"

"Because it seems that self-preservation is often more important than finding solutions to the problem for which the society was founded in the first place. There are, of course, exceptions. One that stands out is the Lung Assocation. Their approach to prevention is not only sincere, but quite integrated. They attempt to incorporate lifestyle factors into their promotions and programs. However, one area they could place more emphasis on is diet - especially in relation to asthma."

"Is everything so self-serving?"

"Unfortunately, it's often the case. Take for instance, dietetic associations. As long as they continue to be backed by processed food giants, the public will never be given objective, unbiased information."

"Even dietetics associations are connected to big business?"

"In my opinion, too many are. I once wrote an article for the local newspaper in which I mentioned these affiliations. The national president of one association wrote back saying they are not 'backed by', but are 'in partnership' with these companies. If that's not a blatant admission of conflict of interest, I don't know what is!"

"So even the people who are supposed to act on our behalf and protect our health have vested interests!"

"Often they do. Just about a month ago, a friend of mine who's a hospital nutritionist, sent me a contest form mailed to all dieticians and nutritionists across the country. It was sponsored by a well-known processed food manufacturer. The main criteria for entry was based on a public endorsement of the company's products through contestants' publications or hospital menus."

"It's just terrible that we've come to this - so driven by money."

"At other times, it's just plain old, honest ignorance. While working on my thesis, I had to research hospital menus. I focused on hospitals that specialized in the treatment of children, heart patients, and cancer. The standard fare was french fries, chicken fingers, ice cream, and Jello. All spokespersons claimed to follow the standard food guide 'to ensure the patient receives adequate nutrients during their hospitalization'. Several nutritionists indicated that they try to follow the Guide, but stated 'if chicken fingers or ice cream is all they [the patients] want, something is better than nothing. As long as they eat, we're happy'. Imagine the fat and sugar content of those meals! And we already had a quick glimpse into the many chemicals contained in these types of foods - hardly conducive to healing!"

"My uncle had a triple bypass a year ago and one of his first solid hospital meals was fries and a milkshake. I didn't know very much about nutrition, but I remember being appalled even then, given the little knowledge I had at the time."

"We have a long way to go in improving hospital nutrition." Eva paused for a moment. "But you know Jillian, ultimately, it's not just the greedy multinational corporations, uncaring politicians, or unaware health care providers who are the primary villains of our demise . . ."

Eva could sense my confusion.

"It's also we, the consumers, who demand these goods and services. In his book *Beating Cancer With Nutrition*, Dr. Patrick Quillin writes: *Americans choose their food based upon taste, cost, convenience and psychological gratification - thus ignoring the main reason that we eat, which is to provide our body cells with the raw materials to grow, repair and fuel our bodies.* Ultimately, the real question is: Are we ready to forfeit our convenient, affluent, quick-fix lives?"

"Usually, it takes illness to make changes . . ."

"Sad, but true," Eva said quietly, shaking her head. "And on that note, let's get back to you."

We returned to the chart on chronic illness and heredity. "I still have such a hard time with the idea that these illnesses can actually be caused by foods."

"They often are, but keep in mind that an underlying factor in many of these sensitivities is yeast overgrowth and other factors that Dr. Rowland will discuss with you later. Remember Jillian, it takes time to assimilate all of this. It's not a religion. You don't have to *believe* in it. You simply have to follow an elimination diet for two weeks and *experience* it. Which brings us to more practical matters - your diet. An hour goes by fairly quickly, and we still have a lot of ground to cover. The next part of our session is primarily instructional. Would you like me to tape it?"

"That would be great."

As Eva walked over to the tape recorder, she stopped, swung around, looked straight at me, and said, "Jillian, don't you ever buy the story that your health has to deteriorate with age! You can look and feel better right now than you ever did in your youth. What's that old saying, "The older she gets . . ."

I finished it for her. "The better she looks."

She laughed and said, "Wasn't that from an old T.V. commercial? Here's an even better one I've always loved by Victor Hugo: *Forty is the old age of youth. Fifty is the youth of old age.*"

"And I'm not even thirty-five yet," I moaned.  "Do you think I'll ever feel and look as good as you?"

"Of course you will.  I *know* you will!  And within a few weeks you'll know it too.  After today, your life will never be the same."

I didn't know it then, but she was right.

*Allergies (sensitivities) are more widespread*

*than most physicians, including allergists, realize,*

*and they can cause*

*far more serious health problems*

*both physical and mental,*

*than is commonly believed.*

*Allergy sufferers don't need to despair, however.*

*Proper diet and nutrition,*

*combined with other alternative approaches,*

*can relieve and reverse allergies,*

*even after conventional approaches have failed.*

**The Burton Goldberg Group**
**Alternative Medicine: The Definitive Guide**

# 6

# Elimination Diet

*Let thy food be thy medicine and thy medicine be thy food.*
**Hippocrates**

*E*va pushed the start button on the tape recorder and turned back to her desk. Out of the blue, she asked, "What's your favorite food?"

"My favorite food?" I stammered, caught a bit off guard.

"And don't say carrot sticks and salad, 'cause I won't buy it!" She laughed. "Seriously, if you were marooned on a desert island, and could eat whatever you wanted, what would it be?"

"Hmm . . . anything sweet, creamy or . . ." I had to think for a moment. "Bagels! Bread! I'd have to have my freshly baked homemade bread." Pizza was another biggie!

"So, sugar . . . dairy . . . wheat . . . and yeast," Eva said, writing it down as she uttered it. She opened my file. "Let's take a quick peek at your diet."

I jumped to the defense. "I always thought I had a pretty healthy diet. When I was pregnant with Max, my youngest, the hospital dietician told me I ate very well. The only thing she advised me was to increase my milk intake . . ."

Eva let out a little chuckle. "And I'll bet that poor child had one ear infection after another."

I was flabbergasted! "How did you know? It's true! He had them almost from birth."

"Because the two almost always go hand in hand. Plus it's all right here in your file!" She laughed. She had a great sense of humor and a very easy way about her. "It's a simple equation - an increase in a problem food equals an increase in chronic symptoms. Where dairy products are suspect, more often than not, the result is an ear infection. Dairy is also implicated in many chronic diseases - from bowel disorders and asthma, to eczema and behavior problems - although any food can cause just about anything."

"You know, I'm amazed that after all my years in nursing, this information is entirely new to me. I feel like I've been living in the Dark Ages, but if it's true, so is everyone else. I just don't get it!"

"Jillian, it all goes back to the fact that this type of nutritional research has no established economic value."

"I still find all this so incredible . . ."

"Well, as I said earlier, it's not a religion." Eva grinned. "Again, you don't have to *believe* it. You need to *experience* it. And I can promise you'll never look back. I can just see it now, you out there converting the masses."

"Well, maybe not the masses right away. What I did say to Dr. Rowland is that I'd do just about anything to get better. Whatever it takes, I'm willing to do it."

Her smile acknowledged my intention to see it through to the end. She continued with the same intensity she'd demonstrated throughout our session, "You see, allergy and addiction are two sides of a double-edged sword. *The food you love the most is probably your worst enemy.* In fact, most people with food sensitivities have either a love or hate relationship with the food that's creating the problem. Foods about which you feel neutral are rarely implicated."

"So in my case, what foods are we talking about?"

"Common foods that North Americans tend to eat every day - dairy, wheat, yeast, corn, sugar, eggs . . ."

This reminded me of the conversation I'd had with Dr. Rowland. "Are you telling me that I also have to stop eating cheese, yogurt, bread and pasta?"

"Do I detect a sense of panic in your voice? Or are you simply hyperventilating?" Eva's eyes twinkled. She was obviously amused. Sensing my concern, however, she added, "Don't worry. You'll likely be able to eat some of these foods later - after you've eliminated them for awhile, and once your gut has healed . . ."

"But these are all considered wholesome foods."

"Yes, for some individuals. For others they can wreak havoc. There are numerous studies that support this as well as hundreds of thousands of anecdotal reports."

"And by eliminating these foods, people can get better?"

"If these foods are causing the problem, yes. In some situations, supplements may be necessary. In other cases, intestinal imbalances could be the underlying cause."

"Like yeast?"

"Yes, that's one example."

"So, what exactly is there left to eat?"

"Don't worry, we won't let you starve. But first, let's clarify what I mean when I say 'dairy'. For a period of two weeks, you must leave out everything that contains any component of dairy products. Reading labels is crucial. It's very important to be able to identify and avoid milk derivatives such as whey powder, casein, lactose, and so on."

"But what do I drink? What do I put on cereal in the morning?"

"Well, the good news is that you can easily find many alternatives to cow's milk . . ."

"Like goat's milk?" I cringed. I'd heard it tasted awful.

"No. Although some people are fine with goat's milk, it's from the same family of foods. And, by the way, good quality goat's milk is delicious. But for now, it would be wise to avoid everything from that family, especially during the elimination phase. Soya, almond or rice milks would serve as good alternatives."

"Dr. Rowland mentioned these as well. Where can I buy them?"

"Health food stores carry them, as do some of the more progressive grocery stores."

"I've never even been to a health food store. Where would I find one?"

"Don't worry, I'll give you a list before you leave. But now for the bad news about breakfast. Unfortunately, most dry cereals not only contain preservatives, but also include loads of sugar. In fact, I often half-jokingly tell people to eat the box instead, since it may contain more nutrients than what's inside."

I laughed at the thought. Eva really was very funny.

"Then," she continued, "if you're sensitive to wheat, it's helpful to know that the majority of boxed cereals are made from wheat or have wheat added in one form or another. Others are made from corn, oats or rice, but nearly all of them contain added sugar - except for two or three varieties. If you're into dry cereals, I can tell you which ones to consider . . ."

"What's wrong with sugar? Don't tell me I can't eat that either."

"You know Jillian, I don't even consider sugar a food. In fact, I call it a non-food. Why, just removing refined sugar alone from most peoples' diets - especially children's - often brings astounding improvements. There are many studies which support this view. You wouldn't believe the cases of colitis and irritable bowel that respond to this one simple measure. Unfortunately, sugar companies go to great lengths to finance studies which 'prove' just the opposite. This confuses the public."

"So are you telling me no sugar?"

"Right. That includes anything that ends with 'ose' such as dextrose, fructose, maltose, sucrose and glucose - inexpensive and commonly used sugars in processed foods. And sugar alcohols such as sorbitol and mannitol, need to be excluded as well. But, remember, you won't have to worry because you'll not be eating anything boxed or packaged."

"Right." I was getting rather discouraged. "But what *can* I eat?"

"Plain rice cakes made from whole-grain rice, rye crackers without yeast, pancakes made from different flours like barley, oats or rye. Or, you could try some of the less commonly known grains like quinoa, spelt and amaranth."

"I've never even heard of those."

"Again, you can find them in health or bulk food stores. There are also some unsweetened dry cereals as well as those that are lightly sweetened with fruit juice, honey or maple syrup. Just make sure the sweetener isn't among the first two ingredients listed on the box. These would be good choices for your children."

"I usually use a mix for pancakes or buy frozen waffles that take only minutes to heat in the mornings."

"But for now, don't forget, anything packaged will have to be eliminated. Eat only things made from scratch, so you know exactly what ingredients you're using. You'll be eating the way we all should - like generations past. Again, your local health food store should carry all these items."

I began to panic at the thought of adding to the burden I already felt. "God, I'll be spending all my time in the kitchen!"

Eva became very serious. "Would you rather be spending it in the hospital? Or, would you prefer to feel the way you have over the past few years?"

"Well, no," I responded sheepishly.

"You'll find ways of cutting corners when it comes to food preparation. A slow cooker goes a long way. You turn it on in the morning and by evening, supper is cooked. Add a salad, and presto, it's all done! Or, turn it on in the evening, and the next day's meal is ready to eat. It's like having your own, personal chef. Incorporating more raw foods into your diet will also make it much simpler. A food processor sure helps. Is your health not worth the extra time it will take in the beginning? Jillian, without it, what have you got?"

I thought about the past three years and knew the answer. "I already know what I have right now - a substandard existence."

"Exactly. What you want to aim for is *quality of life* - to feel good while you're here on earth. Before you know it, your life will be over and you'll not have lived!"

"You're absolutely right. It's been so unfair to everyone around me. "

"Unfair?"

"Well, yes. I've been so sick - useless to everyone. I've been more of a burden than a help."

"Is your husband supportive?"

"Yes . . . and no. He's getting really tired of me not being able to keep up with him or manage the simplest things - like keeping the house organized . . . "

"And does he help?"

"Somewhat. But I think he resents it. Then I start feeling guilty."

"Whoa! Guilty? For what? For being sick?"

"Well . . . yes . . . " I began to cry, feeling the pain of the past three years catch up with me.

Eva reached over and touched my arm. "Jillian," she said softly, "you need to bring your husband in with you to see our counsellor, Leah Irwin. She's wonderful at helping people cope with chronic illness. I think it would be very helpful. Could I have Emily arrange an appointment for you?"

With my eyes still downcast, I murmured, "I'll take any help I can get. I'd really appreciate it." She handed me a Kleenex.

Scribbling a note on her memo pad, she said, "There. Done. Are you okay?"

I nodded.

"Now let's get back to your diet." Eva rooted through my file until she found my three-day diet sheet. She read off a typical day: "For breakfast you had a bowl of bran cereal, a muffin for a snack, a cheese sandwich for lunch, and macaroni and cheese for supper. This adds up to wheat/dairy, wheat/dairy, wheat/dairy and more wheat/dairy. It's a lot healthier than most diets that cross my desk, but it's certainly not a *varied* diet. In fact, it's a typical example of repetitive eating."

"But isn't that how most people eat?"

"Yes, but that doesn't make it right. As we discussed earlier, this is, in part, why so many people develop food sensitivities. Because their digestive tracts are compromised, enzyme systems used to digest the same foods day-in and day-out become depleted. This is one reason why cyclical or cumulative sensitivities arise."

She stood up and turned a page on her flip chart. "This explains the concept of food sensitivity a little more clearly." Pointing to a chart by the door captioned *Diagnosing Masked Sensitivity* (fig. 8), she highlighted the first item. "Here you are, Jillian Stowe, a chronically ill person. You have most of the symptoms listed here."

She pointed to number two on the chart. "So you avoid the irritant or the food that you love the most for seven to twelve days. You'll probably experience a withdrawal, followed by a period of relief. If you're really lucky, you might feel better almost immediately. Either experience signifies you're on the right track."

"What do you mean by withdrawal?"

"Headaches, cravings, fatigue, diarrhea, flu-like symptoms - you name it."

"So I guess I should start this on a weekend."

"That would be wise, considering you have kids to look after. It certainly would allow others to help in case you have a rough time."

"So what happens after twelve days?"

"Normally, you'd be back for a follow-up appointment, but due to the holidays that won't be possible. However, you can begin to test yourself with the foods you eliminated during that time period. Of course, if you were a serious asthmatic or were at risk for anaphylaxis, I would never advise reintroduction as a means of testing. In that case I'd suggest you simply accept that you're feeling much better and continue to avoid the offending foods."

"How do I test myself?"

"Always first thing in the morning, when you're clear of symptoms. And the food must be tested in its purest form. For example, you can't test wheat by using bread. Bread has yeast, egg, and other ingredients which would confuse the results. Instead, use cream of wheat cooked in water, or plain puffed wheat. See how you feel after eating a couple of bowls full. Has your energy changed? Are you more irritable? Wired? Can't keep still? Or are you wiped out? Is your diarrhea back? Also, always wait a few hours before you eat anything else in case you have a delayed reaction."

"How long could that take?"

"Normally less than four hours unless you're one of the more complex cases. A delayed reaction could take several days, then specialized blood tests like the ELISA/Act or provocation-neutralization testing would be

# Diagnosing a Masked Sensitivity
## (fig. 8)

**Avoidance of Irritant**
for 7-12 days
(usually what you love most)

2

1                                                    3

**Masked Sensitivity**                    **Withdrawal &**
(Chronic ill health)                       **Symptomatic Relief**
e.g. asthma, eczema,                        after 5-10 days
migraines, behavioral              (ranges from initially feeling
problems, etc. . .                       worse to feeling better)

6                                                    4

**Tolerance**                              **Hypersensitivity**
but excessive exposure                      12-14 days after
leads to masked sensitivity              avoidance/withdrawal
again

5

**Latent Sensitization**
will tolerate <u>some</u> exposure
(i.e., as on rotation diet and/or bowel
management program)

Based on a chart by Drs. George T. Lewith & Julian N. Kenyon in *Clinical Ecology* more appropriate. But let's not get bogged down with these alternatives until we try the simple, self-test approach first. Remember, the body doesn't lie. You must listen to it carefully."

"Does this mean I can never eat wheat or dairy products again?"

"It depends upon the degree of the original sensitivities. In a few months' time - if you stay away from foods to which you're sensitive and work at healing your permeable gut - you might be able to indulge in them once in a while. But, given your history, likely not on a regular basis."

"No more Friday night pizza," I lamented.

"Don't worry," she reassured me with a smile. "Once you've made the connection between eating it and feeling bad, you won't want it anyhow."

"Why do I get the feeling you've been there!" I smiled.

"I haven't the foggiest," Eva kidded. "Also, keep in mind that if you have wheat only occasionally, you'll probably feel okay. Unfortunately, we have a tendency to think more is better. Just remember, as I said earlier, allergy and addiction are two sides of a double-edged sword. That pizza you may be able to have once a week could quickly turn into a daily habit or rekindle the addiction, only in different forms - bread, pasta, crackers and cheese. Then, before you know it, all your symptoms resurface."

"So, what's the bottom line?"

"For two weeks, you won't eat refined sugar, wheat, yeast or dairy products. Make sure you consult the list I'll give you. It will clarify where these foods are found."

"What do you mean?"

"For instance, wheat is used as a filler in wieners, sausage, cold cuts, canned soups - in just about anything processed."

"I would never have known!"

"That's why it's important to familiarize yourself with these lists. One of the best books on this subject that has the greatest amount of detail is the *Food Allergy & Nutrition Revolution* by Dr. James Braly. You might consider getting it out of the library at some point. And you must drink only clean water, especially during this elimination period."

"Clean water?"

"Yes, distilled, spring, or adequately filtered - never tap water. It's full of chlorine, one of the more common chemical irritants. One of my patients actually cured her chronic bowel problems simply by changing the water she drank. Fluoridation is also very controversial, causing problems for many. It's actually been banned in several countries. There's a growing concern that the risks outweigh the benefits in terms of overall health and safety. Dr. David Collison, author of *Why Do I Feel So Awful?*, cites an example of one busy practice where 1200 patients with a history of intolerance to a variety of chemicals were tested to see if they reacted to fluoride. More than 30% were found to have a significant positive reaction to sodium fluoride, the form in which it is added to water supplies."

"My dentist thinks it's great that our water's fluoridated. He says it's significant in reducing cavities . . ."

"Yes, I have this image of a strong, healthy set of teeth chattering down a street without a body. The body rots away from slow chemical poisoning, but the teeth remain perfect, like a pair of dentures!"

I burst out laughing at the very thought! "Isn't anything safe anymore?"

"Sure, many things are safe," replied Eva. "But in this day and age, you really have to be informed."

She looked at her calendar, frowning slightly. "Hmm. Because of the holiday season, your next appointment will have to be on the fifth of January. That'll give you plenty of time to experiment with reintroducing foods. There are a few cookbooks that you can sign out of our library. In fact one of them was written by yours truly!"

"You've written a book? Wow!" I was impressed. I figured she must really be on top of all this.

"Yes, as a service to my clients, I decided to put it all into a book. There are recipes for every meal imaginable, along with appropriate substitutions. Also," she advised, "we have information on a support group called Back to Basics. They're a group of people with sensitivities who've compiled a terrific collection of their own. They've also started a food co-op. Not only is it considerably cheaper to buy food that way, but many of the foods are free of pesticides, so the quality is much better than you'll find in the average grocery store."

"I'd be interested in pursuing that."

"There are many children in my practice who *must* live on organic food. They can no longer tolerate produce from the regular grocery store."

"How can you tell? What happens to them?"

"They get diarrhea, headaches, or other adverse reactions. In other instances, their behavior is affected. But, when they eat organically, their symptoms subside - as if by magic."

"I still can't believe the government allows this to happen!" I was outraged.

"Sad, isn't it? What's considered safe and harmless often proves to be the opposite in light of practical experience, especially when it comes to children." Eva glanced at her watch. "We still have a bit more to go over, then we'll start wrapping up."

"What about vitamins and minerals? I've always felt I needed them, but was afraid to take them on my own."

"There's no doubt you'll need to take supplements. As I indicated earlier, we'll focus strictly on food elimination for now. Taking vitamins without changing your diet would be like pouring water into a leaky bucket. You must alter your diet first, observe any bodily changes, and then work with supplements to achieve a balance. Please don't forget to record how you feel at the end of each and every day until you return. This is of utmost importance when you start reintroducing the foods you've eliminated."

"Do I need to write down everything I eat?"

"If you could, it certainly would be informative."

"So when I return in January, we'll talk about supplements?"

"Absolutely. By the time you return, you'll have accumulated more information from your experiences at home and from your next session with Dr. Rowland. Without the straight food elimination, we really won't know what's causing what. I'm curious to find out which of your symptoms will subside with elimination alone."

"Will the handouts be clear about what I need to avoid?"

"They should be. If you have any questions between now and your next appointment, don't hesitate to call." Then, with a concerned look, she gently asked, "Jillian, we've covered a lot of territory. It must be somewhat overwhelming. But does it make sense?"

"It all makes sense, but it sounds almost too simple. To be totally honest, it's hard for me to imagine that eliminating a few things from my diet is going to change the way I feel."

Eva handed me the cassette of our taped session. "Well, I appreciate your honesty and fully understand your skepticism. It takes me back to the time when I first met Dr. Rowland and he told me to stop eating wheat, dairy products and sugar. I thought he was out of his mind!"

"I know just what you mean." I was relieved she understood.

"But if you stick to it rigorously, Jillian, I guarantee you'll never regret it. And don't forget to pick up your instruction sheets from Emily."

She reached out and held both of my hands in hers. "You'll make it! It's onward and upward from this day forward."

I felt like I was walking on air. This woman made me believe I was capable of anything! I felt empowered.

It all seemed a bit surreal. Over the past two hours, I'd learned that my environment - the food I ate, the water I drank, and the air I breathed - was making me sick. On top of all this, it seemed that a yeast imbalance, coupled with years of misdiagnosed sensitivities, were at the root of my problems.

It was obvious I had a lot of reading to do. I left the clinic with a pile of books and a new-found optimism.

Eva was right - my life would never be the same.

*The next major advance*

*in the health*

*of the American people*

*will be determined*

*by what the individual*

*is willing to do*

*for himself.*

John Knowles
Former President, Rockefeller Foundation
The Burton Goldberg Group,
Alternative Medicine: The Definitive Guide

# 7

# Back Home

*Do not believe in an authority. Rather examine all that an authority says. Put everything to the test. Let truth be your authority, not authority your truth.*
**Joel Robbins, D.C.**

*T*he drive home seemed far longer than the drive earlier in the day. It was cold and dark. I was exhausted by the time I turned into the driveway. I opened the car door. The first sound I heard was Michael yelling at Nathaniel. "You're going to have to settle down once and for all, young man! This is the second note from your teacher in two weeks - it's just not acceptable!"

I didn't want to go inside. The last thing I needed was another battle over Nathaniel's behavior at school. Basically, he was a good kid and meant well. Often, he'd say or do something he hadn't given much thought to, and would end up regretting it. We'd taken him to the Child Guidance Center and had tried using behavior modification techniques with him. At times they worked, other times they didn't. Some days he was well-behaved, while on others, he was unbelievably irritating and fidgety. It was strange, very frustrating.

For Nathaniel's sake, as well as for our own peace of mind, we had to find a solution to his ongoing problems. Perhaps he did have an attention deficit, but why? And why was it such a problem this year and not other years? There had to be a reason. I was beginning to sound like Dr. Rowland. But it only made sense. I knew one thing for sure - if he were diagnosed as A.D.D., I'd never consider Ritalin as an option. The thought of drugging a child to curb behavior scared me. Not only did the whole idea seem extreme and archaic, but it only masked underlying reasons for such behavior. Then there were possible side effects which weren't too pleasant. Only in extreme situations and for very short periods of time could I see Ritalin being used. I was thinking particularly about situations where children were in absolute crisis and where everyone around them was adversely affected. The idea would be to keep searching for underlying causes for the problems.

As soon as I opened the door, Emma and Max came running. "Mommy! Mommy!" They jumped all over me, Max hugging my legs. Emma could hardly wait to tell me that her brother was in trouble again.

I could smell pizza throughout the house. It was Friday night! The thought that I couldn't indulge after tomorrow was more than I could bear. Michael came over to me, looking frazzled and spent. He shrugged his shoulders and said, "Jillian, *you* deal with him! I give up! I just lose it with him - it's like nothing gets through!" With that, he stormed upstairs and slammed the bedroom door.

Great, I thought. Another crisis for me to handle. I barely had enough energy for myself. I ushered the two younger kids downstairs to watch T.V. and went into the living room to talk to Nathaniel. He sat by the fireplace, his head hung low, obviously not feeling too great about the exchange he had just had with his Dad.

"Hi, Mom."

I rubbed his back and bent down to kiss the top of his head. He began to cry. "Dad's so mad at me. He says I'm grounded for a week and that I'll have to give up hockey if things don't improve at school. Mom, I can't give up hockey . . . I just can't."

Nathaniel didn't have to work at hockey - he was a natural. The thought of giving up something he did so well was ridiculous. One had nothing to do with the other.

"Look, I'll talk to Daddy. In the meantime, I want you to think of ways you might improve your behavior in school. We'll talk about it tomorrow when we're more rested. Go watch a bit of T.V. for now. Where's the note from Mrs. Allen?"

"It's on the kitchen counter . . . Mom, I really don't mean to be bad."

How many times had I heard those words! My heart ached for him. I leaned over to hug him and said, "I know you don't mean it. You're *not* bad! We just need to work on a few things. Nathaniel, it'll all work out, you'll see."

Later, in bed, I told Michael about my visit to the clinic. I told him about all I'd learned - from pesticides and drugs in our food to food sensitivities. "No sugar, dairy, wheat or yeast for fourteen days . . ."

"*You* . . . not eating sugar? *That* I'll believe when I see it!" He paused for a moment. "Actually, no sugar I can see, but no milk, yogurt or cheese? Jilly, who are these people? This doesn't sound right to me."

I had expected this response. "I know, at first I had the same reaction, but then it all started to make sense. When I spoke to a few people at the clinic, including Eva, the nutritional consultant, they all said that everyday foods had caused a lot of their problems."

"Jilly, people have eaten these foods since the dawn of history. I'm sorry, I find this a bit out to lunch - oops, no pun intended!"

He laughed, but I detected a hint of sarcasm.

"Michael," I began to cry from a combination of fatigue and frustration. "I need your support. This is *not* going to be easy."

"But Jilly, what are you going to eat? What's left? Think about it. No more homemade bread, bagels? No cookies, cheese or yogurt? What, may

I ask, are you planning to have on your cereal every morning? In fact, what *are* you going to eat for breakfast?"

"Well, I'm allowed rice cakes, crackers without wheat or yeast . . . stuff like that. Eva gave me a list of alternatives. Tomorrow morning I'm going to a place called Sunshine Health Foods to get everything I need."

"And what about Christmas? Aren't you going to bake all those incredible treats like you do every year? No shortbread cookies? No poppyseed rolls? Jilly, how are you going to survive?"

"You mean how are *you* going to survive!" I snapped. "Michael," I pleaded, "I can't go on the way I've been. I *know* it sounds crazy. I, too, find it hard to believe that food - especially healthy food - can be the cause of my problems. But Dr. Rowland and Eva are convinced that what I eat every day has caused many of my symptoms."

"Well, what have we got to lose? You've already spent good money to see these people, so I guess you may as well follow their program. And it's only for two weeks . . ."

It always came down to money. "Michael, I'm going to need a lot of help. Apparently, people can actually have withdrawal from foods they regularly eat."

"Withdrawal? I don't believe it."

"Seriously, they say it's the same as when you quit smoking or drinking. People with food sensitivities are often addicted to foods. They crave the very food to which they're sensitive. But because they're hidden sensitivities, you have to stop eating the foods you crave and then reintroduce them later to discover which symptoms they cause. This is known as unmasking a masked intolerance."

"So without eliminating these foods, you'd never be able to figure it out?"

"That's right."

"But why do you crave them in the first place?"

"Because addiction and allergy are often the same. That's why when you give up coffee and get a headache, drinking another cup will usually clear it up. The headache is an actual *withdrawal* symptom. The doctor said it's similar to the alcoholic's symptoms that end with the next drink or the smoker's withdrawal that stops with the next cigarette. Only my addiction is to food."

"You do eat a helluva lot!" Michael joked.

"When I sit down to have a piece of pie and have to have the whole pie, I know there's a problem. I wasn't like that a few years ago!"

"That's for sure. But what did this Dr. . . . Dr. . . . what's his name?"

"Dr. Rowland."

"What exactly did he say is your problem?"

"He said I've become sensitive - reactive - to things I eat, drink and breathe every day, and that these sensitivities stem from a weakened immune system."

"A weakened immune system?"

"You know all the medication I've been on for one thing or another? And all the renovations over the past few years? Then three years ago, bingo - I was pregnant with Max. Apparently, I'd exceeded my tolerance, or what he calls the total load, and became ill."

"But I don't get it. You and I eat, drink and breathe most of the same things . . ."

"That's true," I interrupted, "But *you* haven't lived on the birth control pill for the past fifteen years or taken as many antibiotics and other drugs as I have. And *you* didn't have babies or come from a family that's full of sensitivities."

"What's your family got to do with it?"

"Well, there's a good chance that Mom's arthritis and migraines, as well as Dad's chronic depression and long-standing bowel problems, are a result of undiagnosed sensitivities. When Dr. Rowland looked at the health history of my extended family, he connected many of their chronic problems with this whole phenomenon."

"It sounds like these folks believe that everything in life is caused by sensitivities. I find that very one-dimensional, don't you?"

"Well, at first I did, but after having talked to the patients at the clinic, I'm beginning to wonder. They told me that before Dr. Rowland, no one could find the cause of their problems. All they had to offer was drug therapy. Now, they all feel much better. The doctor also said I probably have a yeast imbalance in my gut. Don't ask me to explain that one." I showed him *The Yeast Connection* and told him I planned to read it over the next few days.

We talked about Nathaniel for a while and agreed on some disciplinary strategies based on positive reinforcement techniques. I mentioned how the children had a lot of the same symptoms I had while growing up and how Dr. Rowland and Eva were both convinced that many of these problems were environmentally related.

Michael's back immediately went up at the very suggestion. "Now I suppose you're going to try and tell me that Nathaniel's behavior is caused by what he's eating. Let's not get too carried away!"

"Well . . . if it turns out that all this is true for me, why would our children be any different?"

"I can see them giving up some of the junk they eat, but they aren't giving up milk and bread - I can tell you that right now!" exclaimed Michael, bordering on anger.

"Why are you so agitated?"

"Because I think those people at that clinic out in the middle of nowhere have a few loose screws!"

Fresh tears rolled down my cheeks. That familiar feeling of being alone and isolated came back full force. I began to sob.

In the end, Michael leaned on his elbow, looked at me, and said, "Jilly, I'm sorry about what I just said. I think I'm uptight about the whole situation about you not being well and Nathaniel having so many problems in school.

I'll help you out. I'll do whatever it takes . . . The whole family is affected when you're not well."

"Michael," I sniffled, "I plan on giving it all I've got. I have to! I can barely handle life. In fact, I have no life!"

He held me close and whispered, "Jilly, it'll all work out somehow. I'll help you. I promise.

Tomorrow was shopping day and the first day of my diet.

What I didn't know then was that I would never look back.

*The road to better health*

*will not be found through*

*more drugs, doctors and hospitals.*

*Instead, it will be discovered*

*through better nutrition*

*and*

*changes in lifestyle.*

**William G. Crook, M.D.,**
**Chronic Fatigue Syndrome and the Yeast Connection**

# 8

# A Test of Courage

*Good health does not come easily; you must work for it.*
**Charles B. Simone, M.D.**

*T*he morning was spent shopping at the market for pesticide-free produce and at the health food store for all my other supplies. I bought rice cakes, lentils, brown rice, oats and some of the strange flours Eva had mentioned, like quinoa (pronounced "keenwa"), amaranth and spelt. Then I arranged to have spring water delivered to our home, and picked up a jug to tide me over until Monday morning.

People were friendly and extremely helpful everywhere I went, especially at the health food store. I explained what I needed, and when I mentioned Dr. Rowland and Eva, they knew immediately which products I required and went to great lengths to explain how to prepare these different foods. They also directed me to a section full of self-help books and cookbooks. I browsed for a while, then headed home.

I made a quick lunch - tuna on ricecakes. It actually tasted good. Michael and the kids looked at me with pity as they bit into their homemade bread, happy they weren't part of the program.

Emma thought my ricecakes looked like styrofoam while Max, still unable to pronounce the letter 's', kept repeating, "Oooh! Groth Mommy! Groth!"

After lunch, I opened the bag I'd brought home from the clinic. Inside with the books and instruction sheets, was a box labelled 'liquid stool kit'. Attached were instructions that the sample be couriered within twenty-four hours of completion to the lab noted on the requisition .

By mid-afternoon, I had a headache, felt exhausted and chilled. I excused myself, and trundled off to bed with *The Yeast Connection* in one hand and a hot water bottle in the other.

Near the beginning of the book was a questionnaire and score sheet. The bottom line read: *Yeast-connected health problems are almost certainly present in women with scores over 189 . . .* I scored a grand total of 477! By the time I finished the first section, I knew that yeast had to be a big part of my problem.

I must have drifted off to sleep for several hours because it was dark by the time I awoke. I felt like a zombie and the pain in my head was excruciating. As I made my way to the bathroom for some Tylenol, I heard Michael speaking in a hushed voice and Emma gasping for air.

"Where are you guys?" An all too familiar feeling of panic came over me.

"In Max's room," replied Michael. "Emma's having another attack. This time she might have to go to Emergency." I walked into the bedroom, took a quick look at Emma under her mask, and immediately knew she was in trouble. I held her and rubbed her back.

"Are you well enough to put Max to bed?" asked Michael.

I nodded. "Don't worry about us. Just get Emma some relief. Poor baby . . ." I rocked her while Michael went to get her jacket. We'd been through this so many times. I would have given anything to trade places with her. I worried about all the drugs she'd taken since she was a baby. Some of them were very potent steroids with dangerous side effects.

Holding Max, I gave Emma a quick kiss as Michael carried her out the door. I thought back to the woman in the waiting room at the clinic and what she had said about her asthma and how it was related to foods she ate every day. Could Emma have sensitivities too?

By the time they returned, I was fast asleep. I could feel Emma's little body curling up next to mine and Michael whispering that she was okay. I pulled her in closer to me. Dreading the morning, I fell back into a fitful sleep.

Day two of the diet started out considerably worse than day one. I was too weak to get up. My head felt as if it were splitting apart. Emma, obviously feeling better, peeked at me from under the covers. "Mommy, are you still sick?"

"I have a terrible headache." I tried hard to summon a smile. "But more important, how are *you* feeling?"

"I'm fine. We had to wait forever at the hospital! Daddy was getting mad at everyone."

"He was probably very tired . . . I'm so glad you're feeling better, my sweetie!" I reached over to pull her closer to me.

The smell of toast and coffee wafted up from the kitchen. I began to salivate. Michael called out his usual Sunday morning greeting, "Breakfast everybody! Come 'n' get it!"

I was just wondering where the boys were when I heard Max race down the hall and Nathaniel emit his ritualistic wake up groans. I decided it would be better to stay put rather than tempt myself with bagels, cream cheese, homemade jam and other goodies that Michael normally served with Sunday brunch. After shooing Emma downstairs, I picked up my book again, but I was so spaced out that I couldn't even connect with the words. They jumped all over the page. My arms were so weak I could hardly hold the book! I got up to refill the hot water bottle, curled up in my favorite fetal position, and promptly fell back to sleep.

The next time I opened my eyes, the alarm clock beside me read 2:21

p.m. There was a note beside it from Michael, saying he had taken the kids out for the afternoon and would buy them supper. He had really meant what he said - that he would do everything he could to support me during this period.

I was consumed with guilt - I had robbed my children of a mother for years. Now here I was, needing even more time off. It just didn't seem fair!

When I finally made it to the kitchen, it was all I could do not to eat the cinnamon rolls and bagels sitting on the counter. I could almost hear them screaming 'Eat me! Eat me!' I ended up devouring leftover chicken and crunching on raw vegetables. It was so frustrating!

Deciding that a hot bath might soothe me, I prepared the tub. As the steam rose around me, I began to weep. I felt so depressed. It was pathetic. I would have killed for a taste of anything sweet - even a piece of bread! It was like an obsession. I felt totally out of control. But worse than the cravings was the deep-seated feeling I couldn't shake - that I had let my family down. Climbing out of the tub, I dried off and dragged my aching body back to my room. Still sobbing, I collapsed into bed and went out like a light.

"Mommy! Mommy! We're home! We're home!" were the first sounds to reach my consciousness. I could hear the kids' feet pounding up the stairs. "What time is it?" I groaned.

"Seven-thirty," said Michael looking at his watch. I was shocked! I had slept most of the day. Suddenly I realized Monday morning was only hours away. I knew I would need help once Michael went to work.

"My God, Jilly, you look terrible!" remarked Michael, stripping off Max's clothes to get him ready for bed.

"What do you mean I look terrible!" I snapped. I pulled a small mirror from my bedside table and took a quick look. I did look awful! My face was even more pale and puffy than usual and my hair stuck out every which way. Noises seemed louder than normal and I was on edge. Michael told me he planned to set up an interview with Nathaniel's teacher within the next couple of days. The thought of anything extra like that was more than I could handle. I felt overwhelmed.

Michael read my thoughts. "Jilly, are you going to be able to cope for the next few days? Should I call Beth?" Beth was our neighbor who had baby-sat for us since Nathaniel was born.

"That's not a bad idea. If I keep feeling like this, I don't think I'll be able to handle anything for awhile."

"Jilly, I didn't want to say anything since you're so gung-ho about that clinic, but to be perfectly honest, I'm really getting worried. You're getting worse, not better. Maybe you should phone them tomorrow morning and tell them how you're feeling . . ."

"Michael, I think this is the withdrawal part. I'll wait a while longer. They say it's only supposed to last four or five days. I guess I'm not one of the lucky ones who simply gets better without going through a withdrawal first."

"Whoever said life would be easy, huh?" Michael commiserated. He gave me a lopsided grin, turned off the light, and went to put the kids to bed.

The next two days were a blur.

Symptoms which had bothered me only sporadically over the years came and went. It felt like I had a bad flu. I couldn't decide which was worse - the fatigue or the persistent headache. I also had bouts of diarrhea. One minute I'd be sweating, the next, nearly freezing. I wore two pairs of socks to bed. Thank God for my hot water bottle and Michael's body heat at night. On top of everything else, I was starving. Although I ate non-stop during my waking hours, which were few and far between, I obsessed about bread, cheese, and anything sweet.

Then, an incredible thing happened.

Wednesday morning, the fifth day of the diet, I woke very early - around 6:00 a.m. - stretched, and immediately realized . . . no more headache! It was unbelievable! I felt limber, even somewhat energetic. My joint pains were at an all-time low. I felt more clear-headed than I had in months. The fog had lifted. But the most amazing part was that, for the first time *ever*, I could breathe! Both nostrils were clear and I was no longer congested. Could this be real? I pinched myself to make sure I wasn't dreaming.

I got up quietly, went into the bathroom, looked in the mirror and noticed that the color had returned to my face. The puffiness and dark circles under my eyes were gone. I actually looked good! I felt lighter.

By the time Michael got up, I was whistling in the kitchen, making muffins for breakfast - for everyone but myself. I also noticed my cravings had diminished. I wasn't even the least bit interested in anything sweet!

"Whoa! Who's this we have in the kitchen this morning?" Michael stared in disbelief at my instant recovery.

"A new woman! Michael, I can't believe how much better I feel. Who knows, it may be only a spurt of energy, but I'm going to enjoy it while it lasts. I feel great!"

"Well, you sure look good! Looks like you've lost some weight, too. I guess anyone would, eating the way you've been," he chuckled.

"You're right! I've lost six pounds! I even *feel* lighter. You know, I don't think I'm going to need Beth anymore. I really feel I can tackle the day."

"Are you sure Jilly? Maybe you've just got extra energy this morning because of all the sleep you've had over the past few days. Maybe you had a bug." He thought for a moment and continued. "But then, you haven't been this good for at least a couple of years . . ."

"Three to be precise," I interrupted. "Michael, I think I'm okay . . . Maybe it *is* food that makes me so sick!"

"I wouldn't be too quick to jump to that conclusion. But it sure is nice to see you so upbeat," he smiled. "I'll call Beth to cancel." He returned in a few minutes. Looking at the clock, he said, "I've gotta run. Call me if you need anything. Onward and upward!" He gulped the last of his coffee, shouted "See ya, kids!" up the stairs, and ran out the door.

The kids came down one by one, barely able to contain their usual morning grumpiness. It had become a way of life. When they saw me, they were shocked! In that moment I realized how long I'd been mentally and emotionally absent from the family. These children needed a mother who could fully be there for them. This morning, I felt focussed. My eyes welled with tears of gratitude.

"Good morning, good morning!" I welcomed each of them with a hug.

"Mommy, you're all better!" exclaimed Emma.

"Yeah, you haven't baked muffins for breakfast in ages!" grinned Nathaniel, biting into the largest one he could find.

"Mommy! Mommy! Muffins!" shrieked Max, trying to outdo everyone's enthusiasm.

After the kids left, I took Max to pre-school, picked up a few groceries, and headed home to read. I was amazed. I could actually retain the information! What I read fascinated me. Case histories illustrated both physical and mental illnesses caused by sensitivities to everyday foods and chemicals in our increasingly contaminated environment. Often, people fasted in order to clear their bodies of symptoms, and then reintroduced foods one by one to see which symptoms returned. I was grateful I didn't have to go that far. Symptoms ranged from psychosis, hyperactivity, and headaches, to gastrointestinal problems, arthritis and severe depression. I felt like I was entering a whole new world.

But the process seemed too simple - I still didn't trust it completely. Was it a fluke that I seemed better? Deep down I felt like Cinderella, waiting for the clock to strike midnight. I didn't want to be sick again.

But midnight never came. I felt better and better as each day passed.

Near the end of the second week, Michael began to believe. He admitted it was either the diet, the power of suggestion or both. As long as it worked, he really didn't care. I tried to get him to read at least one of my books, but he wasn't very interested in theory, only in results.

Fourteen days into the diet, I decided to test myself.

I began on a Saturday morning, so Michael could watch the kids in case I had a bad reaction. My first test was sugar. I ate three small cubes. At first I felt racy. My heart beat loud and fast. I began yelling at the kids for no specific reason. Then I started in on Michael - I was definitely out of control. After about an hour, the anger turned into depression. All of my thoughts were dark, negative and hopeless.

Later, Michael said that within twenty minutes, he'd watched me go from the happy, bubbly woman with whom he'd fallen in love years ago to that grumpy person he'd lived with for the past three years - only worse. He couldn't believe it. In his words, it was like watching Jekyll and Hyde.

Now that I'd unmasked this particular sensitivity, I could clearly see it had been the cause of so many of my emotional problems. I recorded the reaction in my journal, and from that point on, swore off sugar in any form whatsoever. It was a deceptive food - dangerous not only for me, but for everyone around me.

It took a couple of days to stabilize myself. Then, with much trepidation, I decided to try dairy products.

I drank two glasses of milk first thing in the morning. Within twenty minutes, my nose was running. For the rest of the day and night, I relived my lifelong battle with stuffy sinuses, which in the past, had routinely developed into chronic infections. The normal treatment had always been broad-spectrum antibiotics. No wonder Dr. Rowland thought I had a yeast problem. The only consolation was that, unlike sugar, milk didn't affect anyone but me.

I had two other foods left to test - wheat and yeast. I was terrified of another cerebral reaction, similar to the sugar test. Just in case, I called Beth to look after the children. Wheat brought back my incredible fatigue, and yeast gave me painful intestinal gas and bloating.

Now I had most of my worst symptoms pegged. I felt like I had a handle on which symptoms were caused by what foods. With this new-found knowledge, I could take full responsibility for my health. I was able to make more appropriate choices. If I chose to eat wheat, then I knew what I could expect. Not knowing had been the worst part. Now I had information to work with and it all seemed more manageable. I could exert more control over my life again.

Over the next two weeks, I prepared for Christmas. Malls, theatres - anywhere where there were large gatherings - were still a problem. At home I felt great, as long as I adhered to my new diet, but in some public places, several of my symptoms reappeared, especially the fatigue and brain fog.

Friends who saw me couldn't believe how great I looked. My face had lost its puffiness. The scales showed I had lost eight pounds. I was met with total skepticism whenever I mentioned the food connection. People didn't understand and felt sorry for me because I couldn't indulge in sweets. They were sure I had truly flipped when I mentioned the 'no milk' and 'no bread' routine.

"But what are you going to do for calcium?" "How can you not eat bread?" "No sugar? God! Our house would fall apart without it!" "My kids would die without their treats!" were all typical responses.

Then an interesting thing happened. On the way to the market one Saturday morning, I noticed a huge sign that read: PESTICIDE-FREE CHRISTMAS TREES. Curious, I turned into the lot. The staff were volunteers for a non-profit group called the Environmental Action Coalition. They told me that most cultivated Christmas trees are sprayed with pesticides that release dangerous residues while we admire them all fancied-up in our homes. They explained that these chemicals could cause serious health problems. Over the years, I had heard of people who couldn't tolerate real trees and had to buy artificial ones. In some cases, the tree itself had been the problem, but how many people had actually reacted to the spray rather than to the tree? I decided to purchase one of them.

I couldn't believe the difference!

Normally, everyone was extremely high-strung and irritable a few days before Christmas. In the past, I had attributed our moods to holiday stress and the increased intake of desserts and junk foods. I still believed that these were contributing factors, but it quickly became apparent that the new tree made a significant difference. Emma, for example, didn't have her usual asthma attack. This year, we were all somewhat calmer and made it through the holidays with flying colors.

There was something to be said about going natural!

I made three New Year's resolutions: to help Nathaniel with his problems at school, to find out what else triggered Emma's asthma, and to discover the cause of little Max's eczema and repeated ear infections. Of course, included in all these good intentions was my commitment to my own journey toward wellness.

Eva was right . . . without our health, what have we got?

*If traditional medicine has no solution
to a medical problem,
the patient is to blame, and then labelled
as neurotic and a hypochondriac . . .*

*The new physicians,
well-trained in allergy and immunology
will actively search for food allergy and
chemical sensitivity in their patients,
and they will frequently find it,
just as I have . . .*

*but more importantly
these allergy educated physicians
will look for the many
underlying
nutritional and lifestyle causes
of food allergy.*

**James Braly, M.D.**
**Dr. Braly's Food Allergy & Nutrition Revolution**

# 9

# The Internal Inferno

*The ecology of your gastrointestinal tract is intimately connected to the health of your immune system.*
**Zoltan P. Rona, M.D., M.Sc.**

*J*anuary fifth was a clear, crisp day - perfect driving weather. I cranked up the music, whistling and singing along with the songs I knew. It was exhilarating! I could hardly wait to see Dr. Rowland and Eva to tell them how much better I felt, thanks to them.

The waiting room was packed when I arrived. Emily looked up at me, her face beaming. "Wow! Are you the same person who was here just a month ago?"

"Are you kidding? I'm a whole new woman!"

"You look terrific!" Then, in an apologetic tone, she whispered, "It's not normally such a madhouse. We're really backed up right now because of the holidays."

"How long?" I asked.

With a worried look, she whispered, "About forty-five minutes."

"No problem. It's certainly worth the wait." I thought of all the help they had given me in such a short time. What was forty-five minutes compared to the years I'd run around trying to find help?

Emily, considerate as usual, reminded me of the things I could do while waiting. "There's lots to read in the reception area, and there's always the library . . ."

"Oh yes, I almost forgot, I have some books to return."

In the library, I went directly to the section on yeast-related books. Titles included *Back to Health* by Dennis Remington and Barbara Higa, *Candida* by Luc de Schepper, as well as a large number of cookbooks. Next was the allergy section. Most of the authors were physicians. Several of these books were written by Doris Rapp, including *The Impossible Child* and *Is This Your Child?* I had just begun leafing through one of them, when a voice beside me said, "I don't mean to be nosy, but I just have to tell you, that doctor changed my whole life."

"What doctor?"

"Doris Rapp, who wrote that book you're holding. I saw her on the Phil Donahue show about a year ago. She had some kids with her who seemed as normal as you and me. The videotapes they aired showed what the kids were like before treatment. You wouldn't believe it! You'd never know they were the same children."

"What were they like?" I was curious.

"Some of them were wild - angry, belligerent, even violent. Others were whiny, clingy and unable to focus. Upon being tested for things to which they were sensitive, their writing would go from being perfect to being completely illegible. Some became dopey and fell asleep at the drop of a hat. Those poor mothers - their stories broke my heart! What they went through with those kids is what I'd been going through for years. I could never figure out why my kids would be fine one day and so bad the next. There were many days I came close to wringing their necks!"

"I know what you mean," I said quietly. "Thanks for the tip. I'll be sure to check these out." Her comment about the change in handwriting struck a familiar chord, since I'd often wondered why the kids' schoolwork was much better on some days than on others. But the part about behavior really nagged at me. I thought back to some of our more difficult days when disciplining the kids was an exercise in futility.

I browsed for a few more minutes. Another book that caught my eye was *Solving the Puzzle of Your Hard-to-Raise Child* by William Crook, the same doctor who wrote *The Yeast Connection*. With Nathaniel in mind, I added it to my growing pile of reading material.

As I walked from the library to the waiting area, I passed a huge room filled with people. Wondering about its purpose, I asked one of the patients to fill me in.

"Oh, that's the testing room."

"The testing room?"

"Yeah, that's where they test for foods, chemicals, and airborne irritants. They stick little needles into your arm all day and watch for different reactions. Go take a look."

I peeked through a window in the door. There were adults and children of all ages sitting around the room, many with one sleeve rolled up. Some of the kids were playing together. Others were quietly drawing or reading. Every few minutes, someone would go into another room for a short time, then come back out to a waiting area.

I thought about the books I'd read over the past few weeks.

"Excuse me," I asked another patient walking by, "but is that provocation-neutralization testing they're doing in there?" I remembered reading about it in *An Alternative Approach to Allergies*.

"Yes, it is. You haven't been tested yet?"

"Well, no. I was told to try the simple route first and follow an elimination diet."

"And are you feeling better, dear?" asked an elderly woman who had overheard our conversation.

"As a matter of fact, I feel much better, except when I go into malls or other places where there are lots of people. Then some of my symptoms return and I don't know why. It's very frustrating."

"Well then, you might need to have some testing done. You'd find out which chemicals make you sick."

"I've had scratch tests before . . ."

Both women laughed, as if I had just said something hilarious.

"Scratch testing doesn't even come close! Furthermore, you can get serums, or, as they call them here, antigens, tailor-made for you which help block reactions. A drop in the morning, a drop at night and presto - like magic, you can cope with life again!"

All of a sudden, a little girl, not a day older than Max, came tearing out of the testing room, wailing like a banshee! No one seemed terribly alarmed. Two women came running after her. One wore a lab coat, the other was obviously her mother.

"Sandra, dear! Come back here, honey. Let's go back and see Linda."

"No! No! No! I hate you! I hate you!" the child screamed.

The mother looked at us apologetically and said, "Peas! Can you believe it? She's reacting to peas!"

Everyone but me seemed to understand what was happening. Several people helped get the child back to the testing room.

"Peas?" I asked the woman next to me.

"Yes. Just about anything can cause a reaction when you have sensitivities. But just think how lucky that child is. Her mom now knows that peas cause her to react in that way and that her behavior is *not* psychologically rooted. No doubt she's been told otherwise by experts in child behavior. *They're* the ones who should be forced to sit here and watch what goes on!"

"I know what you mean. I just went through all that with sugar, wheat and . . ."

"Jillian, Dr. Rowland's ready to see you," announced Emily as she came to escort me to his office.

"Oh, gotta go!" As I stood up, I could feel my heart pound with excitement. I could hardly wait to tell him about my last few weeks!

I had just sat down on the sofa in his office, and arranged my bags and books when I heard a familiar, jovial voice. "Well, hello, Jillian Stowe! It *is* Jillian Stowe, is it not?" It was the man who had saved me! I turned to greet him.

"Dr. Rowland, I owe my life to you! I can't begin to tell you . . ."

"Whoa! I'm flattered, but you don't owe your life to anyone but yourself. And from what I can see, you've done a marvellous job! *You* have taken responsibility for your own health."

"But if it hadn't been for the direction you and Eva gave, I can't imagine where I'd be."

"Knowing people as well as I do, my guess is that eventually you would have arrived at this point on your own. You're a survivor, a fighter. But, I'm glad we were able to set you in the right direction - sooner rather than later."

"Me too! It's been a hard road to follow, but well worth it."

"Shall we tape this session, Jillian?"

I nodded, "That would be great. It really helped last time. I referred to it quite a bit."

He turned on the recorder and leaned back in his chair. "Now, how are you feeling? Let's go over your symptoms one at a time and rate them from one to ten, one being terrible and ten being terrific. Are you ready?"

"I'm ready!"

"Fatigue?"

"Almost gone! I'd give it an eight. And I discovered that *wheat* was the prime culprit. The only time I notice it now is when I'm out in public places like malls . . ."

"Shopping malls are a prime source of pollution. I call them hazardous wastelands. It might be wise to stay away from those sorts of places until we determine what specific chemical sensitivities you have."

"You know, Dr. Rowland, now that I think about it, I always felt kind of strange in malls."

"Strange?"

"I mean tired and cranky. After a few minutes of shopping, I'd always feel irritable. I never thought it could be a *physical* reaction."

"It really is amazing, isn't it? So few people ever attribute their daily aches and pains to environmental factors. How are the headaches?"

"I still have them, but only about twice a week compared to every other day, and they're not nearly as severe. I'd say a six."

"Gas and bloating?"

"Not quite as bad as before, but still a problem. Baker's yeast seems to be the chief culprit."

"So on a scale of one to ten?"

"Probably only a three or four. But I can handle that since so many other symptoms are better."

"Jillian, you'll continue to improve. You have to remember, it took years to get this way. It'll take time to heal. You'll see your recovery process accelerate as soon as we discover more causes and find more solutions. What about your joint pain, brain fog and inability to concentrate?"

"Well, the joint pains are still about a five, but the brain fog is lifting every day. I'd give it a seven - unless I'm out in crowds or in enclosed spaces other than my home. But I have noticed that I feel spaced out in my family room."

"Is it in the basement?"

"Yes. Why?"

"Well, basement areas are often damp, and dampness breeds mold. These molds can be a problem for people with yeast overgrowth and environmental sensitivities. Before you leave today, I'll refer you to a wonderful woman who gives workshops on healthy indoor environments. Sometimes she holds smaller sessions in her home, which is itself a wonderful example of a healthy indoor environment. Now, what about your mood swings, depression and panic attacks?"

"Basically, I feel far more balanced than I have in years. I discovered when I challenged myself with different foods, that refined sugar was the worst. My reaction bordered on violence!"

"Yes, you and thousands of others have that same reaction. In fact, there's a strong link between sugar intake, violence and crime. Jillian, did you know that the average person consumes more than *120 pounds* of refined sugar annually? And the worst part is that people don't even realize how much of it they actually eat. Most of it is well hidden in packaged and processed foods."

"After that appointment with Eva, I read labels on everything I consider buying. It takes me twice as long to get through the grocery store . . . if I can't pronounce it, I don't buy it."

He chuckled. "Eva obviously got through to you! You know, the elimination of refined sugar is, in my view, the most significant thing anyone can do - along with eliminating food colorings and additives, of course."

"Well, I believe it, especially now that I've experienced first-hand what sugar can do."

"And I don't mean only how sugar can affect behavior, but how it can affect overall health in general."

"What do you mean?"

"Eating excessive amounts of refined sugar overstimulates the pancreas, which in turn, produces excess insulin. It can cause hypoglycemia in one extreme and diabetes in another." He opened a book. " Frederick Banting, the co-discoverer of insulin, wrote: *In the U.S. the incidence of diabetes has increased proportionately with the per capita consumption of sugar . . . In the heating and recrystallization of the natural sugar cane, something is altered which leaves the refined product a dangerous foodstuff.* And then, there's the deplorable condition of our teeth due to indiscriminate sugar use. Nearly all American adults are afflicted with tooth decay and many studies have linked sugar to dental caries. Did you also know that high sugar intake depletes the body of essential vitamins and minerals?"

I shook my head.

"I could go on and on about the horrors of refined sugar - obesity, gastrointestinal disorders - you name it, they're implicated. Speaking of which . . . how are your bowels these days? Other than gas and bloating, has the irritable bowel settled down?"

"Much better, although there's still a little problem with occasional diarrhea."

"That will clear up with the next phase of our program."

"Dr. Rowland, you know what amazes me? Not a single doctor ever asked me what I eat or how I eliminate - not one! They didn't even blink an eye when I told them I had bowel movements once a week. They never related my condition to my lifestyle - especially not to my diet. I was sent for every test imaginable, as if there were some phantom cause. And dieticians would tell me to drink more milk to coat my stomach and bowels! One gastroenterologist even advised me to eat more margarine to make my intestinal tract more slippery! Can you imagine?"

Dr. Rowland smiled. "Yes, my colleagues have so much to learn, although I call it a process of unlearning - going back to basics. After all, focusing on what goes in and how it comes out is a *profound* teaching!"

I knew he was being sarcastic, but truer words were never spoken! I thought back again to our earlier conversation about the hazards of eating too much processed sugar. "I'll bet a lot of family dysfunction is tied into faulty eating habits."

"You bet," he replied. "I've worked with entire families who weren't able to relate to one another at all. They were so busy fighting over the most insignificant things, primarily due to their chronic irritability. Many of these families were on the verge of breaking up. Some of them thought I was a genius after they followed my suggestion of eliminating sugar from their diets. That alone, made the greatest difference by far in terms of family harmony. As crazy and simple as it sounds, it works. I've seen it over and over again. This is not just my own experience - these observations are shared by my close associates. Sugar reactivity is consistently implicated in aberrant behavior."

"Are there any studies on this?"

"Yes, but unfortunately, most of them are gathering dust on library shelves. One book that comes to mind right away is by Alexander Schauss called *Diet, Crime and Delinquency*. There are many others, of course, and literally hundreds of research papers that show how harmful sugar can be. In the late seventies, a Dr. Schoenthaller conducted a series of studies which demonstrated that antisocial and aggressive behaviors were reduced by half, simply by decreasing sugar intake alone. Just think . . . most institutional diets are loaded with sugar, and our hospital menus are certainly no exception. Let's put it this way - they're a far cry from the days when Florence Nightingale had recovering patients tending the hospital garden that provided their fresh fruit and vegetables. Fresh air and exercise were a bonus."

"How interesting! What a great idea!"

"In fact, I've often proposed a challenge to physicians and dieticians who work in psychiatric institutions. The program would involve the removal of all processed foods, sugars, dairy and wheat products from the patients' diets, to be replaced with brown rice, vegetables, legumes and fish. I'll bet many of the patients would make major strides in their recovery. Tending a garden would be therapeutic as well."

"Did anyone ever take you up on your offer?"

"Not one."

"But really," I suggested, "if we all just think, even for a minute, about the sugar-behavior connection, it makes sense. Just think how parents and teachers dread Halloween. It takes about a week for the kids to get back to normal."

"That's a great example!" exclaimed Dr. Rowland. "Everyone can relate to that."

"And birthday parties," I added. "I learned very early on to serve the cake and ice cream only minutes before the parents came to pick up the kids. You wouldn't believe the difference in the energy level before and after eating. It's no picnic to deal with a group of hyperactive kids for the whole afternoon."

"Good strategy!" He laughed. "I'll pass it along to other parents. Some families who have made the sugar-behavior connection substitute attractive fruit and vegetable trays and have come up with some unusual recipes for cakes that don't send the kids into orbit. Others, whose kids are dairy sensitive, use a rice-based ice cream as an option."

"But getting back to sugar, if we know all this, why isn't something being done about it?"

"Because there's no profit to be made by eliminating something from a diet. It would be a very threatening proposition to food processing companies. They would stand to lose bundles of money."

"Eva talked about that as well. I guess we always come back to the same bottom line - the almighty dollar."

"Unfortunately it's true. Incidentally, have you noticed that hospitals have recently introduced doughnut franchises? We even have one right here in our own Children's Hospital."

"Now that I'm better informed, it makes me cringe to think about what we're teaching our children."

"If hospitals endorse sugar, fat and caffeine, we're teaching our children that these things must be good for you. We forget that in the long run, this attitude will cost us billions of dollars. Lifestyles like these result in disease. I ask myself repeatedly, are we ever going to learn?"

"Maybe not. Eva suggests as long as dietetic associations and processed food giants mutually support one another, nothing will change. By the way, how do you feel about sugar substitutes like Aspartame and Sugar Twin?"

"In my view, sugar substitutes are dangerous, especially if used on a regular basis . . ."

I thought of all the diet pop we consumed in the run of a week.

"Just look at cyclamates like saccharin for example, which were widely used in the sixties, but banned ten years later by the FDA as potential carcinogens. And the safety of the newer substitutes such as aspartame and sucralose is at best uncertain. In fact, the evidence is still conflicting, but diets high in either product produce a number of negative side effects. According to Dr. H.J. Roberts, Director of the Palm Beach Institute for Medical Research, more than ten thousand people have reported side effects from consuming aspartame. Some of their symptoms include headaches, dizziness, decreased vision, confusion, memory loss, depression, and even seizures. Further research on sucralose is still recommended, especially since the long-term effect of even low-level consumption of these substances is still unknown. Like most other chemicals, they stress the liver. Personally, I wouldn't touch them. I certainly don't recommend that anyone consume them routinely, and I'd never give them to small children. The ultimate goal is to tame our taste buds so we won't crave sweets in the first place."

"What about honey and maple syrup?"

"They're better because they break down more slowly than cane sugar. But neither are appropriate if you have yeast or parasitic infestations."

"You know, as long as I stay completely away from sugar, I don't crave it. It's the first bite that does me in - then I'm out of control. It's like I *have* to have it!"

"That's the allergy/addiction pattern - you crave that to which you are sensitive." He looked down at my file and asked, "How's your bladder these days? Is it settling down?"

"It's improved slightly, but I'm still pretty uncomfortable a lot of the time. It feels like I'm getting an attack of cystitis, but nothing ever develops."

"On a scale of one to ten?"

"I'd say a four."

"Don't worry. That should also resolve over the next few weeks. It looks like we'll have to tailor your diet even further."

"Cut more things out? But . . ."

"Remember, these are *temporary* adjustments that will go a long way towards healing your body. What about your nasal congestion? On a scale of one to ten?"

"Ten. Gone completely! For the first time in my life I can really breathe. I still can't believe I had two nose operations to fix a deviated septum, something I now know I never had."

"I understand nasal surgery is quite an ordeal."

"It's even worse when it doesn't cure the problem."

He chuckled. "Let me guess - it was dairy, right?"

"How did you know?" I was amazed.

"Because dairy products had the same effect on me and on hundreds of other patients who have undergone needless surgeries. By the way, other than airborne irritants, dairy products are the leading cause of congestion. What a joke to find out that I was sensitive to the two litres of milk I drank daily for my health!"

"Yes, and don't most parents insist on it?" I remarked snidely.

"Absolutely. Our society is brainwashed into believing that without milk our teeth will fall out and all our bones will break by the time we're fifty."

"It's true. My family was appalled that I had stopped dairy products. You should have heard their comments! In the meantime, of course, they all have their 'mysterious aches and pains'."

"When you stop and think about it, two thirds of the world's population don't drink milk, and they still manage to have healthy teeth and bones. And, I might add, they sure don't suffer from osteoporosis to the degree we do here in North America. But I think we might have covered that last time we met."

"We did. And I'm still trying to overcome the years of conditioning that milk is a perfect food."

"I don't know if you're aware, but the latest on cow's milk is that an artificial growth hormone, bovine somatotropin - BST, more commonly known as rBGH - has been approved for use in the United States and is being considered by the Canadian government."

"Another hormone! One more thing added to our food supply!" I groaned.

"Outrageous, isn't it? In fact, Eugene Whelan, former Canadian Agriculture Minister and one-time dairy farmer was quoted as saying: *If I were the minister of agriculture today and I caught any Canadian farmer using BST, I would never let them sell milk again.* And a poll taken earlier this year suggested that seventy-four percent of Canadians are concerned about the hormone and would pay more for milk from cows that hadn't been injected with it. In the meantime, the European Community has adopted a seven-year ban on the use of this hormone and has also forbidden the import of BST-derived dairy and meat products into the European Union . . ."

"And the biggest milk drinkers are women and children!"

"That's right," said Dr. Rowland. "They'd be the most vulnerable to the effects of this hormone. And long-term studies of its impact on human health haven't been done."

"So, just another example of consumers being used as human experiments!"

"You're learning!" Dr. Rowland glanced at my file again. "Is your hair still falling out and do you still feel cold?"

"Yes, it's still falling out and I really can't afford to lose much more."

"It looks a bit dry and dull."

"I've changed my shampoo enough times."

"Have you ever had pets?" He caught me off guard with his question.

"Yes, at one time, but not now. Why do you ask?"

"Well, think about it. When an animal's fur is dull and lifeless, you add oil to its diet. The solution is to work from the inside out - to find the internal imbalance in order to correct it. It's the only way true healing can occur."

I ran my fingers through my hair. "It wasn't always like this." I thought back to the thick, shiny head of hair I had in my teens and twenties.

"So, on a scale of one to ten, where are you?"

"I'd say a two."

"Still cold?"

"Yes, but not as bad as before. I feel somewhat warmer and remain that way for longer periods. I guess I'd give it a five."

"Yeast infections?"

"They haven't cleared up yet, but they're not as intense and don't last as long. They're still an ongoing problem though, so I'd say a five as well. I should have been a man!"

"Don't kid yourself. Males have their share of problems too. They can have yeast overgrowth as well. In fact one common manifestation is prostatitis, a condition often caused by yeast, only never identified as such. It's usually treated as a bacterial infection with antibiotics which makes the situation worse. The sad part is that when the tests come back negative, they're often told to go home and live with it. And when it becomes more serious, surgery is the only option offered. No one ever mentions diet or the possible yeast connection."

"How else does yeast affect men?"

"Fatigue, headaches, gastrointestinal problems, depression, irritability-similar to the way it affects women and children." Stroking his chin, Dr. Rowland pondered the information in my file. "It's clear from your history and symptoms that gastrointestinal yeast is a large part of your problem. By the way, did you ever complete the questionnaire in *The Yeast Connection?*"

"Did I! My score was nearly five hundred!"

"That's extremely high. You're lucky to be as healthy as you are with that score! You obviously have a very strong constitution."

"Now I know why my vaginal infections never cleared up! Not one doctor - not even my gynecologist - ever told me to change my diet. They'd just keep prescribing creams and suppositories. I lived on the stuff for the past three years!"

"There have been numerous studies showing the connection between excessive sugar intake and recurrent vaginitis. And as we said earlier, vaginal yeast is usually a manifestation of an overgrowth of yeast in the bowel."

"I understood that from Dr. Crook's book."

"In his newest book, *The Yeast Connection and The Woman*, he cites a study by the St. Jude Research Hospital in Memphis, Tennessee. Thirty-six mice were colonized with gastrointestinal yeast. They were given a drug to suppress their immune systems. The control group was given water; the other, dextrose. Cultures of the stomach walls were carried out and the results indicated that the gastrointestinal growth and invasion of the yeast, *Candida albicans*, was approximately 200 times greater in the mice receiving dextrose than in the control group."

"All the more reason to stay off sugar . . . and keep my immune system strong!"

"Good conclusion - I wish everyone I saw was as quick to catch on as you are! Crook's new book makes even more connections - between yeasts and diseases such as asthma, endometriosis, multiple sclerosis and cystitis. He also makes reference to A.D.D. and recurrent ear infections in children."

"I didn't see it in the library."

"It'll be here by the end of the week. Talk to Bruce, our head librarian. He can send it out to you as soon as it comes in."

As he jotted some notes in my file, I noticed a funny little plaque on the wall:

> *If I had known*
> *I would have lived*
> *this long . .*
> *I would have taken*
> *better care of myself.*

I pointed to it and said, "If only we, naive citizens, had better access to more objective, unbiased information, we might be better equipped to take care of ourselves!

He nodded in agreement. "But remember," he said, "we're also the consumers. Once we're reprogrammed toward a healthy lifestyle, we do have the power to make changes by demanding what we want and need."

This was reminiscent of a conversation I'd had with Eva. "That's quite a job, don't you think?"

"Yes, but persistence works. If you want organically grown produce in your local grocery store, you must keep asking for it. The laws of supply and demand work quite well. Just a few years ago, how easy was it to find a health food store? Was anyone selling organic produce or free-range chickens?"

"I wouldn't know. I was eating the same junk that most people eat. But I suspect the answer is no."

"You're absolutely right. And human nature, being what it is, people have to become quite ill before they're willing to change their lifestyles, especially their eating habits. Personal experience truly is the best teacher."

"So the more sick people there are, the greater the chance of awareness and consequently, the greater the demand for healthy foods. Is that what has to happen to bring about change?"

"With one minor alteration. It may depend upon *who of importance* gets sick. When it happens to individuals who direct or lead major institutions - such as heads of hospitals, marketing boards, corporations and government officials - then things might change. It has to hit close to home."

"A terrible thing to wish on anyone, but I think . . ."

Suddenly, there was a loud commotion. It seemed to be coming from the waiting room. Emily burst in. "Dr. Rowland! Come quickly! Someone's passed out."

As they ran down the hall, I could hear Dr. Rowland ask, "Who is it?"

"She's a new patient. It's her first visit."

I followed the crowd into the waiting area. With an abrupt "Excuse me," Dr. Rowland pushed through the small group that had gathered to help the poor woman. She was quite elderly and frail. Her face was as white as a sheet and her breathing was labored. He knelt to examine her and asked without looking up, "Does anyone know her?"

A thin, middle-aged woman looked up and said meekly, "She's my aunt. Please help her!"

"Is she asthmatic?"

"Yes . . . she is . . ."

He listened to her chest, and glanced up. "Get her on oxygen - get a mask ready immediately!" He motioned to a staff member. "Janice, start her on a drip right away." Other employees scurried about, following orders.

In a few minutes, the color returned to the elderly woman's face. Her breathing changed from short gasps to a more even flow. By this time, several staff members were gathered around.

Janice, obviously in charge, looked around the room at the concerned faces. "Thanks for your help. She'll be fine now. You can return to whatever you were doing."

Dr. Rowland quietly chatted with Janice and the woman's niece. I returned to his office. After a short wait, the door opened and there he was, as calm as could be.

"Wow, that was a scare! Do things like this often happen around here?" It reminded me of my days in Emergency.

"Hardly ever. Apparently she became ill on her way here, and collapsed just outside the door. She'll be fine now. Hopefully, we'll find out what triggers her asthma so she won't have to endure this again."

"You seemed to take it all in stride. How do you manage to stay so calm?"

"Before opening this clinic, I spent many nights on duty in various emergency departments in the city. As you know, acting quickly, but calmly, was the order of the day. What I love about the work I do here is that it truly is holistic in the sense that I can draw upon whatever modality is necessary."

"What do you mean?"

"Well, that woman who just had the asthma attack clearly needed pharmaceutical intervention. Without that, she could have died. Once the immediate situation is dealt with, I can then use my knowledge and experience in complementary medicine to try to find the cause or causes of her asthma. Hopefully, her need for medication could eventually be reduced, or if we're really lucky, eradicated."

"So it's like being a detective . . ."

"Yes, it is. In order to be truly holistic, these approaches to healthcare must be integrated. They really complement one another beautifully, although I certainly prefer to work with the wellness model rather than the disease model. There are enough physicians working exclusively with the latter."

"Some people I've chatted with in the waiting room say you practice *alternative* medicine . . ."

"I really don't like the term 'alternative'. It sounds like we're in the business of excluding certain kinds of treatment. Nothing could be farther from the truth. What we do is truly *holistic* in the sense that we use treatments that complement one another. Sometimes we use pharmaceuticals, although we try to minimize their use. Other times we use vitamins, minerals, enzymes, herbal remedies and in almost all cases, diet. Then, we also have a homeopath, massage therapist and acupuncturist upstairs. It's a very balanced approach."

"And it's most reassuring to be treated by someone who knows when to use what . . ."

"That's good to know!" he laughed. "But on a more serious note, most of the patients I see can no longer be helped by surgery, are unable to tolerate drugs, or no longer choose to take them. Of course, many of those interventions were, and are, unnecessary in the first place."

"All I can say is thank God there are people like you to help people like me."

"Why, thank you."

"Dr. Rowland, I noticed you started an I.V. on that woman. I didn't know you had them here."

"We sure do. In addition to medicated I.V.'s for emergencies like this, we have vitamin and mineral drips we administer to patients who can't absorb oral supplements. We also use intravenous chelation therapy to treat heavy metal toxicity." He walked over to the tape recorder. "Now, where were we? I left this on when I rushed out. It'll only take a minute to rewind."

"Good thing I have that to go by. I'd never remember where we left off.

"Here we are," he said. "Oh, yes . . . we were just talking about what it would take for society to make changes. Anyway, I think we've exhausted that topic."

I nodded in agreement.

"Let's move on." Referring to my chart, Dr. Rowland explained the specialized stool test. "It will tell us how well you're digesting your food; will very likely confirm overgrowth of yeast in your bowel; and indicate whether or not you are low in stomach acid or have digestive enzyme deficiencies. Each, of course, is a strong possibility. It will also pick up any possible parasitic problems . . ."

"Parasites? You mean worms?" I cringed at the very thought.

"According to Dr. Theodore Nash from the National Institute of Allergy and Infectious Diseases, parasitic infections are a major cause of illness in the United States, and Canada wouldn't be any different. Even certain amoebas, previously thought to be harmless, can pose a real problem for people with weakened immune systems. On average, I find parasitic infections in two out of four patients with digestive problems."

I gasped in disbelief. "Yuck! I can't imagine that in this clean, sterile country, we'd have problems with parasites!"

"When you stop and think about it, it's really not all that surprising, and you don't even have to leave home to get 'em! Just consider the year-round availability of foods from all parts of the world, and our fascination with regional foods that are often prepared raw or partially cooked . . ."

"I thought raw foods were the way to go."

"Yes, in terms of enzymes and nutrients, that's true, but they have to be carefully scrutinized in terms of contaminants. Then, of course, there's water - one of our greatest sources of contamination. Do you remember a while back the headline story about the people in Milwaukee, Wisconsin who came down with severe stomach ailments and diarrhea?"

"No, I can't say I do. But then, my memory was shot for a few years."

"Well it turned out that their city water was contaminated with a microscopic organism called *Cryptosporidium*. Apparently, New York City also had a problem with this particular organism, and for people who have suppressed immune systems, it can be particularly dangerous. According to the EPA, *Cryptosporidium* is currently the leading cause of waterborne illness in the United States, found in eighty percent of surface water and twenty-eight percent of drinking water samples. In fact, there's a new countertop filtration system on the market that's specifically designed to remove *Cryptosporidium*, among other contaminants."

"And I suppose, once again, no one connects symptoms to the cause."

"That's right. Many who are infected don't even know it. After the initial infection, which is often misdiagnosed as a virus, it becomes chronic and can last for years. Most doctors don't even think to look for parasites because the symptoms mimic other ailments."

"Like what?"

"Anyone with chronic gastrointestinal complaints, such as gas and bloating, diarrhea, abdominal pain, chronic constipation, unexplained fatigue and especially those with multiple food sensitivities, should all be screened for intestinal parasites. Dr. Leo Galland of New York, author of *Superimmunity for Kids*, reports that nearly half of the people diagnosed with Irritable Bowel Syndrome have intestinal parasites. He says that eighty-two percent of those who suffered from chronic fatigue were relieved of those symptoms too. In fact, in one study, over *one-third* of the Chronic Fatigue Syndrome patients tested were found to be infected with *Giardia lamblia*. Chronic candidiasis is also strongly suspected in these cases."

I was appalled. "Why don't doctors routinely check for them?"

"Partly because they don't connect all the vague symptoms that are often associated with yeast and parasitic problems. The usual course of action is to treat each symptom rather than look for the cause. Again, take the case of patients with Chronic Fatigue Syndrome. Their symptoms include depression, muscular pain and weakness, headache and flu-like symptoms that often span several years. No one makes the connection!"

"And most of these people are told to go home and wait it out!"

"Yes, unless they happen to learn about complementary medicine and its approaches to the illness. Parasites are a far greater problem than we had ever thought. The book, *Alternative Medicine: A Definitive Guide* cites a research paper that appeared in *The American Journal of Tropical Medicine and Hygiene*. It revealed that, in both 1987 and 1991, stool examinations by state diagnostic laboratories revealed parasites in *twenty percent of all samples*."

"That's amazing. So, really, doctors should routinely test for them."

"Yes they should - especially where everything's been tried and the patient is still suffering. But the other part of the problem is that most parasitology labs fail to find the majority of intestinal parasites in the stool specimens they receive."

Dr. Rowland could see I was puzzled.

"According to Dr. Martin Lee, Director of Great Smokies Laboratory in North Carolina, regular hospital labs fail to diagnose parasites because they don't allow the time required for proper analysis. About a year ago, we used to take stool samples over a three-day period and now, the protocol is to take only one sample. These critters ain't gonna appear when you want 'em to! In fact, one naturopath in Portland, Oregon, reported that an AIDS patient had to give *twelve* stool samples before his *Giardiasis* was confirmed."

"So what if nothing shows even in multiple stool samples and the person is still suffering from all sorts of strange symptoms?"

"If everything else has been ruled out, and symptoms are still present, I always put patients on herbal remedies that target parasites. It's similar to yeast overgrowth - you don't always need absolute proof before beginning treatment. When it's almost impossible to identify certain parasites with a lab test, I usually rely upon symptoms to guide me. After two weeks, the results will confirm that we're on the right track - or not. I place a lot of emphasis on patient feedback."

"So can anyone do this on their own?"

"There are enough professionally written self-help books on the market that could provide direction, but it's always best to seek out a practitioner who's familiar with these problems."

"And are these drug-free therapies?"

"Yes, the ones I recommend are. Many years ago, I learned that most of the pharmaceuticals are far too toxic. They upset the natural balance of the body's own immunity even more and often have side effects such as nausea, mental disturbances and stress on the liver. In addition, I never found them to be as effective as the herbal combinations."

"So, shouldn't I start on some of this stuff right away?"

"Let's hold off until we see how far we can go with the yeast therapy."

"Getting back for a moment to parasites . . . would our whole family have to be treated?"

"It would be wise, since family members can pass them back and forth. Pets should also be treated at the same time. According to Ann Louise Gittleman, author of *Guess What Came to Dinner*, there are 240 infectious diseases transmitted by animals to humans. Of these, sixty-five are transmitted by dogs, and thirty-nine by cats. When you think about the 110 million dogs and cats living in American households, it's only common sense to assume that parasitic infection is a very real problem. But then again, they almost always go unsuspected and unrecognized. So, never, ever, let pets lick your face or eat from your dishes. It's a sure way of asking for trouble. The habit of sleeping with them also contributes to the problem. Regular de-worming is essential."

"How else can we become infected?"

"We already talked a bit about water. As for food, never eat raw or undercooked pork, beef, poultry, fish or shellfish. Always wash utensils and your hands thoroughly after handling raw animal protein. Washing and soaking vegetables in a salt or vinegar solution is helpful as well. Grapefruit seed extract that you can buy in healthfood stores is another alternative. And never drink water from a lake or stream. I often see families infected right after a camping trip. They usually think they've caught the flu, but if I listen carefully to their story, I can more often than not detect the point of infection. The most common line is, 'We were all well until we went camping,' or, 'We were all well until that trip to' . . . wherever."

"So is there anything we can do to protect ourselves?"

"The best thing you can do is to build up your immune system so you won't harbor any of these things. Generally, a strong immune system flushes them right through. It's when the system is weakened that yeasts and parasites create problems."

"Again, it all boils down to maintaining a healthy diet and clean environment, doesn't it?"

"That's a good start. Speaking of clean environments, daycare centers are breeding grounds for *Giardia* and other parasitic diseases. Gittleman says that the Center for Disease Control has estimated that every year, day care centers are the source of nearly 20,000 cases of *Giardiasis*. She says that these centers, often called the 'open sewers' of the 20th century, provide a fertile environment for transmission."

I thought about the play-school Max attended. Could he possibly have parasites?

"I could quote you hundreds of studies to prove that parasites are an enormous problem in our society today - and not just here. *Alternative Medicine* cites a study of 900 children and 140 workers in daycare centers throughout Toronto, Canada. It showed an overall intestinal parasitic infection rate of nineteen percent for children and fourteen percent for staff. Of those, the parasite *Dientamoeba* was found in the largest number of people, with *Giardia* a close second. And remember, symptoms can include behavioral as well as physical problems."

"You know, Dr. Rowland, when I think about it, my grandmother used to do what she called 'spring-cleaning' every year. She'd mix up some kind of tonic and would say it was 'time to clean out the critters'!"

He laughed. "Listen, Jillian, those old-timers knew what they were doing. And these days especially, a once-a-year cleanout is a grand idea. But, again, I must emphasize, that maintaining a healthy body and living in a clean environment is the best prevention."

"You mean by being aware of food hygiene and eating unprocessed, whole foods made from scratch?"

"Indeed. We've already discussed the harm that sugar can do in terms of behavior. Not only does it suppress the immune system, but it contributes to yeast overgrowth and parasitic infestation. Both thrive on sugar. Therefore, eliminating sugar from your diet is the single most intelligent thing you can do. I'd include the elimination of excessive amounts of fruit juice in that category as well. Staying away from processed, fiber-depleted foods is also crucial. Constipation is the parasite's best friend. And when the bowel flora has been disrupted, by the overuse of antibiotics for example, anything can flourish in that milieu - yeasts being only one of many unwanted guests."

"Well, I'll take yeast any day over worms!"

"You know, Jillian, when people have multiple food sensitivities, the *underlying problem* is often an imbalance in the gut, known as dysbiosis."

"And you say that an overgrowth of yeast and parasites is often the underlying cause?"

"Yes, but enzyme and hydrochloric acid deficiencies can also be significant factors."

"I still don't fully understand this yeast thing."

"Well, *Candida albicans* is the technical name for the yeast that causes a lot of difficulty, although there are others as well. They live in everyone's gut, quite harmoniously, until there's a disruption. Remember the last time you were here, we talked about how antibiotics kill the good bacteria along with the bad?"

"Yes, it seems so irresponsible." My blood boiled just thinking about all the prescriptions Max had been given. I blurted out, "Utterly irresponsible!"

"I agree, and we must do something about it or the situation will only worsen. Take a look at this." He pointed to a chart titled, *The Yeast Connection . . . A Vicious Cycle* (fig.9). "This is right out of *The Yeast Connection*. You develop an infection and take a broad-spectrum antibiotic which kills the 'good germs' along with the bad. Add to that, diets rich in yeast and carbohydrates; a high sugar diet; the birth control pill; cortisone and other drugs; some mold and chemical exposures; and there's a good chance you'll end up with a full-blown infection again. And what do you take for it?"

"More antibiotics! And then, of course, begin the endless rounds of vaginal creams!"

"Exactly. So can you see how it's truly a vicious cycle?"

"I sure can. I've experienced it for years!"

# The Yeast Connection . . . A Vicious Cycle

### (fig. 9)

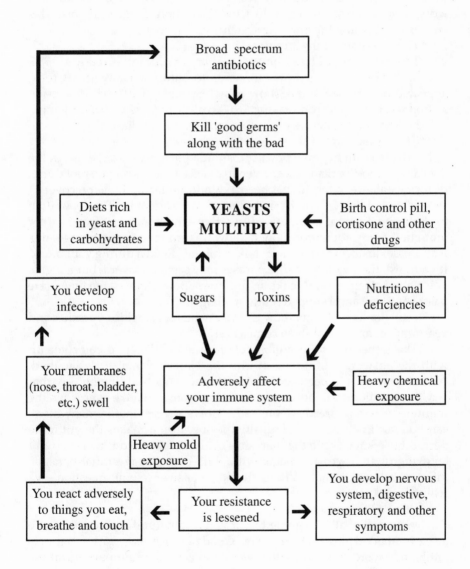

Used with the permission of **William Crook, M.D.**, author of **The Yeast Connection.**

"It should be mandatory for the manufacturers of vaginal creams to print on the containers: *Sugar intake should be eliminated for maximum efficiency.*"

"But how do these yeasts cause so much damage?"

"The theory goes like this: Yeasts overgrow and produce root-like structures called rhizoids, which permeate the mucous membranes of the gastrointestinal tract. This penetration breaks down the boundary between the gut and the circulatory system, allowing all kinds of substances to enter the bloodstream. As a result, we develop food sensitivities. To make matters worse, a yeast overgrowth can block the absorption of vital nutrients. This ends up weakening the immune system even further."

"How common is this problem?"

"Estimates vary, but the numbers are very significant. As early as 1986, Dr. Carolyn Dean, a holistic practitioner in Toronto, and Dr. William Crook, appeared on a phone-in talk show called 'Speaking Out'. The television station received a record-breaking 56,000 calls from people wanting more information and the names of doctors who treat candidiasis."

"That's amazing!"

"It truly is. In my own practice, candida plays a very large role in the ill health of most patients I see. Even in cases where it's not the root cause, restoring balance in the gut has been a significant factor in their recovery."

He rooted through his desk drawer. "Ah! Here it is. This is written by Ephraim Kishon, a famous Hungarian-Israeli author. Eva's father brought it to my attention, knowing how this antibiotic issue troubles me. It addresses just what we've been talking about. Read it during your break. It's a translation, so some of the phrases may seem awkward, but it'll give you a good chuckle - and make an important point at the same time." He passed it to me and I slipped it into my bag.

"I still don't understand how environmental sensitivities, parasites and yeasts are connected. Which comes first?"

"That's the sixty-four million dollar question. Jillian, if you come up with the answer, you'll make it into the Hall of Fame!" He laughed. "Chances are, you'll become rich, too! Some schools of thought say that yeast, or candida, is an opportunistic invader and will take over when the immune system is already depressed. Others suggest that in many cases, candida itself is the cause of sensitivities because it makes the gut more permeable. Some argue that parasites couldn't take hold if there weren't an overgrowth of yeast to begin with. Still others suggest that parasitic infection allows candida to flourish. So, in answer to your question - we really don't know."

"What's the next step?"

"Well, first of all, I'm going to put you on a natural antifungal. There are several good ones on the market. Good old-fashioned garlic - nature's antibiotic - works well to combat yeast and acts as an antiparasitic at the same time. There are products made from grapefruit seed extract that are effective against both candida and amoebas. However, the one I tend to favor is made from caprylic acid, a short-chain saturated fatty acid derived from coconut, combined with a variety of other fatty acids."

"What about some of the pharmaceutical ones Crook mentions?"

"If the natural antifungals are not strong enough, we can progress to more powerful antifungals like Nystatin, or move to more potent ones like Nizoral, Sporanox and Diflucan. They can be very effective in combatting more stubborn cases of candida. At the same time, I'll start you on some good bacteria . . ."

"By good bacteria do you mean aci . . . acidophi . . . however you pronounce it?"

"Yes, *Lactobacillus acidophilus* is the good bacteria your bowel needs in order to restore balance. In your case, we'll use the kind that is dairy-free due to your sensitivity to milk products. Remember, should you ever have to take an antibiotic in the future, always take acidophilus along with it, and for several weeks after. It should be routine protocol for every physician who practices responsible medicine. And if it's not sufficient, a good strong antifungal would go a long way."

"Boy! It's even buyer beware when it comes to doctors! None of them ever suggested that to me. Where do I find this stuff and how do I take it?"

"You can buy these products at any health food store. We also stock them here at the clinic for your convenience. Acidophilus must be taken on an empty stomach. Start with one capsule and increase to a maximum of six per day, three in the morning and three at night. The antifungal, however, should be taken with food - three capsules a day, one with each meal. At first, you might feel worse - similar to the way you felt during your food withdrawal. It's called 'die-off', an exacerbation of your symptoms caused by yeast being killed off."

"Oh no . . . not again. It was so awful . . ."

"Chances are, you won't experience too much die-off, if any, since you've already killed off some of the yeast simply by avoiding certain yeast-provoking foods. Some patients find that psyllium seed powder helps."

"Is that a laxative?"

"No, it's a bulking agent that provides fiber and gently sweeps debris through the intestinal tract. Pharmacies stock it under the name, Metamucil. It's critical to increase your water intake during this period. Sometimes I recommend adding Bentonite - a clay mixture - to this concoction. Its job is to absorb toxins as the yeast is being destroyed."

"It all sounds rather complicated. Do you have written instruction sheets explaining all of this?"

"We sure do. I have all the information you need with respect to candida protocol right here, in my hand. Continue to stay away from sugars, dairy products and any other foods that promote yeast growth such as mushrooms and fermented products . . ."

"What do you mean by fermented products?"

"Vinegar, soy sauce, sauerkraut, things of this nature - even wine. Also, limit fruit intake during the first few weeks. Following the caveman diet outlined in either *The Yeast Connection* or *The Yeast Connection and The Woman* for two weeks *before* going on the antifungal and acidophilus can minimize die-off reactions. The trick is to keep even complex carbohydrates to a minimum, but only for the first two weeks. And last but not least - take three plant enzyme capsules before each meal."

"Why? How will that help?"

"Efficient digestion is the foundation of good health and enzymes are essential for the proper digestion of food. You see, it's not always the food that's the problem, but rather, that your body is unable to break it down and utilize it without reactivity. So while your permeable gut is healing from candidiasis or a parasitic infestation, it's a wise step to supplement with plant enzymes. Also, enzymes give your body a chance to preserve its own internal enzyme supplies which can be better used to strengthen internal body systems."

"So is it like giving the body a break so it can focus on healing?"

"Yes, well put. Enzymes also enable your body to absorb more efficiently from the foods you eat every day. Hopefully, your diet is now based on whole foods and not denatured junk."

"After what I've read over the past few weeks, I wouldn't even dream of going back to some of the garbage we used to eat."

"You know, Jillian, about 20 million Americans have digestive disorders. Billions of dollars are spent on both pharmaceutical stomach medication as well as over-the-counter antacids and laxatives, not to mention what's spent every year on costly and invasive gastrointestinal testing. I've had patients of all ages whose chronic long-standing bowel problems were helped simply by changing their diet to whole foods, by eliminating problem foods, and by using plant enzymes or hydrochloric acid on a regular basis while their digestive systems healed."

"What's hydrochloric acid?"

"It's an acid, naturally excreted by the stomach that aids in digestion. Hypochlorhydria, or low stomach acid, leads to dozens of nutrient deficiencies, particularly B12 deficiency, which in turn can lead to pernicious anemia. Often, those with heartburn, gas, bloating and repeated bouts of candidiasis, suffer from this condition. The sad thing is that many physicians treat these symptoms with antacids - the opposite of what the body really needs."

"How do I know if I need enzymes or hydrochloric acid?"

"Good question. I usually start patients on plant enzymes. Most of them respond well. If we get minimal results, then I supplement with acid - but there's a protocol that goes along with this. Still others may need pancreatic enzymes. If we're really stumped, I order what is known as a CDSA or comprehensive digestive and stool analysis."

"I've never heard of that before."

"There are specialized laboratories that do these. Often, they help to determine the exact cause of the gastrointestinal upset."

"So, do I find enzymes in the health food store?"

"Yes, or here, at the clinic. It's another item we stock regularly. Your next step would be to listen to your body very carefully . . . hear what it's telling you."

"You mean notice if my symptoms get better or worse?"

"Exactly. An environmentally ill woman, Dawn McLaughlin Mongillo, once said, *I began listening carefully to my body with compassion and love. It began whispering to me and the whispers became clearer the more I listened.* I thought she said it so beautifully."

"Well put . . . but how do I learn to listen?"

"Through getting in touch with yourself. There are many ways to do this, such as yoga, t'ai chi, meditation . . ."

"Meditation? It sounds kind of far out to me."

"I see here you have an appointment set up with Leah Irwin, our clinic therapist. She's the very best person to talk to about getting in touch with yourself - how to access your inner teacher."

He could see I was puzzled.

"But for now, listening to your body will suffice. Take a moment or two out of your busy day and stop everything. Close your eyes and ask yourself, 'how do I feel?' The answers will come. This is where meditation, yoga, and t'ai chi would help you connect to your body's signals. We have a list of classes posted in the reception area. Emily has information that describes each technique and its benefits. Now, getting back to the initial two-week caveman diet . . . you can reintroduce complex carbohydrates, one at a time."

"Like whole grains?"

"Yes. But preferably grains without gluten, like rice and millet . . ."

"What's gluten?"

"It's the protein component of grains such as wheat, oats, barley and rye - the stuff that holds it together. That's why these flours bake so well."

"So I'm to avoid these grains?"

"Yes, but only for the first few weeks. And you must chew all grains thoroughly. Digestion begins in the mouth. Using a variety of grains so you're not eating the same foods day in and day out is also wise. It's easy to become sensitized to things you eat every day when the gut is permeable. Another important step is to increase your intake of raw foods so your body won't have to expend as much energy on digestion. And take your enzymes! This will all help the body to heal."

"When you say raw foods do you mean salads?"

"Yes, or just plain raw vegetables. But make sure you clean them well."

"You can bet on that!" I was vividly reminded of an earlier discussion about the two 'p factors' - pesticides and parasites.

"Platters of raw vegetables with a homemade dip work well. After the initial transition, you'll find that with this way of eating, your body will require less volume. Later, Eva will show you how to set up a rotation diet so you can avoid developing sensitivities to other foods . . ."

"A rotation diet? This is a bit overwhelming. I think I need a summary."

"Don't forget," he said pointing to the recorder, "it's all being taped. And I wouldn't let you leave without a copy of the protocol. I'll go over it with you now. When we're finished, you'll have a few minutes to take a short break and maybe get a bit of fresh air. How does that sound?"

"Great. I could sure use the break."

He smiled and began. "You've already done the first two steps but it never hurts to hear it again. Ready?"

I nodded.

"Here goes . . .

1. Identify your major food sensitivities by following an elimination diet.
2. Re-introduce foods one at a time. To establish cause and effect, always test first thing in the morning when you're least reactive.
3. Expand the elimination diet into a yeast-free diet by avoiding all foods that promote yeast growth.
4. Increase your intake of raw food - well washed, preferably pesticide-free.
5. Ten days after beginning the yeast-free diet, start taking acidophilus and an antifungal.
6. Introduce supplements, such as plant digestive enzymes, hydrochloric acid, vitamins, minerals and essential fatty acids. (Some of these you'll be discussing with Eva)
7. If symptoms don't subside within the first four weeks, begin an herbal anti-parasitic (you can check back with me for this).
8. If your progress is slower than anticipated, a CSDA will be in order.
9. Do an environmental checkup of your workplace and home - especially the bedroom where you spend much of your time. (I understand you'll be doing a workshop soon)
10. Begin provocation-neutralization testing for other foods, but particularly for chemicals and airborne irritants.
11. Begin detoxification therapy if symptoms have not abated.

Jillian, I hope this is helpful. Does it make it any clearer?"

"I'm glad it's all written out. By the way, what's detoxification therapy?"

"Detoxification is the body's natural process of eliminating toxins through the major organs such as the skin, liver, kidneys, bowels and lungs. This is done through deep breathing, sweating, urination and bowel function. The problem is that toxins often accumulate in the body more rapidly than they can be eliminated. We already went over the sources of pollutants to which we're exposed every day . . . "

"You mean like auto exhaust, cleaning products and pesticides?"

"Yes. Most people can handle a great deal of exposure. But if there's been damage from acute or chronic exposure to these pollutants, we need to use more aggressive detoxification measures in order to restore full function in these organs."

"Like what?"

"Detoxifying baths, sauna therapy, fasting, homeopathic and herbal remedies, massage, aerobic activity . . . to name a few. You know, some patients are so toxic, we can actually smell chemicals leeching out of their bodies during sauna therapy."

"How awful! What kinds of chemicals?"

"Pesticides, diesel fuel, gasoline, formaldehyde, paint . . . we've smelled them all."

"That's incredible!"

"Incredible, but very real. Jillian, remember when I suggested to you during our first meeting that illness is the best teacher? At the time I'm sure you thought I was crazy."

I smiled, remembering how I had thought both he and Eva were really quite off the wall.

"It'll all come to light in time - trust the process. See you in a bit. The fresh air should pick you up for round two."

I put on my jacket and grabbed my bag. As complicated as it sounded, it was all beginning to make sense. I knew that truth resided here - in this clinic.

I also knew that slowly but surely, my whole family would find their way to wellness.

---

# Newer Alternatives for Allergy Sufferers

Since the first printing of *Free to Fly*, several alternative approaches to the testing and treatment of allergies and sensitivities have gained considerable attention. I hope to cover them in detail in either a revised edition of this book or in an entirely new book. However, space in this update only allows for a brief description of these alternatives.

For additional information on alternative testing methods, including Muscle Response Testing (MRT) and Electro-acupuncture Bio-feedback systems (EAV) please refer to page 279 at the end of the chapter on *"Testing"* (Chapter 17).

Information on newer methods of treatment, such as Enzyme-Potentiated Desensitization (EPD) and the Nambudripad Allergy Elimination Technique (NAET), is located on page 141 at the end of Chapter 10.

To obtain detailed information about EPD and NAET, the Internet is likely your best resource. It can also provide you with lists of practitioners who administer EPD and NAET treatments. See also the *Reading List* at the end of *Free to Fly*.

*It is our children who pay*
*the severest penalities*
*for consuming our modern diet -*
*over-refined, unbalanced, highly allergenic -*
*and for the constant assault*
*by chemical pollutants*
*in food and in the environment.*

*Today more children than ever before*
*suffer from asthma, hay fever, eczema*
*inflammatory bowel disease,*
*and migraine headaches.*

*There is a marked statistical increase in*
*hyperactivity, learning disorders,*
*motor skills impairment,*
*childhood depression, and, most alarming,*
*teenage suicide . . .*

*All these problems can be traced, in large part,*
*to overconsumption, dietary deficiencies,*
*sedentary life-styles, and environmental pollution . . .*

*Nutritional abuse is a subtle form of child abuse.*

**James Braly, M.D.**
**Dr. Braly's Food Allergy & Nutrition Revolution**

# 10

# And the Children?

*Children suffer needlessly. One common source of their distress is improper food and drink.*
**Stephen J. Gislason, M.D.**

$T$he sun peeked out from behind the clouds as if awaiting my arrival. I sat on a bench sheltered from the wind and took a deep breath. My head was spinning. At the same time, I felt like I was on a journey from which there was no return. Two young mothers walked slowly toward me, chatting, keeping an eye on their children as they played in the snow. I caught bits of their conversation.

"Mandy and Jonathan were on so many antibiotics last year," said the woman in the red jacket, "we thanked God every day for our drug plan. And the number of diapers we went through! Mandy's diarrhea was so bad, at times she was literally pooping water. At one point, Jim and I were sure she had some terrible disease. And if that wasn't enough, Jonathan's tonsils were so enlarged, they wanted to remove them."

"I know just what you mean," replied the other woman. "Gregory lived on puffers and steroids most of the winter. It cost a fortune! He spent more nights at the Children's Hospital than I care to remember. And how many times were we told that his diet had absolutely nothing to do with his asthma!"

"Yeah, right, I know. I've been there. I honestly don't know where we would have ended up had we not met Dr. Rowland. Within just days of stopping dairy, wheat and corn, Mandy's ears cleared up and Jonathan's tonsils shrank to the point where the idea of surgery was history." Her voice choked a bit. "When I think of what my poor Mandy had to go through, week after week, month after month - because she was sensitive to foods I assumed were good for her! She's been fine ever since."

"Gregory! Thane! C'mon! Time to go!" called the other woman. They disappeared around the corner. The fresh cold air had perked me up. I took out the piece of paper Dr. Rowland had given me.

It was entitled *The Antibiotic Relay Race:*

---

*It started on the staircase. Suddenly I felt a slight itching in my left ear lobe. The wife nagged me to see a doctor. One should never be careless about such things.*

*I went to a specialist for internal diseases. He crawled into my ear, rummaged about in it for maybe half an hour, then came out and announced that apparently my ear was itching.*

*"I advise you to take six penicillin pills. That ought to clean out your ears."*

*I swallowed the pills and, indeed, two days later the itch was gone and my lobe felt newborn. My joy was somewhat marred only by the fact that crimson, itching spots had appeared on my stomach and were almost driving me mad. I went to the specialist. He only glanced at me and straightaway knew what had happened.*

*"Some people are oversensitive to penicillin and get an allergic rash from it. But don't worry, take a dozen tablets of aureomycin and in a few days it'll be gone."*

*I took the aureomycin and the spots disappeared. On the other hand, I ran up a high fever and my knees became swollen. I dragged myself to the specialist.*

*"Well, yes," the specialist said, "Aureomycin often causes unwanted side effects in the joints."*

*He prescribed thirty-two terramycin tablets and my problems disappeared as if touched by a magic wand. The fever dropped, and my knees returned to normal. We called the specialist to my bedside, and he said that the agonizing pain in my kidneys was caused by the terramycin. I should not make light of this - after all kidneys were kidneys.*

*I was given sixty-four shots of streptomycin by a registered nurse and the bacteria died in droves inside my body.*

*At the hospital I had to submit to a long series of laboratory tests, and it was found that not a single living microbe was left inside my body, the only trouble being that my muscles and nerves had shared the microbes' fate. Only an extra-strong chloromycetin shock could save my life. They gave me an extra-strong chloromycetin shock.*

*My admirers turned out in force at the funeral, as did thousands of curious idlers. In his wonderful eulogy, the rabbi dwelt on the heroic and losing battle which medicine had fought against my disease-ridden organism.*

*Really, it's a pity that I had to die so young. Only in Hell did I remember that my ear had itched because a mosquito had bitten it.*

---

I burst out laughing. It was hilarious - yet, so true! How modern medicine tended to complicate things - all he would have had to do was scratch his left ear lobe! The humor and fresh air was just what I needed to prepare myself for the second half of my session with Dr. Rowland.

When I got back to the office, I noticed a stack of flip charts and began to leaf through them. One in particular caught my eye - a line drawing of a figure captioned *Is This Your Child?* (fig. 10). It was very similar to a chart I had encountered when I first entered his office back in December - the

# Is This Your Child ?
## (fig. 10)

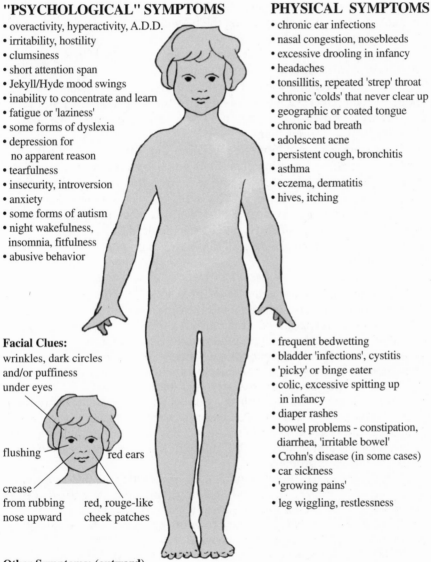

**"PSYCHOLOGICAL" SYMPTOMS**
- overactivity, hyperactivity, A.D.D.
- irritability, hostility
- clumsiness
- short attention span
- Jekyll/Hyde mood swings
- inability to concentrate and learn
- fatigue or 'laziness'
- some forms of dyslexia
- depression for
  no apparent reason
- tearfulness
- insecurity, introversion
- anxiety
- some forms of autism
- night wakefulness,
  insomnia, fitfulness
- abusive behavior

**PHYSICAL SYMPTOMS**
- chronic ear infections
- nasal congestion, nosebleeds
- excessive drooling in infancy
- headaches
- tonsillitis, repeated 'strep' throat
- chronic 'colds' that never clear up
- geographic or coated tongue
- chronic bad breath
- adolescent acne
- persistent cough, bronchitis
- asthma
- eczema, dermatitis
- hives, itching

**Facial Clues:**
wrinkles, dark circles
and/or puffiness
under eyes

flushing            red ears

crease
from rubbing    red, rouge-like
nose upward    cheek patches

- frequent bedwetting
- bladder 'infections', cystitis
- 'picky' or binge eater
- colic, excessive spitting up
  in infancy
- diaper rashes
- bowel problems - constipation,
  diarrhea, 'irritable bowel'
- Crohn's disease (in some cases)
- car sickness
- 'growing pains'
- leg wiggling, restlessness

**Other Symptoms: (outward)**
Pale face, anemic-looking, glassy or 'dull-looking' eyes, body overly thin or overweight,
mouth breathing, runny or stuffy nose . . . **or he or she could look perfectly healthy, yet
have environmental sensitivities.**

**... and (s)he may live on broad spectrum antibiotics, ventolin,
ritalin, decongestants, etc... etc... etc...**

one that so accurately described me. On one side was a list of *Physical Symptoms* - chronic ear infections, infantile colic, asthma, eczema . . . It was déjà vu! But instead of me, it described my kids! What really struck home were the *Psychological Symptoms* - overactivity, attention deficit disorder (A.D.D.), Jekyll/Hyde mood swings, short attention span . . . It described Nathaniel to a tee! I immediately thought of the years of guilt, feeling like an inadequate mother, shouldering the blame for his poor behavior. And all those years trying to find help - anywhere I could.

"So, you think your kids have sensitivities too?" asked Dr. Rowland as he walked in carrying two glasses of water.

"My worst nightmare is that they'll end up like me. In fact, I was just about to hand over $2,000 to a company that specializes in stopping bedwetting. I'd do anything to save Emma the embarrassment I experienced as a young child."

"Bedwetting is certainly one symptom that often resolves with the identification and elimination of problem foods - and it sure costs a lot less than $2,000! From what you've told me, your kids certainly have their share of sensitivities. On the positive side, it's been my experience that children are the easiest to work with when it comes to lifestyle changes. Adults have the most difficulty - old habits die hard."

"I can't see Nathaniel eating all this weird stuff . . ."

"He's how old?"

"Twelve."

"It can be challenging, but it's workable, especially once the child sees the connection between what he eats and how he feels. It's very experiential. A reward system, especially during the first few weeks, goes a long way. A non-food treat he's wanted for a while might work quite nicely. After the two-week period, he'd have to accept some of the responsibility himself. Remember, *everything in life is a choice*, even when they're that young."

"Peer pressure seems to be everything these days."

"Yes, I understand," he replied. "At that age, it's easier to work with highly visible problems like acne or obesity since they affect their self-esteem in a more direct way. Somehow, they'll live with behavior problems, stomach upsets and headaches, but not with something that's as obvious as a skin or weight problem."

"Maybe when it comes to behavior, it's harder to make the connection. Even I have difficulty comprehending that certain foods can actually cause psychological symptoms and I've already had first-hand experience."

"Good point. I'd like, however, to comment on your choice of words - your reference to healthy food as 'weird'."

"What I meant was that it's quite different from what I used to eat . . ."

"I understand. But it never ceases to amaze me that people who eat a junk food diet constitute the norm in our society, while individuals who try to live a healthy lifestyle by adopting a sound, natural diet are classified as extremist, or to use your expression, 'weird'. Society accepts disease states such as alcoholism and drug addiction, but when we eat healthy foods, take vitamins, or visit holistic practitioners, we're regarded as fringe-as if it were some kind of disdainful practice. Some of my patients have even been called 'healthaholics'!"

"You know, you're absolutely right. My family and friends think I'm being ridiculous. They see significant changes, but deep down they believe my problems are emotional and have very little to do with what I eat."

As we spoke, I thought of our 'normal' household. Dinnertime was usually chaotic. I'd be exhausted and cranky. Michael was often irritable, searching for Tylenol or Tums the moment he walked through the door. Lately, he always seemed to have a headache or an upset stomach. Nathaniel would drive everyone nuts by constantly aggravating the two younger ones. Michael and I were increasingly concerned over his behavior at school. Emma, who spent far too much time on asthma medication, was still unable to have sleepovers due to her bedwetting. Her constant whining was getting to us. And then there was little Max, congested, scratching himself silly from eczema, and screaming from the pain of those never-ending ear infections. *This* is what I'd accepted as normal.

"Are there any families who are functional, healthy and happy?" I asked.

"I suspect you won't find too many. Because of the nature of my practice, I certainly don't come across such families very often . . ."

"Neither do I. The only one I can think of is the Stuart family down the street. They eat as much junk as we do, yet all four of their kids combined don't even come close to one of mine in terms of behavior. Come to think of it, those kids aren't sick much either. It just doesn't seem fair!" I was beginning to sound like a pouty child.

"Well, it's quite possible they don't have the genetic history that's often part of the equation."

"I guess some of us are destined to have to work harder at our health!" I sighed.

"Jillian, we're all walking time bombs, waiting to explode. Sooner or later, poor lifestyle habits catch up with most of us. Have you looked at children in a typical preschool class - pale faces, drippy noses and dark circles under their eyes? Or, next time you're at the grocery store or standing in a bank line-up, take a close look at those around you."

"Why?"

"Do they look happy, healthy and vibrant?"

"Far from it. In fact, too many look quite the opposite, with pasty, puffy or scowly faces. On the whole, people don't look like they enjoy life."

"Maybe it's because they're broke," grinned Dr. Rowland. "Or, because they're living like you and I once were - on one medication after another. Think about it - Americans spend about $680 million a year on over-the-counter medications alone and proportionately, Canadians are not too far behind."

I shuddered.

"These individuals, along with those who regularly use prescription drugs for chronic conditions, are the ones who fall between the cracks of sickness and wellness. You see, Jillian, we've come to accept this as normal. Even though we're tired, cranky, suffer from headaches, and constantly take something to relieve our constipation and insomnia, we don't really think about what we're doing - not until we're so sick that we're forced to make changes. Only then can we see there's an entirely different way of being, a way of life that's available to each and every one of us."

"How true!" I exclaimed. "How many times have I heard, 'That's just the way I am,' or 'I've had a sensitive stomach since childhood' or 'I'm just a headachy sort of person'. We really *are* quick to accept these conditions as normal. And it's all because we don't know any better."

"And you wouldn't believe how many people I've seen over the years who come to me with a specific condition which they believe is their only problem. It's not until I interview them that I discover the needless surgeries they've had and the multiple medications they're on at any given time. I'm not sure why people accept this as normal, but I think you hit the nail on the head - they just don't know any different. Education is the key to bringing about societal change."

"But Dr. Rowland, it has to be truthful, unbiased education, not propaganda imposed upon us by those with vested interests."

"Ah, Jillian, you're catching on. You and I now know this to be true, but it takes time to learn. More and more people are slowly realizing that optimal health is available to them. They're starting to acknowledge that it's possible to be symptom-free and full of vitality - at any age."

"I want my kids to live happy, healthy lives. I'm really worried - they're already sick far too often. I'm afraid they'll only get worse. They get an infection, we run to the doctor for medication, they get another infection and back we go for more. It's a vicious cycle!"

"You took the words right out of my mouth. Take a look at this, Jillian. He flipped the chart over to a page entitled *Vicious Cycle of Ill Health* (fig. 11).

He pointed to each step on the chart. "Here we have a child with a masked sensitivity to something he's eating, drinking or breathing. And he's likely developed some nutritional deficiencies as well."

"Why would that happen?"

"If the digestive system isn't properly breaking down foods to which the child is sensitive, he won't be able to obtain all the nutrients from that food. As I mentioned earlier, I've noticed that children with sensitivities who drink the most milk are often the ones with the most cavities. They're also the same kids who show very low calcium levels on their mineral analyses. Their bodies are so busy warding off the daily assaults from whatever sensitizes them, that they can't absorb the nutrients."

"And that could lead to malnutrition?"

"Absolutely. Also, keep in mind that while the body is busy fighting the effects of foods to which it's sensitive, it loses the ability to fight more important invaders like viruses and bacteria. This is how sensitivities can weaken the immune system."

"And then I suppose eating a nutritionally deficient diet would only make matters worse . . ."

"You're right about that! Although we're an overfed society, we're undernourished. It's hard to believe, but subclinical malnutrition is an increasing problem right here in North America."

He moved down to the next section - *Ill Health*. "Then, the child develops

# Vicious Cycle of Ill Health
## (fig. 11)

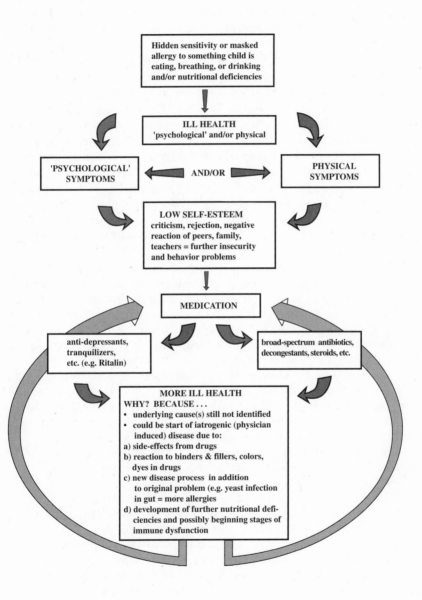

chronic problems, which manifest themselves as physical or psychological symptoms. Both can create low self-esteem. After all, it's hard to feel good about yourself when you're sick all the time, isn't it?"

I nodded. "I know only too well. When you feel lousy, it's impossible to function well."

"It sure is," he replied. "Then, operating within the typical framework of western medicine, we medicate. If the child has physical symptoms, we use broad-spectrum antibiotics, steroids, decongestants and broncho-dilators. If he exhibits behavioral problems, we use drugs like Ritalin or anti-depressants."

I cringed at even the thought of putting Nathaniel on a drug. I vowed right then and there that I would get to the bottom of his problem.

Pointing to the lower box on the chart, he continued, "So, what have we got? We have more ill health. And why? Because the *underlying cause* is still not identified. It's often the beginning of a drug-induced disease, due to a reaction to the drug itself, or a reaction to the binders, fillers or colors in the drug. It could also be the start of a new disease process *in addition to* the original problem. One example of that is the overgrowth of yeast in the gut. Finally, further nutritional deficiencies can develop which could end up causing more serious immune dysfunction or auto-immune disease. As a result, the child's ill health intensifies and we're back to more medication." With the pointer, he traced the thick broken line on the chart. "Do you see the cycle?"

"Do I see it? I live it! And just think about the message we're giving our kids about drugs - hey, you've got an ache or a pain? Just take a drug and everything will be okay. It's sick!" I exclaimed in disgust.

"And to make matters worse, if the reaction happens to result in poor behavior, the child is labelled 'a problem' - a stigma that may haunt him throughout his school years. In the meantime, he really can't change his behavior until the cause is discovered."

"Dr. Rowland, my kids are always sick! One's hyperactive, especially at school; another's asthmatic and drives everyone around the bend with her whiny disposition; and my little one's constantly medicated for ear infections - not to mention the sleepless nights we've endured due to his eczema." I could feel myself becoming upset all over again.

"Well, I strongly suggest you eliminate the same foods from their diet as from yours and consider bringing them in for testing."

"I'll book an appointment today."

"The last I heard, our testing room is backed up about two months. In the meantime, do exactly what you've done with yourself up to this point."

"Two months! Why such a long waiting period?"

"Well, the testing we do is very labor-intensive," he replied. "It takes about four to five days to complete, but it's well worth doing. It provides us with invaluable information. We can provoke reactions from foods, chemicals and airborne irritants, similar to those you experience every day. It helps to pinpoint sensitivities. But Jillian, I can't emphasize this point enough - diet, diet, and more diet will provide at least half, if not more, of the answers to the puzzle."

"Do you mean an elimination diet?"

"Yes, including all refined sugar and junk foods, especially those with additives and colorings. But I also mean some of the foods we consider to be healthy - foods to which you were sensitive such as wheat, yeast and dairy products."

"Dr. Rowland, is there anything I could have done to prevent the problem in the first place?"

"It's easy to find answers in hindsight," he replied. "But, yes . . . we ought to start before conception. Although heredity and environment play an important role, a healthy diet usually means healthy kids. Now, if sensitivities run in the family, one has to be extra careful not to sensitize the fetus. Research shows that the fetus begins to produce antibodies against allergic substances as early as eleven weeks into pregnancy. You know that baby who kicks and punches incessantly *in utero*? Or that baby who barely moves? Chances are, those are the babies who'll have sensitivities at birth."

"According to my doctor, the most active ones are the babies who are supposed to be strong and healthy; the punching and kicking are supposed to be good signs."

"It was more than likely a signal to his mother to stop eating the foods that affected him. Toxins in a woman's diet can do irreparable harm during pregnancy. Eric Jansson, coordinator of the National Network to Prevent Birth Defects says that a *fifty percent* reduction in birth defect rates could be achieved through an improved diet and a reduction in the levels of toxic exposure. To a sensitive fetus, allergenic foods can be toxic as well."

"And I was told to increase my intake of milk, cheese and yogurt!"

"Very common advice, and to many, potentially one of the most damaging. No wonder so many babies are born sensitized to dairy."

"So, suppose some of the damage was done *in utero* . . . was there anything I could have done to prevent problems after they were born?" I listened intently as he described the journey from birth to adolescence.

"Many things - namely, that you provide them with clean air, water and food. Let's look at the baby's first few weeks. First, we bring this precious newborn home to what's often a contaminated nursery . . ."

"Contaminated?" I asked. "How?"

"Chances are, the well-meaning parents have painted or papered the walls, carpeted or refinished the floors, and purchased a fresh-from-the-store crib with a plastic mattress and bumper pad that slowly emit toxic gases. If that's not enough, often the baby's covered with a new polyester comforter and fastened into a plastic, disposable diaper. Remember, an infant's breathing rate is far more rapid than an adult's. Therefore, you can well imagine the rate at which that baby inhales or absorbs that chemical brew. I've often wondered if there's a connection between Sudden Infant Death Syndrome (S.I.D.S.) and environmental factors, such as formula feeding and the synthetic world into which babies are thrust."

"Speaking of chemicals and babies - they actually moved our newborns into the newly constructed maternity hospital when the paint was barely dry! Who knows what effect it had on the babies and their mothers. Mind you, they were only in there for a few days, but the impact on the full-time hospital staff has been dramatic - and tragic. Many became ill and quite a few are still off on worker's compensation."

"I've seen several of them over the past few months," Dr. Rowland said quietly. "All I can say is, it was a preventable tragedy." His expression changed to one of sadness. "When are we ever going to learn?" He gazed out the window for a moment. Taking a deep breath, he continued. "Now, getting back to baby. If Mom decides to breast-feed, great! If not, the baby is put on formula. I called our local maternity hospital to ask them if they would consider using an alternative brand - one that's easier to digest than their regular formula. Even after I explained the health benefits, they refused to consider a change - not even on a trial basis. The bottom line is, they're tied into a long-term contract with a particular company whose formula, by the way, is known to cause the greatest number of health problems."

"That's a disgrace!" I exclaimed.

"Yes," he sighed, "but it's reality. In any case, then solid feeding begins, but far too soon in my opinion, and often with the wrong foods. Grains like rice, oats and wheat shouldn't be introduced until the baby can chew. Digestion of grains occurs primarily in the mouth. So vegetables would be a more logical place to begin, followed by fruit. But, Jillian, what's in any of the commercial baby foods we feed our children?"

I whispered, "Pesticides?"

"That's right. But I'm sure Eva's gone over the dangers of chemicals in our food supply."

"She certainly has - it's appalling!"

"Just the other day I read an article in *The New York Times*, listing the twelve fruits and vegetables that have the highest levels of pesticides. Strawberries ranked as the most contaminated. Bell peppers and spinach tied for the second-highest ranking, while the following were listed on the 'to avoid' list: cherries, peaches, Mexican cantaloupes, celery, apples, apricots, green beans, Chilean grapes and cucumbers."

"So what's left to eat?" I gasped.

"Alternatives were provided, as were the principal nutrients found in each. For example, alternatives to spinach would be broccoli, brussels sprouts, romaine lettuce and asparagus. The conclusion was that if consumers avoided these twelve fruits and vegetables, they could reduce their health risks from pesticides by half and still get the significant nutritional and health benefits that alternatives provide. Did Eva mention the number of allowable pesticides for each item?"

"Not specifically."

"On apples alone, *forty* different pesticides are allowed. It's the same for tomatoes - and on top of that, they're often gassed to give them color; on citrus fruit, it's twenty-seven; on green beans, twenty-four; on grapes, thirty-two; and on that healthy-looking head of cabbage, they can use up to twenty-two different sprays. And these are the fruits and vegetables that are supposed to help fight heart disease and cancer."

"What a joke! If we *don't* eat them, we risk heart disease; if we *do*, we're slowly poisoned by pesticides and could likely end up with cancer. What a no-win situation!"

"Now, just think for one moment how many apples it takes to make up one can of juice. And most babies are given apple juice from morning till night - one of the worst fruits for pesticides."

"I never really thought about it that way! Come to think of it, I don't recall drinking this amount of juice when I was a child."

"You probably didn't. It's a fairly recent practice - one I discourage, not only because of the risk of pesticide exposure, but also because that amount of juice contains so much sugar."

"But if it's one hundred percent natural, it wouldn't contain added sugars."

"That's quite correct, but in such large quantities, the naturally occurring fructose is still far too much. It creates imbalances. Children tend to fill up on it and miss out on other vital nutrients they would normally get from other sources. And then of course, there's the issue of yeasts and parasites which we've already discussed."

"Because of the sugar?" I asked.

"Precisely. Parasites thrive on sugar. And so do yeasts. These organisms don't differentiate between natural or processed sugars."

"Can children have yeast imbalances?"

"Absolutely. In fact, many children born with thrush already have gastrointestinal yeast imbalances - often from yeasty moms. So the cycle perpetuates itself."

"What are the symptoms?"

"Colic and chronic ear infections are first on a long list. Other symptoms are the same as those on the chart you were looking at when you came back from your break. But remember, yeasty or not, limiting the total intake of sugars, whether natural or processed, is the best policy. So instead of massive amounts of juice, offer the whole fruit, peeled, of course. That way, they get fiber and far fewer pesticides."

"So what should they drink?"

"They should be encouraged to drink clean water."

"When you think about it, apples have historically been linked with wholesomeness - *an apple a day keeps the doctor away*."

"Ah, but life in the nineties just isn't quite what it was in the forties and fifties. It's more like the Snow White tale. Remember the wicked queen giving Snow White the poisoned apple?"

"I sure do. The only difference is that *she* wakes up from her poisoning and lives happily ever after. In real life, it's not quite that simple, is it?"

"It certainly isn't," he replied grimly. "We're all fast asleep - totally unaware of what goes on around us."

I felt a sudden sense of urgency. "We really do need to wake up! If not for our own sake, at least for our children's."

"The good news is that some people have. There are organic baby food businesses sprouting up all over the country and it's high time. It's interesting to note that these entrepreneurs are looked upon as 'fringe' by the establishment. In fact, anyone who questions the safety of the food supply is considered an alarmist. Dieticians are forever locking horns with Eva when she speaks to the public about the hazards of the foods we eat. They've accused her of being a fear-monger, simply for reading aloud the list of ingredients found on the packaged foods we eat every day."

"I think I know what you mean. When I mentioned Eva's name to my neighbor who teaches nutrition at the local college, she just rolled her eyes and immediately began to discredit her. In the meantime, this woman is at least fifty pounds overweight, still has acne, and her kids are holy terrors! Come to think of it, they always have at least five or six cartons of milk a week delivered to their doorstep, and their kids eat ice cream and chocolate covered granola bars like they were going out of style - and not homemade ones either!"

"Need we say more?" Smiling, Dr. Rowland continued. "So, getting back to babies . . . we do our best for the first two years. We feed them what we think is right, pure and wholesome. We're very lucky if the infant makes it to his or her first birthday without several rounds of antibiotics. Next, we're out and about in public places, especially malls. Then the onslaught of junk begins - anything to keep the child quiet while we shop. Cinnamon rolls, doughnuts, chocolate, fruit drinks, even pop. I'll bet more often than not, these contribute to the crankiness. It's not just the boredom of shopping. And you wouldn't believe how many parents allow their children to dictate what goes into their grocery carts! Parents often use the excuse, 'Well, at least he'll eat these'."

I thought about what Dr. Rowland was saying. I was no better than all those other parents. The kids often picked their favorite junky cereal, instant soup or canned spaghetti - the kind that stained their faces orange for hours. I was one of those parents he had just described. I'd reached the point where I was happy they'd put at least something in their bellies - anything. I now realized what a mistake that was.

"And they fill up on junk," he continued, "leaving little, if any, room for important foods - foods that could provide valuable nutrients."

"Like nuts, seeds, vegetables, fruit and whole grains?" I asked.

"Right. How many children in your neighborhood eat that way?"

"None that I know."

"Is it any wonder why kids have problems? Think back to your own school days. There might have been a couple of kids who were fidgety and acted up. Perhaps one, or at most two, were real troublemakers. Ask any teacher about classroom behavior today and you'd be shocked by their reply."

"I know that's true. Several friends of mine are teachers and they're burning out - fast. They spend more time disciplining than teaching. Their colleagues who've been in the system for twenty or thirty years will attest to the difference between kids today and back when they began their careers. There's no comparison."

"And observe what they bring to school for snacks and lunches - fruit chews full of coloring ; fruit drinks that contain far more processed sugar than fruit; and even chocolate bars! One mother told me the funniest story. Her little guy had just started kindergarten and she sent him to school with a huge pile of carrot sticks so he could share them. One of the children asked for a third helping and said, 'Can you get your mom to tell my mom how to make these'? Sad, isn't it?"

I had to laugh, while at the same time, acknowledging the gravity of the situation. "But how can we make changes for the better when we're inundated with junk?"

"It's not easy," replied Dr. Rowland. "But in my experience, most children are open to learning. Facts, figures and anecdote seem to capture their interest. For example, they never fail to respond when told about a study using rats, conducted in a private school in California involving groups of students with behavior problems. The study was originally set up to show students how their poor behavior was influenced by what they ate and drank, as well as to reinforce the reasons for the implementation of stricter nutritional guidelines. Kids who hear this story, often end up feeling so sorry for the rats, that change becomes relatively effortless."

"Isn't it sad that we give more credence to experiments performed on animals than we do to our own personal experience? But I guess if a story can grab their attention and helps bring about positive change, then we should keep telling stories."

"I agree. If it works, do it. Anything as long as the message gets through. In this particular study, the first group of rats was fed natural food and clean water. They remained alert, curious, calm and social. The second group was fed natural foods and wieners. They became violent, fought, and bit off their own tails. Some even severed their own tongues."

"How horrible!" I cried.

"The third group ate sugar-coated cereal and drank fruit punch . . ."

"That would be equivalent to many children's breakfasts!" I couldn't resist the comment.

"Exactly. But listen closely and see if you detect any similarities with the rats' behavior. They ended up running around the cage, nervous, hyperactive and aimless. Some hung upside down from the ceilings of their cages."

"Boy! It does sound like my kids at times - but even more like my nephews, nieces . . . and definitely like many of the neighborhood kids. They seem so hyper, unfocused . . ."

"I thought you'd see the parallel! The fourth group was fed sugared doughnuts and cola. They were unable to sleep and sat quivering alone in corners, unable to function as a social unit. Parents often come into this office and describe their children's behavior in very much the same way - particularly that of their teenage children, some of whom are even suicidal."

"Dr. Rowland, it's a tragedy. We reward our kids with synthetic ice cream, popsicles, flavored chips and chocolate, then wonder why they turn into basket cases."

He nodded. "There is good news, however. When the agitated rats were switched over to natural food and clean water, they became sociable, and their interaction was calm and normal. Their coats went from dull and thinning to sleek, full and furry."

"So it's never too late."

"Never. And humans are no exception. But here's the real clincher. Some of the rats had babies, and their offspring displayed similar behaviors. So, when you asked earlier what one could do to prevent sensitivities, there's your answer."

"Just like Pottenger's cats! And a lot like your colleague's daughter, who gave birth to a healthy son by monitoring her diet throughout pregnancy."

Dr. Rowland laughed. "Jillian, you do connect things quickly. Those are perfect examples!"

"Where could I find this rat study? I'd like to read it to the kids."

"In *Diet for a Poisoned Planet*. Even though it portrays reality, it's not a book I'd recommend you read from cover to cover to children as it could cause them to become fearful. But sharing that study and the parts about processed foods, certainly would be an eye-opener. Read the rest yourself. It will change the way you look at things - forever."

"Is it in the library?"

"Yes, we have several copies. You know, a friend of mine compares the terrible two's with adolescence. Although both stages are times of growth and independence, they're also times when diets deteriorate drastically. We do our best to feed our infants the purest foods possible - given the information we have - but between eighteen months and two years, their diets often begin to go downhill, rapidly. The same happens during the teen years."

"Don't I know it!" I exclaimed. "Nathaniel lives on packaged soup, flavored chips, pop and chocolate bars, wherever and whenever he can sneak them."

"And, I'll bet he drinks loads of milk - to keep Mom happy that he's at least getting *that* amount of nourishment. Right?"

"Right."

"In *Dr. Braly's Food Allergy & Nutrition Revolution*, there's a study that concludes that juvenile delinquents drink three times more milk than non-delinquents, consume 30 to 100 percent more sugar, and live on coffee and packaged sweets. When put on a more natural, low-sugar diet, the incidence of repeat offences was reduced to one-sixth. Another study published in the *International Journal of Biosocial Research*, looked at twenty-four inmates aged twelve to eighteen. Sugar and cola were removed from their diet. After three months, when compared with the control group of thirty-four youngsters at the same institution, they had a 45% decrease in disciplinary actions, an 82% reduction in assaults . . . and a 77% drop in thefts. Horseplay was down by 65% and there were 55% fewer refusals to obey orders."

"Those figures are astounding!"

"There are many other studies that draw similar conclusions. But the best study is the one you do on your own. Within a few short weeks, you'll pinch yourself to make sure it's not all a dream, the changes will be so dramatic."

"After my own experience with sugar and dairy, I'm ready to have the whole family jump on board!"

"Good for you!" All at once, he became somber. "It really is a very serious matter. I've seen kids go from being violent, depressed, and even suicidal, to happy, well-adjusted and productive - simply by altering their diets. Yet, society continues to treat aberrant behavior as if it were a Ritalin or Prozac deficiency. We're still on the same old bandwagon - ignoring diet and environment, often the two most significant underlying causes. It's bad enough that these foods can cause poor behavior, but what's even *more* alarming is that bad dietary habits can lead to disease."

"We already talked about how sensitivities can cause chronic illness. Now you're saying that the typical North American diet can cause serious disease as well?"

"Yes. A processed diet is a disease diet. Far too many teenagers and even younger children already have cholesterol levels over 200. The American Heart Association reports that in a recent seventeen-year period, obesity in children aged twelve to seventeen increased a whopping *thirty-nine percent*, while obesity in the younger group, aged six to eleven jumped a staggering *fifty-four percent!*"

"That's frightening!"

"Unacceptable might be a better word. And how long are we going to ignore the rise in cancer and heart disease by merely chalking them up to 'less reliable detection methods' used in earlier years or to 'a lack of reliable statistics back then'?"

"You're right. By putting on blinders, we refuse to take responsibility for what we've created."

"That's about the gist of it, but we can't continue to ignore the National Cancer Institute's figures." He picked up the Steinman book. "Between 1950 and 1985 the incidence of cancer among children under the age of fifteen increased *thirty-two percent*. And more specifically, throughout the population, urinary/bladder cancers increased fifty percent, testicular by eighty-one, kidney and renal/pelvis by eighty-two percent, while non-Hodgkin's lymphoma increased by an astounding *one hundred and twenty-three percent!* These cancers have been linked to toxic chemicals in our drinking water and to pesticide exposure. Something is very wrong somewhere."

"And how many of these and other cancers are linked to the bad fats and additives in our foods," I wondered out loud.

He quickly leafed through some pages. "Ah! Here it is! The 1988 *Surgeon General's Report on Nutrition and Health* estimated as many as 10,000 cancer deaths annually could have been caused by chemical additives in food - chemicals *intentionally* added! And as early as 1965, the World Health Organization concluded that at least half of all cancers in humans are due to environmental factors, while The International Agency for Research on Cancer estimated that *eighty to ninety percent* of all cancers are caused by environmental, rather than genetic factors."

"Where did you get all this information?"

"Once again, two of the best resources for the layperson are *Diet for a Poisoned Planet* and a Canadian book, *Additive Alert*. And the worst part, knowing all this, we still continue to allow big business to dictate to us. Even worse, we allow our children to be brainwashed."

"Saturday morning T.V. is full of ads, especially cereal ads."

"And what a captive audience! In 1991, the Center for Science in the Public Interest analyzed food ads on Saturday morning T.V. *Ninety-six percent* of them were for candy bars, sugary cereals, salty canned foods, fast foods and chips literally dripping with fat - all nutritional disasters. Many studies have been conducted that repeatedly prove that the standard North American diet is a sick one. What happens when people change from their native diets to our diets? Disease strikes - osteoporosis, arthritis, heart disease, cancer . . ."

"You know, Dr. Rowland, what you're saying all makes sense. I've lost two friends over the past year to breast cancer. My mother recently commented that when she was my age, she was losing her friends' *parents*, not her friends."

"I'm hearing that more and more, he murmured, "Steinman says that the incidence of breast cancer increased by *fourteen percent* between 1973 and 1985 - in only a twelve year period! That's a phenomenal jump - more than one percent per year."

"Imagine projecting those figures into the future!" I declared.

"And he goes on to say that another study found that cancerous breast tissue contained abnormal levels of industrial pollutants and pesticides compared with normal tissue."

"It's sure a far cry from our grandparents' day! They could eat whatever they wanted, even smoked and drank, and still managed to live relatively healthy, productive lives."

"Ah, yes, those days are long gone. They had clean food, water and air, and didn't spend their time in front of televisions, computers and video games. Their total loads were much lower, so they could afford a bit of abuse!" We both laughed. "You know Jillian, adults are one thing, but children are really innocent victims - like lambs being led to slaughter."

"I've never heard it put quite so bluntly. But you're right. At every family restaurant, there are kids' menus - french fries dripping with reheated fats; hot dogs full of nitrites; pop, laden with caffeine, sugar or artificial sweeteners; and to finish off the meal, good old Jello, which is little more than sugar with chemical dyes and flavorings."

"I understand it's also standard fare in most school cafeterias."

"And let's not forget hospitals," I added. "Just a few weeks ago, we decided to take the kids to a 'fun-filled' weekend at a resort. The first night was bragged up to be Kool-aid night. Imagine over a hundred little kids after a few drinks loaded with dyes, sugars and artificial flavors!"

"I'll bet you had fun," he said wryly. "These so-called foods are all around you. The best you can do is to set a good example at home."

"But how do you get them to stick with it? Peer pressure is everything."

"First of all, if they don't eat junk in their first few years, they aren't as apt to develop a taste for it."

"It's a little too late for that!" I blurted out.

He smiled. "I understand. But then there are many things you can do at home to help them make wiser choices."

"What, for example?"

"The most important thing is to have only wholesome foods at home, yet not be dogmatic about it. In our house, we allow a junk food day once a week, but never consider or label any of it as 'treats'. One of my patients aptly calls their junk day 'Pig-Out Day'."

"Hmm. Great name!"

"So we still occasionally indulge in french fries, but when at home, they're *à la Rowland*."

I was curious. "How do you make them?"

"We peel and slice our own potatoes, coat them with a bit of olive oil and bake them in the oven. It's several steps safer than the frozen stuff coated in hydrogenated fats or the ones you get in fast food joints."

"I'm beginning to see there are healthier alternatives to almost every food. But how do you convince a twelve-year-old to eat differently from all of his friends?"

"It's not easy. They hate being lectured, particularly by a well-meaning parent. It hardly ever works. But children at any age respond well to factual information, especially when found in a book."

"But as you've stressed, even foods we consider safe like fruit and vegetables aren't free of harmful things."

"That's true, but they're a considerable improvement over processed and packaged foods. Organically grown is obviously the preferred way to go. Living in a large center that offers a variety of these foods is a decided advantage and by supporting organic farmers, you're making a statement to the food industry - that you don't want another mouthful of their poisons."

"And what if you live in an area where you can't get pesticide-free food?"

"Then you do the best you can with what you've got. We've already talked about peeling and soaking in terms of preventing parasites. It's equally important in terms of protecting yourself from harmful residues - and molds. Did Eva go over this with you?"

"Yes, she did."

"In larger centers, another option would be to frequent stores or markets that have sections with organically grown foods. You can also pressure the meat and produce managers at your local grocery store to list all the chemicals found in their products. Encourage them to carry free-range eggs and chickens."

"What do you mean by free-range?"

"It means the chickens are allowed to run around and peck freely instead of being cooped up and force-fed processed feed. It keeps them healthier, thereby reducing or eliminating the need for antibiotics. They are also hormone-free. If you've never tasted one of these birds, it's time to try one. The taste is incredible!"

"Are they more expensive?"

"Yes, but remember, the greater the demand for organically-grown food, the lower the price, both in terms of dollars and health."

"I suppose getting several people together who are like-minded would be a good strategy."

"It would be a great start. In fact, there are names of people who want to do exactly that on the bulletin board out front. Add your name to the list. Another step, which we've already discussed, is to eliminate junk food in your home, and always keep a variety of wholesome foods around. Continue to explain, patiently and consistently, why you choose to eat the way you do. Letting children help prepare food makes it more fun. Be creative! A vegetable or fruit platter can become a work of art. Sprouting kits are also something kids seem to love."

"Sprouting kits?" I wondered what on earth they were.

"You know the alfalfa and mung bean sprouts you can buy in the grocery store?"

"I must admit, I've never tried them."

"Sprouts are full of valuable nutrients, including enzymes. Getting involved in sprouting is like having an indoor garden, only without soil. We have brochures at the front desk outlining the process. In fact, there are several batches growing in the kitchen on the way to Eva's office. Take a peek before you leave."

"Are they expensive?"

"No, they're very cheap and fun to make. Juicers also go a long way in making healthy eating more enjoyable. Kids love to watch solids turn to liquid. Another step in the right direction would be to discuss the merits of foods advertised on television, reminding them that T.V. networks' first interest is in profit, not health. Eva was just telling me the other day how much she enjoys speaking to young children about nutrition. After those sessions, she always receives calls from parents who tell her it now takes them twice as long to get through the grocery store - their children insist they read all the labels!"

"I suppose it's somewhat like the no-smoking campaigns - pressure put upon parents by their children."

"Exactly. Then Eva always suggests that the children and parents together look up the names of some of these chemicals in *A Consumer's Dictionary of Food Additives* by Ruth Winter, or in *Additive Alert*. It'll teach them to be discriminating - it's also very educational."

"What about all those boxed cereals?"

"Some of the leading ones contain the highest levels of sugar and artificial colors. In fact, several have been analyzed and found to contain as much as fifty-four percent sugar! Robbins likens the labels on these boxes to something from a chemistry laboratory rather than from a kitchen. And he's right. I must read you a few lines from this article I clipped from the Toronto *Globe and Mail* called *Sugar-laden Cereals Making Comeback:*

> How sweet it is: that could well be the theme song for some of the recent success stories of Canada's leading cereal makers.
>
> Despite consumers' professed concerns about eating too much sugar, the cereals showing the most sales growth are among the sweetest . . .
>
> Tony the Tiger and Toucan Sam are doing their bit too. The cereals that these cartoon characters tout - Frosted Flakes and Froot Loops, respectively - are considered among the most sugar-laden cereals around and two of the fastest-growing brands over the past year . . .
>
> A lot of these purchases are driven by kids, says Christine Lowry, senior manager of nutrition and consumer communication for Kellogg Canada Inc., the maker of Froot Loops and Frosted Flakes. They like the taste, they like the texture, they like the color. Parents like the fact that their children are eating at least something for breakfast.
>
> 'For my son Matthew, my 2 1/2 year-old, if he eats the food, I'm happy,' said Lowry, a dietician and mother of two young children who eats Froot Loops regularly. 'If it doesn't end up on the floor or in the garbage, I'm happy'."

"Another clear example of our health being governed by big business."

"Right. And I suspect if its effects are not already taking their toll, how about ten or fifteen years down the road?"

I nodded in agreement. "So we work on our diets and try to drink clean water. What about the air we breathe?"

"Good point! I believe you'll be seeing Jane Harding fairly soon. Am I correct?"

"Jane Harding?"

"Yes, the woman who gives the *Creating a Healthy Home* workshops."

"Oh yes. I'm scheduled to see her in a few weeks' time. Emily booked it a while ago, but I can't remember the exact date."

"You'll learn a great deal about your indoor environment from her. Did you know that over 1.2 million Canadians and more than *nine million* Americans suffer from asthma? It's the leading cause of disease and disability in children between the ages of two and seven. The head of the Children's Hospital emergency department recently stated that ten years ago they had one asthma emergency a week. Today, it's nearly one per day!"

"That's close to what I saw when I worked there."

"Although food sensitivities, candidiasis and food additives account for much of our ill health, poor indoor air quality is also a very significant factor. It costs us millions of dollars annually and is largely preventable."

"The scary part for me," I added, thinking of Emma, "is that acute asthma is responsible for an increasing number of hospitalizations, even deaths."

"I was just talking to a spokesperson for the Lung Association. He told me that it's not uncommon to find asthma rates as high as *thirty-five percent* in schools located in, or surrounded by, new subdivisions. New homes are often toxic homes."

"Because they're so poorly ventilated?"

"That, and because of outgassing from new carpeting, building materials, fabrics . . . Add to this, swimming lessons in chlorinated indoor pools plus hockey two or three times a week in a rink full of ammonia fumes, why should we be so surprised at these high rates of asthma?"

"I understand that skating rinks are notorious for causing lung irritation in increasing numbers of children."

"Just one more item to contribute to the vicious cycle of ill health."

"Dr. Rowland, you must find that families who live with chronic illness are under an inordinate amount of stress."

"Absolutely. The saddest part is that the very parents who need the most patience and energy to deal with their overly active or sick kids are often unable to cope themselves, because they, too, are frequently unwell. This results in sick parents trying to look after sick children. If these symptoms result in negative behaviors, you can wind up with a very dysfunctional household - with everyone overreacting to just about everything."

"I can relate to that!" I exclaimed. "It also reminds me of a story Eva told me about how she watches her diet in order to avoid conflict with her family during her visits home."

"Yes, isn't that a great story? It certainly illustrates the point."

He pointed to a chart entitled *A Link Between Environmental Sensitivity and Dysfunctional Families* (fig. 12). "You wouldn't believe just how many families I've counselled over the years whose basic problems were environmentally triggered, foods being a significant part of the total equation. "

"I'm still so disgusted that so much of the medical community refuses to acknowledge any of this . . ."

"Well, slowly but surely, some of this information is creeping into mainstream medical literature. *Lancet*, the prestigious British medical journal, published a study illustrating that out of eighty-eight children who suffered from migraine headaches, ninety-three percent recovered after following elimination diets. Not only did their headaches clear, but other chronic symptoms improved as well . . . "

"Such as?"

"Asthma, eczema, gastrointestinal symptoms, behavior problems, just to name a few. . . and the saddest part of it all is that hyperactivity and other kinds of behavior problems can have lifelong repercussions. Dr. Lendon Smith, author of numerous books on children's health, estimates that *seventy percent* of people in jails were once hyperactive kids."

I couldn't help but think of Nathaniel and Emma's classmates who were on medication. What was the world coming to?

"I don't think we should ever abandon the search to better a child's life. There are always solutions - if we look deep enough. Recent studies that support this view were published in *The Journal of Pediatrics* and *The Annals of Allergy*, two reputable medical publications. They concluded that symptoms can be controlled through a simple elimination diet and that removing the *causes* of ADHD is preferable to the pharmacological therapy for this condition. Then there are the studies by allergist Marshall Mandell, who believes that at least half of all patients in mental hospitals suffer from what he calls 'cerebral allergies' caused by food or chemical intolerances. Among the schizophrenic patients tested, 64% reacted to wheat, 52% to corn, and 50% to milk - three staple foods of our Western diet. A substantial number reacted adversely to tobacco smoke as well. I can't emphasize enough how critical it is to deal with sensitivities at a young age. Masking them with drugs is not the solution."

"But why don't doctors pay more attention to this, especially when it's reported right in their very own journals? What's wrong with them!" I was almost shrieking.

"Again, Jillian, it's because anecdotal and clinical experience are not generally accepted as hard evidence within the medical community. Dr. Richard Mackarness summed it up best in his book *Not All In The Mind* by saying: *I will not wait until the men in white coats with their white rats tell me what I can see every day to be the truth.*"

"There's more than a bit of truth in that!"

"Sadly, there is, but I also suspect an underlying factor is money. It governs our lives far more than we would like to admit. There's not a whole lot to be made by changing lifestyles. In fact, industry and pharmaceutical companies stand to lose. Even doctors fall into this category.

# Link Between Environmental Sensitivities
## and
## Dysfunctional Families
### (fig. 12)

| DYSFUNCTIONAL | FUNCTIONAL |
|---|---|
| • unidentified sensitivities to foods, chemicals and airborne irritants | • no sensitivities or known sensitivities, or<br>• treatment via avoidance and/or desensitization |
| • nutritional deficiencies develop | • supplementation to compensate for deficiencies |

**DYSFUNCTIONAL — PARENTS & CHILDREN**

1) unable to deal with everyday stresses
2) either physically and/or mentally unwell and exhibit following behavior:

- depression
- mood swings
- overly critical
- low frustration tolerance
- anger
- aggression
- lack of self control

**FUNCTIONAL — PARENTS & CHILDREN**

1) able to deal with everyday stresses
2) physically healthier, stronger:

- mentally more positive
- calmer
- more self-esteem
- more even-tempered
- increased humor

• strained or severed relationships
• families full of denial, criticism, shame, and often abuse

• happier, more positive environment conducive to spending more time together
• more intimate, loving

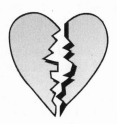

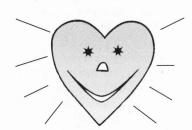

Who knows, many of them might be out of work in a relatively short period of time . . ."

"You think?"

"It's already happening in Europe. I read an article just the other day that stated that over 3,000 conventional medical doctors are unemployed as a direct result of the rapidly growing interest in complementary medicine. In fact, an elderly colleague of mine who has always been very traditional, steeped in orthodox medicine, is now studying homeopathy. The tide is turning. We have to keep up with public demand. Informed patients, who are told by their doctors that natural remedies are nonsense, simply thank them and go off to the naturopath down the street or seek the services of a physician who practices complementary medicine."

"But there are so few of you . . ."

"The politics of complementary medicine is another story in itself. Unfortunately, time just doesn't permit a discussion right now. But keep in mind, only three groups stand to gain in a significant shift from traditional to wellness medicine - patients, the government and insurance companies. Millions of health care dollars would be saved if people were properly educated."

"So why doesn't the government do something?"

"The government, because of the current crisis , has started to focus on public education. Unfortunately, the groups involved in education are still very much in the dark about the nature and magnitude of the health issues we face today. In fact, this in itself, is an enormous, deeply-rooted problem."

"I can tell you, as soon as I'm well enough, I'll be out there spreading the message!"

"Again, human nature being what it is, people won't make appropriate changes until they themselves, or someone close to them, becomes sick. So, while you're out there trying to educate the masses, don't get discouraged if you're confronted by apathy. We need people like you, passionate, with personal experience, to educate and inform the public, but it can be a slow process."

"This illness must create serious rifts between couples . . ."

"More often than not, it does. This illness puts an enormous burden on entire families already overloaded with the stresses of day-to-day living."

"I know all about that," I sighed. "What blows me away is that I had thought all along that we were a typical, normal family and that our health problems were just a part of life."

"Yes, you and thousands of others who accept their numerous aches and pains, prescriptions and trips to doctors as routine. You see, Jillian, our present system is oriented toward sickness care, not healthcare. We're not focused on prevention, only intervention - once someone is already sick. Drugs are covered by most health plans. Only in the last couple of years have a few insurance companies seen the advantage of paying for complementary healthcare. In the short run, staying healthy may cost a bit more. Quality foods tend to be more expensive. Fresh produce - especially those free of pesticides - costs substantially more than processed foods, particularly in colder climates; free-range poultry and meats are higher priced; and to alter our homes, we need to use more expensive, high quality, non-toxic materials. But in the long run, people who make these changes no longer burden the system because they remain healthy."

"It makes so much sense!"

"You know, the ancient doctors of China were paid to keep their patients well; if the patients became ill, the doctors received nothing. It was their job to keep people healthy."

"Maybe we need to adopt a similar system, but instead, put the job of staying well back in the hands of the patient - return more of the responsibility."

"Perhaps you're right. What few realize is that the short-term costs are insignificant compared to the long-term outlay precipitated by our current approaches to chronic illness. Modern medicine has a very important place in crisis intervention and acute care. But it fails miserably in its approach to chronic illness. All we do is medicate symptoms. I believe the future lies in marrying orthodox and complementary approaches - in the promotion of both prevention and the wellness model. Then, and only then, will we have a truly effective medical system."

"With escalating healthcare costs, we may be forced to go this route sooner than later, unless of course, the almighty dollar wins once again!" I exclaimed. I thought of how the pharmaceutical companies pushed drugs through doctors' offices and how the processed food companies used television commercials to hook children. Even the dairy bureaus' sponsorship of milk programs was beginning to irk me.

He continued. "Not only does this type of illness create financial stress, but families often become divided in terms of diagnosis and treatment. The sick person usually ends up getting the most help from holistic practitioners, whereas his or her partner listens to traditional medicine dismiss the problem and often remains in denial."

"I know what you mean. Michael didn't fully believe I was sick because my tests were always negative. I must confess, he originally thought I was crazy for coming here. Now that he's seen the changes, he's becoming more supportive."

"I assure you, when you bring the kids in for testing, he'll become a convert. To watch those you love go in and out of reactions can be quite alarming, but it does bring theory into the realm of human experience."

"True, there's nothing like personal experience. I just saw a little girl about Max's age have a terrible reaction to peas. Not a pretty sight! Still, it'll be quite a job to try to convince Michael to follow a diet over the next few weeks . . ."

"Jillian, I'd let that go for a while. He won't be ready to make changes until he sees the whole family feeling better. For now, I would concentrate on the children."

Dr. Rowland walked over to his bookcase and took out a couple of videos. "These tapes are by Dr. Doris Rapp - *How You Can Recognize Unsuspected Allergies*, and *Why an Environmentaly Clean Classroom?* "

"Is she the one who wrote *The Impossible Child* and other books on children with environmental sensitivities?"

"Jillian Stowe, you've been doing your homework! Dr. Rapp's been relentless in spreading the word . . ."

"A woman in the library says she's been on the Phil Donahue show."

"She's been on many shows, including Larry King Live. She's quite amazing - so dedicated. In these tapes you'll see children react to specific substances found in their everyday environment, whether it be something they're . . . they're what?"

I smiled. "Something they're eating, drinking or breathing . . . It always boils down to that, doesn't it?"

He nodded. "Almost always. After all, what else do we do all day? You'll see in the tapes that even simple airborne irritants like dust and dust mites can cause violent behavior in some children - a far cry from a stuffy nose. One child loses it due to chlorine, another from peach juice. You'll see that the quality of their handwriting and drawing changes during testing. Make sure you and Michael watch the tapes together. It may open him to new possibilities . . ."

A gentle knock at the door signalled the end of our time.

I put the tapes into my bag. Dr. Rowland looked at his watch, gathered up my file and said, "Now I'm going to send your file up to Eva. She should have your Red Blood Cell Mineral Analysis (RBC) back. It'll give you a better idea of your mineral status. Also, we'll need detailed information on each child to make their testing more specific."

"Jillian, you've done remarkably well. Start the yeast-free diet and work with the products we discussed earlier. Eva will go over supplements and the basic principles of rotation. And don't forget, soon you'll see Jane Harding about your home environment. In the meantime, now that you feel better, get more exercise - especially outdoors. Fresh air and deep breathing are fundamental to good health."

"Is there a good book you could recommend that deals with children and health?"

"There are many. Any of Dr. Lendon Smith's books are well worth reading."

"What are some of the titles?"

"*Feed Your Kids Right; Improving Your Child's Behavior Chemistry; Foods for Healthy Kids,* to name a few. Then there are two great books by William Crook - *Solving the Puzzle of Your Hard-to-Raise Child* and *Help for the Hyperactive Child.* Steven Gislason also wrote one dealing specifically with food sensitivities called *Core Diet for Kids.* And, of course, there are Doris Rapp's books. And for a general overview of keeping children healthy, *Superimmunity for Kids* by Dr. Leo Galland is great because it takes you right from infancy through adolescence."

He noticed me frantically jotting down the titles and handed me a thin little booklet. "They're all on this book list. Just tick them off."

As I got up to leave, he said, "You know, you're the type of person holistic practitioners love. You're taking charge of your life, and you're about to help your family take charge of theirs. You're a true warrior." With his usual warmth, he shook my hand and went off to his next patient.

It was great to have my feelings confirmed: This illness was no longer in charge of me - I was in charge of my illness.

Moreover, I was taking charge of my life.

# Alternative Treatments for Allergies and Sensitivities

## Enzyme-Potentiated Desensitization (EPD)

This technique of desensitization was developed in England by Dr.Len McEwen and is becoming increasingly popular among physicians specializing in Environmental Medicine. It involves a series of injections given in eight week intervals that combine small doses of allergens with the enzyme beta-glucuronidase, which is present in all parts of the human body. When beta-glucuronidase is combined with an allergen mix, it provokes an immune response by stimulating the body to produce suppressor T-cells that can turn off allergic reactions. Careful protocol must be followed before and after each treatment to ensure success. Note that it can take up to two years to derive benefits from EPD, but those benefits can be permanent.

## Nambudripad Allergy Elimination Technique (NAET)

"I felt as if I was let out of jail, that I escaped from allergy hell!" is one comment from an NAET patient who experienced the transformation from an allergic body into one which is healthy and balanced. No more strict avoidance! Goodbye rotation diets!

Developed by Dr. Devi Nambudripad of Buena Park, California, this technique is an integrated system using methods adapted from the disciplines of Applied Kinesiology or muscle response testing (MRT), Chiropractic and Acupuncture. NAET is natural, drug-free, painless and non-invasive - and can be used safely from infants to the elderly.

The principle of NAET lies in the energy pathways throughout the body that are known in acupuncture as meridians. Allergens cause blockages in these meridians; the energy flow becomes blocked; the body becomes unbalanced; symptoms begin; and gradually the organs are affected and illness results. NAET unblocks energy pathways, enabling the body to heal itself. The brain re-learns what it once thought of as an allergen and interprets it as a harmless, acceptable substance. The nervous system learns an entirely different response to the same stimulus and you become allergy free - permanently!

For 25 hours following each session, the client must abstain from contact with the item being treated, allowing the treatment to create an energetic change that will circulate through each of the meridians. Since it takes two hours for energy to pass through each of the twelve meridians, there is a 24 plus one hour safety margin or waiting period before the client can resume his or her normal lifestyle habits. However, it is important to understand that NAET treatments are not an overnight success story. It takes multiple treatments for most people to derive benefits.

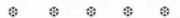

For detailed information about EPD and NAET, the Internet is likely your best resource. It can also provide you with lists of practitioners who administer EPD and NAET treatments. The *Reading List* at the end of this book also lists additional references for various treatment methods, including NAET. For additional information on testing methods, please refer to page 279 of this book.

**Please note that there is a small percentage of individuals who will not respond to either therapy.**

*We need a paradigm shift,*
*and I think it's beginning to occur.*
*Nutrition needs to be looked at,*
*not as a means of preventing specific*
*deficiency diseases,*
*but as a means of contributing*
*to the overall health of the person*
*and his or her*
*resistance to chronic diseases.*

*We have to start looking for the*
*optimum levels of nutrients necessary*
*for optimum health instead of the*
*minimum amount needed*
*to prevent diseases.*

*This is going to produce a big upsurge*
*in human health in the next twenty years.*

Richard P. Huemer, M.D.
Alternative Medicine: The Definitive Guide

# 11

# Expensive Urine

*In over 3000 nutritional evaluations, I have yet to find
anyone without vitamin or mineral deficiencies,
even in those following excellent diets.*
**Zoltan P. Rona, M.D., M.Sc.**


*Y*ou look absolutely terrific!" exclaimed Eva as I walked into her office.
"Why thank you! I can honestly say I don't think I've *ever* felt this
good. I can't thank you enough."

"And you survived the diet! Was it as difficult as you thought it would
be?"

"Well . . . the first few days were pure hell. I came close to calling you
several times but kept reminding myself that I was probably experiencing
withdrawal. But, you know what? In the end, those first few days were
well worth it."

"Life is often a series of trade-offs. A bit of suffering now and again
may be necessary - especially if it improves the quality of your life in the
long run."

"Like that saying *no pain, no gain?*"

Eva smiled. "I'm so glad you're feeling better." She opened my file.
"Aha! Here's the latest instalment. So Dr. Rowland wants you to modify
your diet further by eliminating foods that promote yeast growth."

"Right. I think I'm pretty clear about that, but I need some help setting
up a rotation diet. I read a bit about it in *An Alternative Approach to Allergies*
where some people had to eat one food per meal. I couldn't handle that -
I'd die of starvation!"

Eva laughed heartily. "Don't worry, we only use that stringent kind of
rotation in extreme situations and for very brief periods of time. But let's
focus on supplements right now. Before we do, I'd like to ask you if a
young woman, Elisabeth Proctor, could sit in on our session. She studied
dietetics at Albion University and has worked in one of the county hospitals
for the past three years. She's chosen to focus on orthomolecular nutrition
and environmental health . . . but I'll let her explain the rest - if it's okay
with you."

"That's fine with me."

Eva picked up the phone. "Elisabeth? Eva. Come on in. We'd love to have you join us."

No sooner had she hung up, there was a gentle knock at the door. In walked a tall, willowy young woman, her jet black hair cascading to her shoulders in loose waves. Her dark skin was flawless. She had an infectious smile which put me at ease instantly. Extending her hand, she introduced herself. "Hello. I'm Elisabeth Proctor."

There was a warmth, a very natural way about her. "I'm Jillian Stowe."

"I really appreciate your letting me sit in on your session."

"I hope you don't mind me asking, Elisabeth, but what made you decide to explore this approach to nutrition? It's such a major departure from your training."

"Well, the first thing that helped shift my focus was my little boy, Eric."

"It's hard to believe you're a mother! You look so young."

Elisabeth smiled broadly. "Hey, thanks! Gee, I'll have to come here more often. I could get to like this." Blushing slightly, she continued her story. "From the beginning I knew something was wrong with Eric. He was so active throughout my entire pregnancy, I seldom slept through the night. It felt as if there was a miniature war going on in there. My doctor kept telling me it was a sign that he was strong and healthy. Colleagues suggested that I increase my daily intake of dairy products in the hopes that the extra calcium would have a calming effect. Nothing worked. Eric was born with colic. We lived the nightmare of a screaming baby. After several months, the colic subsided but infections, one right after another, began . . ."

"Just like my Max!" I blurted out. This I could relate to!

"I was puzzled about his ongoing ill health, given that I was doing the best any mother could do - breast-feeding. I had a few episodes of mastitis for which I was given antibiotics with the assurance that none of it would get into my milk. After numerous rounds of antibiotics for both of us, I began to worry. I discussed my concerns with a friend who urged me to see a naturopath, Dr. Nancy Farrington up in Newbury. She told me to immediately remove all dairy products from my diet. Within days, my son's ear problems abated, as did his crankiness - and my long-standing constipation! She had us eliminate other foods, including sugar and yeast, and treated us both for candida. To my amazement, not only did the constipation and mastitis clear up, but so did my fatigue, depression and mood swings - conditions I was told I'd have to live with."

"I still find it difficult to believe!"

"And who would ever have thought constipation could be linked to dairy intake! Or that fatigue and mood swings could be related to foods we eat every day! Since then, I've definitely seen these connections with my clients as well. So . . . having experienced my own, as well as my son's recovery from illness, my interest was piqued. I spent months reading, researching, and learning as much as I could about environmental health. I read stacks of books that focused on holistic nutrition, herbal medicine, homeopathy - you name it, I read it. To make a long story short, my goal is to be more effective in helping others by learning more about this approach to health - it works!"

"I'm just curious . . . Did you learn about these connections in any of your nutrition courses at university?"

"An interesting question - glad you asked. The dieticians' bible, *Food, Nutrition, And Diet*, a textbook by Krause and Mahan, has an entire chapter called 'Nutritional Care in Food Allergy and Food Intolerance'. It makes very clear connections between foods and chronic disease. It even lists these disease symptoms: abdominal pain, asthma, rhinitis, dermatitis, arthritis, colic, cancer, otitis media [ear infections], migraines and even personality changes!"

"Better known in the field of environmental health as brain allergy," commented Eva.

"And this list of symptoms dates from 1973!" exclaimed Elisabeth.

"But if it's all there, why do most of your colleagues miss the connections in clinical practice?" I couldn't understand it.

"Unfortunately, very little class time was spent on this most important chapter. We were left to read and understand it on our own. Another reason might be that dieticians are fearful of contradicting a medical diagnosis. That's just a guess. And then there's the lack of focus in this area during the four years of academic study. Whatever the reasons, it's a sad state indeed. Just think about how many could be helped if only this information were put to use more often. In fact, many of my colleagues think this whole phenomenon is all in people's heads. They think I'm crazy for exploring alternatives."

"You'll see that shift over time," added Eva, "as the public begins to educate their doctors and dieticians. They won't have any choice but to listen - if they want to be effective."

"Just look how pharmacies have changed in the past few years," mentioned Elisabeth. "Not only do they carry a wide assortment of nutritional supplements, but recently they have begun to stock homeopathic remedies for anything from colds and flu to warts. When I complimented one pharmacist about this progressive move, he replied, 'If ya can't lick 'em, join 'em! We did it largely due to customer demand'."

Eva glanced at Elisabeth. "But now, we must continue with the results of Jillian's Red Blood Cell Mineral Analysis (R.B.C.) or we'll run out of time." She picked up a document from my file. "It appears that several of your mineral levels are right off the map."

"Which ones?" Although I was curious about the results, I also felt somewhat anxious.

"For starters, your calcium and magnesium are extremely low. If you weren't feeling and looking as good as you are right now, I'd recommend injections or intravenous drips."

"I read about those in several books on environmental health. They say that it's the only way some people can absorb nutrients when their digestive systems are compromised."

"That's right," said Eva, "And I would say that the majority of problems stem from an inability to absorb - either from chronic yeast overgrowth, food sensitivities, parasites or enzyme deficiency. That's why we have to give I.V.'s to some of our clients. Sometimes the lining of their gastrointestinal tract is so impaired that nutrients can't be assimilated."

"By the way," Elisabeth interrupted, "malabsorption was one of the symptoms listed in the chapter on food sensitivity in that dietetic textbook."

"In all my years of nursing I'd never come across anyone getting injectable vitamins and minerals, let alone I.V'.s. - with the exception of B12 of course - save for this clinic. The only other situation would be with post-operative patients or nutritional feeds in Intensive Care Units."

"No wonder," said Eva, "medical training emphasizes drug, not nutritional therapy. A few years ago, a sub-committee of the National Research Council surveyed 45 of the 127 medical schools in the U.S., and found that barely one quarter require even *one* full course in nutrition. Yet, that same institution connects nutritional factors to six out of ten of the most serious life-threatening diseases today. Heart disease and cancer are, of course, the most significant of these."

"What's even more worrisome," added Elisabeth, "is that traditional university nutrition and dietetic courses don't come close to addressing the issues that our twentieth century lifestyles impose upon us. The curriculum is still largely based on outdated concepts. Not only are we still taught we should be getting all our nutrients from foods, but the *quality* of those foods is never addressed; nor is the relationship of the foods we eat to the way our bodies assimilate them - or to the underlying factors that often compromise assimilation."

Eva smiled, agreeing with Elisabeth's assessment of the situation. "Because of all the problems that accompany life in the nineties, I foresee nutrient therapy on the leading edge. I predict it will become commonplace in the very near future - perhaps in only a few years' time. In fact, it'll be disorders such as chronic fatigue, multiple food and chemical sensitivities, and candidiasis that will pave the way to a more universal acceptance of nutrient therapy by the mainstream medical community. The way I look at it, better to see a patient upright, pushing an I.V. pole loaded with nutrients, than lying in a hospital bed pumped full of medication. The object is to reverse the deficiency state before it becomes a life-threatening disease."

"You know, there would have to be some pretty substantial changes in attitude - in focus - before I'd ever consider returning to nursing. Their world operates from the perspective of a disease model, and I'm shifting toward what Dr. Rowland calls a wellness model."

"That's very true," nodded Eva. "Paradoxically, as more people - especially our youth - succumb to chronic twentieth century disorders, you'll find greater progress in the area of wellness medicine. Orthodox practices are great for acute care, but often are no longer effective for people with chronic conditions. In fact, more often than not, they create more toxicity. And then there's the cost . . . But right now, let's look at your results . . ."

"Eva, I can't understand how I could be so low in calcium. Dairy products were always such a big part of my life."

"But remember Jillian, when you're sensitive to a particular food, you often have difficulty absorbing nutrients from that source."

"Yes, Dr. Rowland mentioned that in one of our sessions. He suggested that it's often the person who drinks the most milk who has the greatest number of cavities. I'm living proof - despite the fact that I brush and floss regularly and avoid sugar.   I was told I had soft teeth by virtually every dentist I ever visited."

"It only makes the point . . ."

"I know calcium is important for healthy teeth and bones, but what symptoms would I experience with a magnesium deficiency?"

"Actually, calcium is responsible for a lot more than just healthy teeth and bones," replied Eva.   "One of your symptoms of premenstrual syndrome is cramping . . ."

"Some months, I think I'm going to die from the pain!"

"Well, I'll bet after a few weeks on a calcium-magnesium supplement, your pain would be greatly reduced, perhaps non-existent."

"That would be a godsend."

"A lack of calcium and magnesium is also responsible for much of the 'growing pains' children experience, joint pain in adults, heart palpitations, irritability, anxiety and insomnia."

"I can vouch for the insomnia bit," added Elisabeth. "I used to drink milk like it was going out of style and suffered from all of the above. It wasn't until I switched to other forms of calcium, including taking supplements to make up for lost time, that I slept well for the first time in years."

"And to answer your earlier question," commented Eva, "magnesium deficiency by itself can cause similar symptoms, such as depression, dizziness, constantly feeling cold and chocolate craving . . ."

"Then I definitely have a serious magnesium deficiency!" I laughed. "I *love* chocolate!"

"So do I," empathized Elisabeth.

"You and many others!" chuckled Eva. "Calcium and magnesium have often been called nature's tranquilizers.  They're important for optimal neurological function.  And we really should take magnesium to heart - quite literally.  Studies suggest that patients who've suffered acute heart attacks often have low magnesium levels.  Usually they're from areas where the concentration of magnesium in the water supply is minimal.  So-called 'soft' water is great for washing clothes and will leave you with shiny hair, but it's lousy for your heart.  So always remember to take a calcium supplement that has magnesium combined with it.  And one of the most common symptoms of magnesium deficiency is neck, shoulder and back pain . . ."

"I'd agree with that," Elisabeth interjected. "After I stopped dairy and added calcium and magnesium to my diet, my physiotherapist said it was like working on a whole new person. My body was looser, more relaxed, limber."

I thought of Michael who always complained about various nondescript aches and pains. Could he be low in these minerals? "Although my doctors always scoffed at the very suggestion of supplements, they did at least recommend I take calcium - but in a chewable antacid form."

"Bad idea," said Eva. "Taking an antacid every day can interfere with natural acid production in the stomach which is needed for mineral assimilation, as well as for the proper digestion of food. Second, there's an important connection - a balance - between calcium and magnesium in the body. They both help regulate the constriction and relaxation of the blood vessels, and if too much calcium is present, that balance might be altered."

"And if it's altered, you could have a heart attack?"

"It's possible. Better to be safe than sorry. Too much calcium is also implicated in kidney disorders . . ."

"I had an uncle," interrupted Elisabeth, "who suffered from kidney stones regularly. He never had the problem again once he cut back on his calcium intake and added magnesium to his diet."

"That's a good example of what can happen when these two minerals are imbalanced. The two really should be taken together. Most supplements from health food stores are sold as a combined formula."

"In the more progressive hospitals," added Elisabeth, "magnesium is given intravenously to heart attack victims to help speed up their recovery."

"Yes, that's right," replied Eva. "In fact, Wrenfrew hospital is beginning to use some nutrient therapy . . . By the way, these minerals are also involved in the metabolism of carbohydrates, fat and proteins."

"Could these deficiencies be one of the underlying reasons for my food sensitivities?"

"Absolutely. Over the years, I've come across several patients whose health difficulties originated from a single mineral deficiency. However, in the majority of cases, it's not quite that simple. But I will say, I've yet to see a single person who's not been low in several very important nutrients."

"Such as?"

"Vitamins A, B complex, C, E, plus calcium, magnesium, iron, chromium, zinc, selenium and essential fatty acids. You name it, they lack it." Eva looked a little closer at my results. "Hmm, speaking of zinc, you're quite low in this essential mineral . . ."

"What does it do in the body?"

"Among it's many functions, zinc is involved in all new cell growth. It's essential for wound recovery and enhances immunity. Zinc is known to have remarkable effects on prostatitis, acne, alopecia, eczema, psoriasis, hyperactivity, learning disabilities - even the common cold . . . In fact, one double-blind study showed that patients whose colds were treated with zinc were sick for only 3.7 days, as opposed to 10.8 days for the placebo-treated patients."

"What would some deficiency symptoms be?"

"Frequent infections, bizarre food cravings in pregnancy, stretch marks, abnormal cravings for sweets, excessive tooth decay, hair that falls out or that's prone to split ends, high cholesterol levels - the list is quite extensive."

"I have almost all of those symptoms."

Eva rolled her chair toward me and examined my nails. "These white spots signify a zinc deficiency." She showed them to Elizabeth, and continued, "It's important to know that this mineral forms an integral part of the composition of at least 160 different enzymes which are involved in multiple bodily functions - digestion being only one of them. It's also needed in the production of collagen and in the metabolism of essential fatty acids.

Even more important, zinc is known to assist in the restoration of the skin as well as the mucosal linings of air passages. It also helps to heal the gastrointestinal tract, thereby decreasing the permeability of the gut. As you can see, it's a mineral that's often underestimated. It's vital to our well-being and would be essential in your particular case. The RDA for zinc is woefully inadequate for you ... and for many others."

"How do you test for it?"

Eva waved my test result. "The best way is with this R.B.C. A hair analysis can often detect it as well."

"What about regular blood work?"

"Blood serum levels are not accurate."

"For years I was told by both doctors and dieticians that supplements are a waste of time and money - that all they do is create expensive urine. It was suggested that if I eat a normal, well-balanced diet, I'd get all the vitamins and minerals I would need from my food."

Elisabeth groaned. "That was the standard line in my dietetics courses, too."

"In an ideal world," said Eva, "that would be true - if you were to eat organically grown food all year round, drink clean water and breathe clean air. But I'd venture to say that even if you were to find that perfect world right this moment, you'd still need supplements, at the very least temporarily, to make up for all the years you were lacking - partly from diet and partly from your inability to absorb nutrients due to underlying conditions." I could see Elisabeth nod in agreement.

"Can we ever catch up?"

"We certainly can, but always keep in mind that even healthy people vary in their nutritional needs, depending upon their genetic make-up and lifestyle."

"So you're saying that in the world as we know it right now, it's virtually impossible to obtain all the nutrients we need for good health from our diet."

"Right ... for all the reasons we discussed during our first meeting."

"Such as our contaminated food supply, artificial fertilizers, pesticides, hormones and antibiotics?"

Eva smiled. "Whew! That was a mouthful!" She searched through some notes, obviously looking for something she wanted to share with me. "Aha! Here it is! As far back as 1978, the *Nationwide Food Consumption Survey*, in its most extensive review to that point, revealed widespread malnutrition greater than that found in all previous studies. Here, in the land of plenty, it was found that one-third of Americans were low in vitamins A and C, and iron, while one-half were low in vitamin B6, calcium and magnesium. And I might add that those with high incomes were only slightly better nourished than the lower-income groups."

I was aghast. "And here our healthcare providers have been telling us for years that no one needs to exceed the Recommended Daily Allowances."

"That's absolute and utter nonsense - totally outdated, naive thinking. In fact, here's a study right out of the *Journal of the American Dietetics Association* ..." She waved the journal in the air.

"And you couldn't get a group more conservative, more legitimate than that!" exclaimed Elisabeth. "I ought to know. I spent the past few years studying and working with them."

Eva continued. "Dr. Jean Pennington analyzed the trace mineral content of more than 200 foods and found most of them to be well below eighty percent of the Recommended Daily Allowance for most essential trace minerals - and let me tell you, the RDA's are extremely low - very conservative minimums to begin with. They're based on the average, healthy individual who lives in near-perfect environmental conditions - that is, an ideal diet, with virtually no pollution of any kind and absolute minimal levels of urban stress. Do you know anyone who fits this picture?"

"No, quite honestly, I don't," I replied. "Do such conditions even exist?"

"In some cultures that haven't been overly influenced by Western civilization - perhaps. Or, in situations where an individual comes from a particularly strong genetic background, has great absorption and lives a relatively stress-free, healthy life. In general, the RDAs fail to take into account all the factors that real life today presents - you know, such as our denatured food supply and our nutritionally deficient diets."

"Including indoor and outdoor pollution?"

"Yes. As you've learned over the past while, we live in a very toxic world. We really can't get away from pollution, so the next best thing is to protect ourselves any way we can. Recent studies suggest that vitamin E, for example, may be a potent lung saver, warding off the ravages of air pollution."

"And then there are lifestyle factors," suggested Elisabeth, "such as the use of socially acceptable drugs including alcohol, tobacco and caffeine, combined with fad diets, sleep deprivation and not spending enough time outdoors. These all contribute to our increased need for supplements."

"Thanks for mentioning that," said Eva. "We also have to remember that along with our increasingly toxic world, we have a large aging population, including the baby boomers, of which you and I are a part. And we all want to stay youthful and healthy - to keep up with Elisabeth!"

"You both look pretty good to me, but you'd better stay healthy. It's my generation that'll be nursing you in your old age!"

"We plan on it, right Jillian?" winked Eva.

"Here, here! And those of us who had our kids later in life definitely want to be around to see them grow up."

"Because of the changing demographics," continued Eva, "we're already seeing a shift that has caused health care costs to skyrocket. Now we have to take a serious look at prevention. Part of that is to address the question: Do we take supplements merely to prevent deficiency diseases or to maximize good health? In many respects, the public has already begun to answer that question."

"How?" I wondered.

"By the popularity over the past few years of self-help and health books as well as by the enormous increase in health product sales."

"And you wouldn't believe the number of my clients who question conventional practices that no longer work for them," added Elisabeth. "They're starved for information about approaches that might be more effective than the ones they presently use."

"Which is one of the reasons why this clinic is so busy," observed Eva.

"Although they've been conditioned to believe almost exclusively in medical experts, the public has become skeptical, and they feel that by taking vitamins and minerals, they're at least hedging their bets. Did you know that an estimated forty-six percent of adult Americans take nutritional supplements? *Newsweek* magazine reported that in 1993 alone, consumer sales of vitamin E grew by 39%, and those of beta carotene by 31%. Multi-level marketing within the health industry is growing by leaps and bounds. Products range from herbal tonics to bottled greens, most of which are aimed at boosting the immune system so it can better withstand environmental assaults."

"People wouldn't be using them," suggested Elisabeth, "if they didn't benefit from them."

"Are there any dangers in supplementing?"

"There are rare exceptions," replied Eva, "but I would say that the danger lies more in *not* supplementing. We really need a nutritional safety net in an increasingly contaminated world which, as we mentioned before, is further complicated by a large, aging population. But what puts supplementation into proper perspective is that to my knowledge, there's never been a death as a result of any supplemented vitamin or mineral. Compare this to the ever-present dangers of drug overdose - whether prescription or over-the-counter. Zoltan Rona points out that there continue to be numerous deaths as a result of tranquilizers, anti-depressants, analgesics such as ASA and then, last, but not least, the pill . . . "

"The birth control pill?"

"According to the Physician's Desk Reference (PDR) and the Compendium of Pharmaceutical Specialties (CPS), the birth control pill alone has over two hundred potential side effects, which include stroke and heart attack."

"That's terrible! And women take them daily for years on end."

"That's right, and usually without a second thought! Compared to this, the risks of using nutritional supplements are slim. For example, excessive intake of vitamins A, D and the mineral selenium can be toxic, but is reversible once you stop taking them. One would have to take massive quantities to cause irrevocable harm. There are rare instances in which people with underlying genetic predispositions can have a problem with certain nutrients, but families who have these conditions are usually aware of them. Again, when compared to even slight overdoses of most over-the-counter medications, it's not very significant. Of course, there are cases where caution should be exercised, such as during pregnancy."

"And in other cases, supplements are essential. One vitamin which attracts attention even within the confines of conventional medicine is folic acid. This B vitamin appears to guard against two of the most common and devastating neurological defects that afflict newborns today - spina bifida, in which there's incomplete closure of the spine, and anencephaly, in which the brain fails to develop fully. Other studies have linked deficiency of this same vitamin to cervical cancer. So, the literature is coming, slowly but surely."

"That's encouraging," I replied. "I've also heard that certain brands of supplements are better than others, while some say it doesn't make any difference."

"Actually, it does make a difference," countered Eva. "Usually, the cheaper the variety, the more binders, fillers and colors are added. People can be sensitive to these excipients." Eva paused, looked at me for a moment and asked, "Have you ever heard the terms free-radical and anti-oxidant?"

"Vaguely, but I don't really understand them."

"Free-radicals are atoms or groups of atoms that can damage cells, impair the immune system and slowly erode our youth by hardening arteries and causing other chronic, degenerative disease. Anti-oxidants help protect our bodies from the formation of these free-radicals. Many researchers are convinced that their cumulative effects also underlie much of the gradual deterioration of the body, better known as aging."

"Give me some of that stuff right away!" I joked.

"I'll take some too!" chimed Elisabeth, smiling. "Seriously, knowing what I now know, I wouldn't go a day without my anti-oxidants."

"It's apparent that the general public would agree," Eva affirmed. "Statistics show that for millions of health-conscious North Americans, anti-oxidant supplements are a way of life."

"What exactly are they?"

"Nutrients such as betacarotene, vitamins A, B, C and E, bioflavonoids, selenium, zinc, silicon, amino acids, enzymes like superoxide dismutase, co-enzymes and essential fatty acids. It's these nutrients that help protect us from radiation, food additives, drugs, pesticides, smoke - you name it."

"But why don't doctors catch up with the times?" I could feel my frustration mount.

"Good question," Elisabeth responded. "Over two hundred medical studies in the past decade alone have reported that anti-oxidant vitamins, minerals and amino acids can help prevent some forms of cancer."

"That's very true," remarked Eva, "but the person who has the best answer to that question is James Braly in his *Food Allergy & Nutrition Revolution*. According to Braly, the kindest answer is that doctors are too caught up with their long-standing, deeply entrenched protocols - drugs and surgery - to pay attention to other alternatives. There's a growing body of scientific evidence that shows that nutritional deficiencies are rampant and that supplementation could actually improve, if not cure, many of their patients' ailments. The less than kind answer is that too many North American doctors don't like nutritional supplements because people aren't legally obliged to visit their offices in order to obtain them - prescriptions are not required. Even more unkind, but all too often true, it poses a direct threat to their livelihood or, at the very least, might require them to keep their knowledge base up-to-date."

"You know, Eva, what I think ultimately threatens them the most is the lessening of their sphere of control - that they'll have less influence over their patients. I sure saw a lot of that when I worked in different hospitals." I looked at Elisabeth. "Have you had that experience working in dietetics?"

"Without a doubt."

"As with most things," Eva pointed out, "there's an upside to all this.

First, there's the rapid growth of the health food industry, and second, by asking questions, people are more willing than ever to take greater responsibility for their own health."

"Maybe this is the quantum leap that Dr. Rowland talks about," I mused.

"You could be right. I do know that the pharmaceutical industry is lobbying hard to get governments to make many of these supplements available by prescription only." Eva held up two bottles. "I could cite several examples of highly effective supplements that were on health food store shelves not so very long ago that are currently available only by prescription. The problem is that if those who are able to authorize their use don't believe in their efficacy, they won't prescribe them or recommend their use. There's an ongoing turf war between the American FDA and the Health Protection Branch of Health Canada on one side, and the health food industry on the other."

"I understand the concern for public safety," I said, "but at this point, I have a hunch that it's more a matter of control and big business."

"You may well be right." Just then there was a knock on the door.

"Yes?" said Eva. The door opened and Emily poked her head in. "Dr. Rowland needs Elisabeth down in the testing room, but only if you can spare her."

Eva gestured to Elisabeth. "You're always in demand. Whatever will we do without you when you go back to Strickland?"

Blushing slightly, Elisabeth grinned. "I've never been anywhere where I felt so wanted and needed - it feels great!" Gathering up her binder, she stood up to leave. "Jillian, it's been a pleasure to meet you. You'll do just fine - I can tell. You're so eager to learn. I really appreciated your letting me sit in on your session." I smiled, thinking about how lucky she was to have become involved at such a young age in the leading edge of healthcare.

"I'll see you in the meeting room at five." Eva turned to me and commented, "Sweet, isn't she?"

"Very nice. Her sincerity shines through."

Eva nodded. "Now, where were we?"

"We were discussing reasons why we should take supplements . . ."

"Your memory is definitely improving. That's a great sign! So another reason for supplementation is that it can compensate for inborn errors of metabolism which can only worsen over time as our food supply deteriorates. The rise in sensitivities and auto-immune disorders may reach epidemic proportions if doctors and nutritionists don't recognize what constitutes a truly healthy diet, keeping in mind, of course, that there's no such thing as a single diet for everyone. That holds true for supplements as well."

"But shouldn't we work at reversing the reasons why we need supplements in the first place?"

"Ultimately, that's where the answers lie. But while we work on long-term issues - cleaning up the food we eat, the water we drink, the air we breathe, as well as curtailing the overuse of medication, we certainly need the extra support to at least protect ourselves right now."

All of a sudden, a funny image came to mind. I had to laugh. "I can foresee us all living on a Jetson diet, feasting on nutritional pellets that contain all the nourishment a twenty-first century citizen would ever want or need."

"Yes, somewhat like a picture in an issue of *Time* magazine. It depicted a woman holding a bowl full of nutritional supplements, just about to devour a spoonful of colorful tablets, capsules and caplets."

The image cracked me up. "I sure hope we never reach that point. I still prefer real food, thank you very much!"

"Actually, that scenario may not be too far off in the future," chuckled Eva. "But I'd still rather eat my spinach and beet greens than a bowl full of betacarotene tablets and folic acid capsules. How about you?"

"I agree. Not to mention how much more filling real food is!"

"In any case," continued Eva, "I predict that anti-oxidants will revolutionize healthcare. In that same issue of *Time*, biochemist William Pryor, of Louisiana State University, envisions simple urine, blood or breath tests that would assess levels of cellular damage caused by free-radicals - somewhat like patients today are screened for cholesterol."

"Someday we might even have home self-testing kits that use dipsticks!" I said jokingly.

"It may not be that far-fetched. But seriously," suggested Eva, "wouldn't it be wonderful to halt disease in its early stages - before it turns into something life-threatening?"

"It sure would." I thought again of all the pain and suffering I had seen throughout my nursing career.

"It's estimated that over fifty percent of the population suffer from at least one potentially serious vitamin or mineral deficiency. Then there's a study by Dr. Rajit Chandra at Memorial University in Newfoundland, where seniors who took a multi-vitamin supplement for one year, were sick only about half as often as those who didn't. As well, their consumption of antibiotics was only half that of the group who were given placebos. You know, Jillian, I could spend days citing studies that prove supplements can help the body defend itself from further damage, as well as assist it in repairing some of the damage that's already occurred."

"Are environmental sensitivities another reason we need supplements?"

"Yes. As we discussed earlier, we need to make up for lost nutrients and strengthen the immune system in order to allow sensitivities to die down. In fact, people with sensitivities often have impaired detoxification pathways. That alone is reason enough to take supplements. It all serves to help the immune system."

Eva stood up and walked over to an open window. Taking a deep breath, she declared, "And there's no such thing as an 'average' person. Each of us has very different nutritional requirements due to genetic predisposition, environmental history and individual lifestyle. People differ in age, size, body type and the ability of the digestive tract to absorb and utilize nutrients. Some have allergies, others are on medication. We vary in our levels of physical activity. The bottom line is that individual variability renders phrases such as 'the average person' and 'average RDA's' practically useless, almost silly. How can we responsibly say that the RDA's are right for everyone?"

"It sounds about as bizarre as saying one diet works for all - and we know how far from the truth that is!" I exclaimed.

"Right. It was Dr. Roger Williams who coined the term 'biochemical individuality' to describe these differences. Outwardly, we have different voices, fingerprints, hair color and skin tone. Internally, we vary as well, depending upon our genetic predisposition and lifestyle. The simple fact is that we all have different needs for specific nutrients."

"For example?"

"Take a smoker for instance. Again, according to Rona, just one cigarette can destroy about twenty-five milligrams of vitamin C in the body. Obviously, that person requires much more vitamin C than his non-smoking counterpart. A second example is alcohol. It destroys most of the B vitamins, zinc, selenium, vitamins E and C. Of course, the ideal solution is to stop drinking and smoking, but in the meantime, the deficiencies must be addressed. Those on birth control pills need a greater intake of most B vitamins, especially B6, as well as folic acid and zinc in order to prevent biochemically induced depression. We're finding that when specific nutrients are supplemented, long-standing ailments often disappear. I really think anyone who suffers from chronic illness should have a baseline Red Blood Cell Mineral Analysis done. That way you can be sure of your nutrient status."

"You mentioned that people might differ in their ability to utilize nutrients."

"Absolutely. Almost any bowel dysfunction can lead to malabsorption. And due to the widespread practice of repeatedly prescribing broad-spectrum antibiotics beginning at a very young age, these problems have now reached staggering proportions. Both parasites and yeast overgrowth increase the production of mucus on the intestinal walls, making it very difficult for nutrients to get through. I suspect this to be a big part of your problem. Eradicating parasites and getting yeast under control is the first step. Nutrient therapy would be the next."

"Eva, I find all this so fascinating. I feel as if my brain is on overdrive, making connections by the minute - like explosions going off in all directions. How on earth did you amass all this information?"

She looked at her watch. "Got all day? Good thing you're the last appointment."

I laughed. "No, really - I do want to know."

Eva sat back in her chair, reminiscing. "When I first became ill, I was studying to be a pharmacist. I was immersed in organic chemistry, biochemistry and, of course, pharmacology. At the end of my second year, I landed an internship with a drugstore specializing in alternatives - Reese's Apothecary. It was old Mr. Reese who started me on my journey, one from which I've never looked back. Then I formalized my training, studying at a holistic school that specialized in orthomolecular nutrition. Needless to say, I dropped out of pharmacology, although I'm grateful for the background in science it gave me."

"How was Reese's drugstore different?"

"I'd see elderly people who had been on drugs for years - often five or six at a time - confused, unable to concentrate, complaining of numbness and tingling, as well as chronic depression. After a few short weeks of B12 injections, many made remarkable recoveries - a new lease on life - even though their regular bloodwork showed normal B12 levels. I began asking questions. I'd see young people who swung between pep pills and anti-depressants switch over to a more wholesome diet and B complex vitamins. They felt better and more energetic than they had in years. I began to ask more questions. Then there were babies with chronic ear infections and teenagers with acne living on antibiotics for months on end. Reese would refer them to a holistic physician who'd get them off of dairy products and sugar. I'd see them transform before my very eyes. For teenagers, he'd also recommend multi-vitamins with extra zinc, calcium and magnesium, and their skin would clear up. To their surprise, so did their lousy moods and bad breath!"

"My God, we have a long way to go! We really *are* living in the dark ages."

"Without a doubt. I saw young women with carpal tunnel syndrome and severe P.M.S. respond beautifully to B6, calcium and magnesium therapy. I saw many asthmatics recover within weeks of removing specific foods to which they were sensitive from their diets - dairy products being first and foremost. They'd also be advised to change their indoor environment at home. It was like watching one small miracle after another. I saw mentally ill patients, especially schizophrenics, become functional again with elimination diets, vitamin and yeast therapy. Fibrocystic breasts would become a thing of the past for those who followed an anti-yeast diet, iodine supplementation, and oil of evening primrose, combined with vitamin E. Heart patients swore by the latter, along with co-enzyme Q-10."

"You must have been amazed by the testimonials."

"I was. Every day, I'd hear at least five or six stories of people who were helped through a change in diet and supplements. People with circulatory and life-threatening heart problems are alive and well today - without surgery or conventional medication. Their doctors used chelation therapy . . ."

"What's chelation therapy?" My interest was aroused, thinking of Dad and his heart condition.

"It's the infusion into the bloodstream of E.D.T.A., a synthetic amino acid, which moves through the vessels, removing excess metals implicated in disease."

"Metals? Like what?"

"Like mercury, aluminum and lead - all of which, in excess, are toxic to the body. It can also remove minerals such as iron and copper if they're in excess of their normal levels. At the same time, it decreases plaque in the blood vessels. When that happens, overall blood circulation improves. It can also help heart patients, people with diabetes and Alzheimer's, stroke patients and those with circulatory problems. Apparently, it also provides greater anti-oxidant activity, reducing free-radical damage to our tissues."

"Does Dr. Rowland do chelation therapy?"

"He used to - until the government clamped down on all physicians doing it for reasons other than removal of heavy metals. Chelation would cut into bypass surgery - big business in this country! The good news is that the health care system is in such a crisis that controlled clinical trials are currently being conducted. I still remember those poor, debilitated patients, who at the beginning, would be wheelchair-ridden and several treatments later, would be able to walk."

"Just from chelation?"

"Dietary changes and exercise would also be important parts of a total program."

"So once again, lifestyle plays a critical role."

"Always. It's the key to good health. Then there were the cancer patients . . . it seemed that everyone would confide in old Mr. Reese. He'd refer them to all the right people who would, in turn, guide them in changing their diets to ones which often included large amounts of carrot juice, concentrated green food and high doses of vitamin C - all of which helped them regain a quality of life. Many would even go into remission. I just knew that there had to be more than drugs. And there is - a *lot* more! Then, when I began to apply some of the principles to my own life, I, too began to heal."

"Is that how you met Dr. Rowland?"

"Yes, he was one of the practitioners who routinely prescribed nutritional therapies for patients."

"You mentioned green drinks. What exactly are they?" I thought back to an earlier discussion with Dr. Rowland where he'd mentioned them in passing.

"They're chlorophyll-rich foods derived from algae, alfalfa, barley or wheat in concentrated form. They're potent sources of enzymatically alive, alkaline-forming foods, full of vitamins, minerals and essential amino acids. They're also exceptionally high in betacarotene, which, as you now have learned, is an important anti-oxidant. They help strengthen the immune system, increase energy and cleanse the cells and bowels of toxins. They come in powder, capsules as well as tablets."

"Where can I buy this stuff?"

"Here or at any health food store. Even some pharmacies carry them, and many are sold under multi-level marketing plans. You should read up on the different ones. They ensure that you at least get your minimum quota of greens every day, in instant form - without pesticides."

"What foods would contain these nutrients?"

"Deep green, leafy vegetables like swiss chard, spinach, beet greens and kale. Do you know many people who eat these nutritious foods on a regular basis?"

"Not really. My kids certainly won't touch them. And the only time I eat these foods is during the short time they're in season. Up here, that could mean only a few months per year."

"That's about right for people living in colder climates. Ideally, we should eat them all year round. The beauty of these concentrated greens is that even kids will take them. My teenage daughter refused to comply with most of my dietary suggestions, but the one thing she did faithfully every morning during the winter months was take her green drink. She claimed it energized her and at the same time helped her stay calm. And I was reassured in knowing that she was getting nutrients equal to several helpings of salad each day."

I thought of Nathaniel and made a mental note to try him on at least one of these products.

Eva looked at my mineral results again. "Jillian, although your hemoglobin and ferritin levels appear to be in the normal range based on your regular bloodwork, your Red Blood Cell Mineral test indicates that your iron is very low."

"What foods contain iron?"

"Dulse and kelp are among the highest vegetable sources of iron and many other minerals. Other good sources in the plant kingdom include rice and wheat bran; pumpkin, squash and sesame seeds; wheat germ and beans. Notice that much of the iron content is found in those parts of the grain that are milled out when processed, leaving us with little more than empty calories. And paradoxically, we call them enriched."

"I'll never forget your story about the 'enrichment' of foods!" We both laughed.

"Of course, as you are probably already aware, red and organ meats and eggs are good sources of iron as well, but I couldn't recommend them unless I was assured my clients would buy products guaranteed to be free of pesticides, hormones and antibiotics."

She referred to my chart again. "By the way, your chromium is also low."

"What's chromium?"

There was a knock. The door opened a crack. It was Elisabeth. "Missed us already?" teased Eva.

"Marianne's helping Dr. Rowland, so he suggested I finish the session with Jillian. Is that okay with you?"

"Great." Eva motioned for her to sit down. "We were just discussing the significance of chromium."

"Ah, yes! Chromium was one of the most significant minerals that I lacked according to my R.B.C. Working with my food sensitivities was one part of the equation; the other was taking a chromium supplement. Once I began taking it, my blood sugar returned to normal."

"Thanks," replied Eva. "Chromium is one of the minerals more recently recognized to be essential for humans. In certain cases, it's also effective in lowering blood cholesterol, and as Elisabeth just mentioned, it's required for maintaining normal blood-sugar levels. In fact, chromium deficiency can be a significant factor in age-onset diabetes."

"What would be some symptoms of chromium deficiency?"

"Craving sugar would be an obvious one . . . high cholesterol is another."

"And where's chromium found?"

"In brewer's yeast, whole grains, meats and cheeses. Unfortunately, most chromium is removed from grains when they're refined. So, once again, processing is a key culprit in not being able to obtain enough of this vital mineral from our diet."

"It's frightening to think that I'm deficient in all these minerals when I've been eating relatively well compared to the diets of my friends and relatives."

"But again, don't forget that you've been sensitive to many of these foods. Not only is the food quality important, but so is the way in which you metabolize your food. What you eat may actually have very little to do with what finally reaches the tissues."

"So what do you do about it?"

"In your case, work with the yeast imbalance in your gut. As Dr. Rowland outlined, you then deal with the possibility of parasitic infestation. At the same time, you take a couple of digestive enzymes with each meal until we improve your nutrient status. Proper digestion of food is essential to overall good health. Dr. Aubrey Katz, a gastroenterologist from Harvard, once said *a good set of bowels is more important than a good set of brains.*"

"Then let's fix 'em up!" I kidded.

"On a more serious note," suggested Elisabeth, "Isn't there a similar expression in holistic health - something to the effect that *death begins in the colon?*"

"I've heard that before - from several people. And it's right on. Proper digestive function is the key to good health. That's where the use of digestive aids comes into play. When the digestive tract is impaired, absorption is also hindered. You can eat the best diet in the world and take large amounts of vitamins and minerals, but if you don't have the proper enzymes, they won't be as effective."

"Eva, I'm somewhat puzzled. I'm not entirely clear about the relationship between vitamins, minerals and digestion."

"Well, it's these substances that activate certain enzyme systems. For example, I've observed that when certain food-allergic individuals take high doses of vitamins B-complex and C before a meal, their typical food reactions are somewhat lessened. Nutritional deficiencies underlie many sensitivities and in turn, food sensitivities often create nutritional deficiencies. It's a vicious circle."

"Most of which originated in poor dietary habits to begin with, right?" asked Elisabeth.

"Definitely. And as Jillian and I had previously discussed, when we were talking about Pottenger's cats, it may take several generations for these weaknesses to be fully corrected."

"But do I need to take large amounts of these supplements?"

"Only temporarily. It's essential in the beginning, to compensate for all the years you didn't absorb them and to make up for what you currently can't assimilate. Then, as absorption improves, the dosage can be gradually cut back."

"So it isn't enough to work with my yeast problem, clear out parasites, avoid eating foods to which I'm sensitive, and take enzymes with my meals?"

"No, because you have so much catching up to do for years of malnourishment." She leaned over. "Let me look at your nails." I held out my hands. Both she and Elizabeth looked at them intently. "Just as I thought. Brittle, pale, chipped and ridged - all signs of malabsorption." Still sensing some hesitation on my part, Eva asked, "Do you have reservations about taking supplements?"

"I guess I've just been brainwashed to think that we don't need them and . . . I hate taking pills . . ."

"Consider them compressed foods. They're a far cry from medication."

"I suppose you're right. God! I can just see Michael watching me pop all these vitamins and minerals. He's going to croak!"

"Just wait until he sees how healthy you'll be. You might even catch him sneaking a few here and there!"

Somehow I had a hard time imagining Michael popping vitamins! "I need to read more. What book or books would you recommend in particular?"

"One of the very best is by Shari Lieberman and Nancy Bruning called *The Real Vitamin & Mineral Book. The Vitamin Bible* by Earl Mindell and *Minerals and Your Health* by Dr. Len Mervyn are good too."

I jotted down the titles. "Are they available in the library?"

"They are, but of course, like most good books, they're always in circulation. Reserve them before you leave. By the way, for the convenience of our patients, the library mails books back and forth within quite a wide radius of this clinic."

"I didn't know that. That's great!"

"Another book that I found most helpful," suggested Elisabeth, "is a book called *Prescription for Nutritional Healing* by Dr. James and Phyllis Balch. You might even want to buy a copy for yourself. It's one of the most comprehensive and up-to-date self-help guides covering just about every ailment imaginable. It suggests natural therapies, using vitamins, minerals, herbs and food supplements. There are a few copies for sale in the front lobby."

"Thanks for mentioning that book, Elisabeth. My clients rave about it. For many it's become their primary guide - their bible."

"I'll check that one out. Is it very expensive?"

"From what I can remember," said Elisabeth, "the price was very reasonable - certainly worth every cent."

"Jillian, getting back to RDA's for a moment . . . a few years ago I decided to use the acronym ODA, or Optimum Daily Allowances instead of RDAs."

"What do you mean by Optimum Daily Allowances?" queried Elisabeth.

"A dose that's both preventative and curative. Let's take vitamin C as an example. Humans are unable to produce ascorbic acid in their livers the way other mammals can. Ideally, we should get enough from our diets. In practice, that doesn't happen. The RDA for humans is only sixty milligrams per day, yet research shows that animals that are able to produce ascorbic acid internally do so at an equivalent rate for humans of between 2,000 and 12,000 milligrams a day. This would mean one would have to eat forty or more oranges a day to produce an equivalent amount of vitamin C. It is, therefore, far more reasonable to consider supplements as a way to increase our intake of vitamin C, especially in cases where the immune system is depressed."

"So we really can't possibly get all the vitamins we need from our diet?"

"Certainly not vitamin C. And judging from the thousands of R.B.C.'s I've studied over the years, it's apparent as well that the mineral status for most people is very low. It would be interesting to test people who manage to eat an optimum diet that's locally and organically grown all year round."

"We should all live in a warmer climate!" I exclaimed.

"I'm certain it would make a difference," replied Eva. Returning to my file, she commented, "Ah yes! I made a note last time to discuss essential fatty acids with you. Dr. Rowland suspected that you were sorely lacking EFA's based on your symptoms and physical . . ."

"What symptoms?"

"Hmm. Let's see." The papers rustled as she dug through them. "Here we are. Feeling cold all over, hair falling out, excessive thirst, dry skin and scalp, dandruff, P.M.S., little bumps on the backs of your arms . . ."

"I always wondered about those."

"And last but not least, multiple food sensitivities."

"How are they connected to fatty acid deficiency?"

"Fatty acid deficiency has been linked to an increase in the permeability of the mucosal membrane of the intestinal tract."

"And then undigested food particles have a better chance of entering the bloodstream?"

"Jillian, you're really up on all this. You must be doing quite a bit of reading."

"I am!" I was proud of sounding somewhat knowledgeable. "But what exactly are fatty acids and why are they essential?"

"As you know," explained Eva, "there are good fats and bad fats. The media has been telling the public to cut down on saturated fats and to eat more unsaturated ones. So people have switched from butter to margarine and other vegetable oils. The problem with many of the unsaturated fats, however, is that most of them are either fully or partially hydrogenated in order to make them into a spreadable product or to prolong shelf life. These altered fats or trans-fatty acids, are very damaging to the blood vessels. Just about every box of crackers, chips, pretzels and corn chips are made with hydrogenated fats."

Elisabeth added, "Even most supermarket variety breads are made from these fats. You just can't win!"

"These fats are everywhere. Anyway, now that you know a bit about saturated and hydrogenated fats, let's look at essential fatty acids. There are at least two kinds of EFA's - omega 6 and omega 3. Because it's trendy to use vegetable oils in cooking and salad dressings, most people today get enough omega 6. However, many people have problems utilizing these oils due to specific vitamin and mineral deficiencies, B-6 and zinc being just two of them. It's somewhat of a Catch-22 situation."

"Boy! It sounds complicated."

"It is, because we've not only milled the roughage out of the whole grain, but also the vitamins, minerals and essential oils."

Elisabeth shook her head. "We've completely damaged our food chain, right from the bottom up."

"Yes, and we're paying dearly for it," acknowledged Eva. "For years, we've known that butter is a much more stable fat than margarine. Finally, a Canadian researcher came to the same conclusion , but within one week of publication of this finding, margarine companies were taking out whole page ads that touted the safety of their products!"

"You know Eva," said Elisabeth, "the best description of margarine is in Rona's *Return to the Joy of Health*." She took a book out of her briefcase. "Here it is. He quotes health writer John Finnegan describing margarine as a *lifeless, devitalized poison, packed with carcinogens (cancer-causing chemicals), fit only for lubricating the front wheel bearings of your car*. Then Rona goes on to say, *Why well-intentioned doctors and dietitians continue to recommend edible plastic as a butter substitute may depend more on financial and political considerations than on science*."

"It's frustrating - always an uphill battle against companies that wield the big buck!" I snorted with disdain.

"But we must never give up the battle, as difficult as it gets at times. So, although butter is better, the cream of the crop - if you'll pardon the pun - the very best are olive oil, flaxseed or canola oil. The one drawback to butter is that it's often high in pesticide content. Animals, like humans, store pesticide residues in their fatty tissues."

"I never would have thought . . ."

"No, most people don't. But getting back to EFA's . . . these fats are called essential because the body doesn't manufacture them. They perform two critical roles - they help to maintain lubrication and resiliency of cells and are responsible for prostaglandin production."

"Prostaglandins?"

"Yes, these chemicals are found in every cell of the body. Certain prostaglandins help protect us against sensitivities, cancer and heart disease. They also keep our bodily thermostat regulated, help control the inflammatory process and the immune system in general . . ."

"Heart disease? How?"

"By controlling cholesterol levels."

"And the only way of obtaining these fats is from foods?"

"Right. And our foods no longer provide enough of them . . . unless of course one were to eat a diet of sardines, salmon, and other oily fish, nuts, seeds, and whole grains on a regular basis and stop eating hydrogenated oils which interfere in the metabolism of these essential fats . . ."

"But in the meantime, would you have to supplement them?"

"Yes. By far the most prevalent deficiency seems to be omega 3, so I suggest you start taking flax oil."

"Where do I find it and how much do I take?"

"Your healthfood store carries it in the refrigerated section. Start with one tablespoon a day. If your skin becomes less dry, then increase to two tablespoons and maintain that for a month. You can stay on one tablespoon as a maintenance dose. If your symptoms become worse, then you need to stop the oil altogether and switch to an omega 6 oil. And you must keep it refrigerated, since it's cold-pressed and unprocessed."

"What about my weight? I sure don't want to regain what I've lost."

"You won't. In fact, you'll see that it will actually help you lose weight. For those who are underweight, it can help them gain."

"Where could I learn more about essential fatty acids?"

"Wow!" remarked Elisabeth. "I wish more clients were like you!"

"I'll give you a really comprehensive list," said Eva, "that will summarize all the books to which we've referred during our session - and more. Would that be helpful?"

"That would be great! I plan on becoming an expert on my own body by the time I'm through."

"That's the object. In order to take responsibility for our health, we need to be educated. If only more people would be as eager. Don't you agree Elisabeth?"

"Hey, we might be out of a job in no time!" she teased.

"My only wish is for my family to be healthy. It was a commitment I made to myself for the new year."

"Are you going to do elimination diets with the children?" asked Eva.

"Definitely. I'm starting at the end of this week. I hope Michael will support me."

"Well, he should come and watch some young children being tested. That would go a long way toward increasing his understanding of the problem."

"That's what Dr. Rowland suggested, but the testing room is backed up for the next two months."

Eva sighed. "It's an ongoing problem. If more doctors would see the benefits of antigen therapy and incorporate more of these modalities into their own practices, there wouldn't be such a long waiting list here."

"And when do you think that'll be?" My voice was full of sarcasm.

"When hell freezes over!" blurted Elisabeth. Apologizing, she said, "Just kidding folks!"

"What she really means is when enough of them become ill or when their families and friends become ill."

"Exactly!" remarked Elisabeth. "Had my son not become ill, I'd probably still be depressed, exhausted and living on Ex-lax. Even worse, I'd still be preaching milk, cheese and yogurt as the cure for most problems, keeping myself and those around me in the dark about food sensitivities. I still can't get over the fact that this information was actually in our primary reference book in university, yet hardly any of my colleagues address it!"

"And that's only food sensitivities. What about the increasing numbers who are sensitive to chemicals?"

"What people don't realize," mused Eva, "is that we're like the canaries of long ago that were taken into the mines to warn workers of lethal gases. Many of us have become sensitive to levels of pollutants so minute that even sophisticated instruments can't detect them. What everyone fails to understand is that these same pollutants probably affect everyone to one degree or another."

"Dr. Rowland suggests that we're lucky to have these warnings. What's your take on that?"

"He may well be right," replied Eva. "Some people never get a warning. They simply wake up one day with a rapidly spreading tumor or some other potentially fatal disease."

"Are you still sensitive to things?" I asked Eva.

"Far less than before, but I still need to be careful. After all, what's the goal? To go back to the lifestyle habits we had prior to becoming sick? To go back to eating butter tarts and drinking five cups of coffee every day?"

"How 'bout just one cup!" I joked.

"Well, that day will come, but the real question is: what quality of life do you want, and in order to have it, what changes do you need to make, and are you prepared to make them?"

"You're right. Sometimes I just miss my comfort foods . . ."

"Yes," she smiled, "the ones that were making us sick for all those years." Again, I hate to sound repetitive, but everything in life is a trade-off."

"It's true. But I still can't help feeling jealous of the person who isn't affected and can eat, drink and breathe garbage all day. It's so much easier."

"Yes, perhaps it is easier, but I can tell you now they may be among those who suddenly discover that they have a serious illness."

"You know," suggested Elisabeth, "It's like all our relatives who choose to live in denial, popping pills instead of looking for the underlying cause."

"You mean those with headaches, irritability and mood swings - the ones with kids plagued with tonsillitis and chronic ear infections?" I thought of so many around me who fell into one or more of these categories.

"They're the ones," nodded Eva. She looked at her watch. "Elisabeth, my watch says 2:30, but I know it's much later. Looks like it's on the fritz again. Do you have the right time?"

"It's almost 3:30."

"Gosh! We still have to go over rotation. Jillian, are you up for it?"

"Kind of, but the thought of doing anything more to my diet is a pain!"

"Don't fret. You won't have to start immediately. And you may not have to adhere to it rigorously. A loose rotation might work for you. I just want to plant the seed, so that when the time comes, you'll have a handle on it - especially where you plan to work with the entire family. Do you understand why it's a good practice to rotate foods?"

"It's to prevent new sensitivities from arising, isn't it?

"Right. In the past, we put people on straight elimination diets for extended periods of time. Before too long, we realized that many of them simply replaced one addiction with another and ended up developing new symptoms from foods to which they were previously non-reactive - due to their permeable gut."

"Why is it called a rotation diet?"

"It's official name is the Rotary Diversified Diet. It was first developed by Dr. Herbert Rinkel in 1934. Remember when we discussed sensitivities that are cyclical as opposed to fixed?"

"Yes. Are they also called cumulative sensitivities?"

"That's right. Either term is appropriate. Most sensitivities are cyclical. Overconsumption of a single food can cause this type of sensitivity. Rotation helps preserve the body's enzyme system. If you eat the same food repeatedly, the same enzyme is constantly called into action, exhausting that particular body function. So by rotating food families every four days . . ."

"What do you mean by food families?"

Eva turned to Elisabeth. "Would you do the honors?"

"I'd be glad to." Elisabeth began, "Foods, whether plant or animal, come in families. For example, grains like wheat, barley, oats, rice and corn are part of the grass family. You might never suspect that sugar - cane sugar - is also of the same family. So if you're sensitive to wheat, you may have a cross-sensitivity to sugar or even to rice. Or . . . take potato as another example. It's related to tomato, green pepper, tobacco, eggplant, all members of the nightshade family. So, if you're sensitive to tomato, you may well be sensitive to potato. In other words, you can cross-react to the 'relatives' of food to which you're sensitive."

"Well put!" exclaimed Eva.

"So how does a rotation diet help? And why four days?"

"Did you want me to answer that?" asked Elisabeth.

"Sure, go right ahead," replied Eva. "You're doing a great job!"

"It takes about ninety-six hours, or four days, for most foods to pass through the gastrointestinal tract. So the four-day rotation allows three full days between each food. This ensures that no food is ingested more often than once every four days. For extremely sensitive people, four days isn't nearly enough. They need to rotate every five, seven or ten days."

"That's correct," commented Eva. "This diet is also quite therapeutic in that it serves three functions:

1. by exposing the body less frequently to a problem food, there are fewer chances for a reaction;

2. it reduces the possibility of new sensitivities developing;

3. it acts as a diagnostic tool, helping you to identify reactive foods. It keeps the problem foods unmasked."

"I don't understand the last one."

"Well, if you only eat a certain food on a given day, you can be quite sure that if the food becomes a problem, it'll usually make itself known on that day, unless, of course, you have a delayed reaction."

"Oh yeah! I see what you mean. So if a specific food reveals itself to be a problem, I simply drop it from the rotation."

"Right! You're onto it! Take a look at this simple example of a rotation diet, eliminating wheat, yeast, sweeteners and dairy product (fig. 13). But to grasp it completely, you really have to understand the food families. I'll give you a chart to take with you."

"There are several books that helped me understand how rotation diets work," offered Elisabeth. "One of the best is a book called *If This is Tuesday, It Must be Chicken* by Natalie and Frances Golos. Another is *Rotational Bon Appetit!*, available through the Environmental Health Center in Dallas, Texas. Some support groups also sell them. The meals are very simple - easy to prepare."

"Both of these, by the way, are included on this list," said Eva, waving what appeared to be a small booklet. "And then there's Sondra K. Lewis' recent book, *Allergy and Candida Cooking - Rotational Style*, which is loaded with information, including helpful hints, meal planning for each day and 200 pages of recipes.

# Sample Rotation Diet
## fig. 13

|  | DAY ONE | DAY TWO | DAY THREE | DAY FOUR |
|---|---|---|---|---|
| PROTEIN | *fish*<br>salmon<br>sardine<br>trout, cod<br>haddock<br>carp, tuna<br>mackerel | *fowl/eggs*<br>turkey<br>chicken<br>goose<br>duck<br>pheasant and<br>their eggs | *legumes*<br>lentil<br>bean<br>alfalfa sprout<br>soy<br>chickpea<br>bean sprout | *shellfish*<br>scallop<br>crab<br>shrimp<br>clam<br>oyster<br>lobster |
| VEGETABLE | *mustard*<br>*family*<br><br>cauliflower<br>turnip<br>broccoli<br>cabbage<br>kale, chinese<br>cabbage | *gourd*<br>*family*<br>cucumber<br>pumpkin<br>squash<br><br>*goosefoot*<br>*family*<br>beets<br>chard<br>spinach | *carrot*<br>*family*<br>carrot, celery<br>parsnip<br><br><br>*separate*<br>*families*<br>sweet potato<br>kelp & dulse<br>avocado<br>corn | *nightshade*<br>*family*<br>potato<br>tomato<br>pepper<br>eggplant<br>*composite*<br>*family*<br>lettuce<br>*lily family*<br>aspargus<br>garlic<br>leek, onion |
| FRUIT | *rose*<br>*family*<br>apple<br>pear<br>peach<br>plum & prune<br>berries | *gourd*<br>*family*<br>canteloupe<br>watermelon<br>honeydew<br>*separate*<br>*families*<br>pineapple<br>rhubarb | *separate*<br>*families*<br><br>grapes<br>raisins<br>bananas<br>kiwi | *citrus*<br>*family*<br><br>orange<br>grapefruit<br>lemon<br>tangerine<br>lime |
| NUTS<br>& SEEDS | almond<br>sesame &<br>tahini | pumpkin<br>seeds<br><br>macademia<br>nut | peanut<br>soynut<br>cashew<br>pistachio | sunflower<br>seeds |
| OILS<br>&<br>FATS | sesame<br>almond<br>canola | flax<br>olive | peanut<br>soy<br>corn | sunflower<br>safflower |
| GRAINS &<br>SUBSTITUTE | almond meal<br>sesame meal<br><br>arrowroot<br>starch | *goosefoot*<br>*family*<br>quinoa<br><br>buckwheat | *grass*<br>*family*<br>rye, oats<br>barley<br>corn, rice<br>millett<br>kamut | sunflower<br>meal<br>tapioca<br>amaranth |

"Recipes I'll definitely need! I must say, it all sounds awfully clinical."

"It is somewhat, but once you set it up, it actually gives you far more variety than most conventional diets. It also provides much more nourishment from a wider variety of foods. The one thing you don't want to do, though, is to include any of the foods you've eliminated. . ."

"Ever?"

Eva laughed. "No, definitely not forever! After about three months of elimination, you might want to reintroduce a particular food into one of your days. If it continues to be a problem, eliminate it again. Try in six months, then a year. If it's still a problem, it may be a fixed sensitivity. Then you simply do without that particular food and compensate with a substitute that provides similar nutritional value."

"Do I have to be on this diet indefinitely?"

"Well, some people would have you think so, but in my experience, as the gastrointestinal tract heals and sensitivities gradually lessen, you can lighten up on the strictness of the rotation. But I must say, it really is a good idea to always be diversified in your food choices for all the reasons we've already discussed."

"So when do I start this? I'm already on two other diets."

"Stay with those for now - especially since you're going to be working with your children. Introduce this one later, once you've established which foods affect you adversely."

"Boy, I have so much reading to do! I feel like my whole world has done a 180 degree turn. At this rate, I'll have to start looking for another career. I can't go back to nursing - not with all this information."

"I suspect you probably won't be able to," replied Elisabeth. "No more than I can ever go back to practicing regular dietetics. And it seems that the more I learn, the less I know. I can't seem to keep up with all the new information. It's certainly never boring."

"I can vouch for that," added Eva, "even after all the years I've been in practice. And the beauty of it is that everything is dealt with in such a harmless manner - using medication only in the more extreme cases. And the other aspect that never fails to amaze me is that people get results fairly quickly. Just think, after years of suffering, most obtain some level of relief in a few short weeks. It's so rewarding!"

"Simply change the diet, incorporate antifungal and antiparasitic herbs where needed, take a few supplements and enzymes and you're on your way!" Elisabeth sounded just like Eva - full of enthusiasm and passion.

They both made it sound so simple. This information had to become public knowledge! Everyone deserved to hear unbiased, objective information in order to make educated choices about their own healthcare.

I knew right then and there that an important part of my life would be dedicated to helping others in the same way Eva, Elisabeth and Dr. Rowland were helping me.

I left the clinic knowing that it all had to begin where it counted most - at home.

*Many victims of Environmental Illness
don't know they have it.
The symptoms can accumulate
slowly and quietly
until one or many parts of the system
break down.
But once a label is given, such as arthritis,
colitis, or depression, then it is assumed
that no cause should be sought;
only drugs and surgery should be used.
Fortunately, control of this disease is
within the grasp of the victim.
If you choose, you can create
an internal and external environment
where you are able to return
to your normal function.
It's not easy being your own doctor. . .
that is what is required.*

**Sherry A. Rogers, M.D.
The E.I. Syndrome: An Rx for Environmental Illness**

# 12

# All Aboard!

*Many adults are totally unaware that some of their children's or their own medical or emotional complaints could be solely due to an allergy.*
**Doris Rapp, M.D.**

*I* kissed the children goodbye. Grabbing my purse, I gave last minute instructions to the sitter and ran out the door. Michael was going to meet me at the school. Our appointment with Mrs. Allen was long overdue. We had cancelled twice before due to my illness. Finally, I felt well enough to start dealing with problems other than my own.

I opened the front door of the school and headed down the hall to Room 121. I couldn't help but notice a strong chemical odor. My heart began to race, my face flushed and I could feel myself become agitated. "Great!" I thought to myself. "All I need is to be spaced out while I'm trying to make sense of my son's situation."

Just then, Michael came through the front door, newspaper in one hand, briefcase in the other. He gave me a quick kiss. A strange look came over his face. "Jilly, you're as white as the wall. You haven't looked this pasty in weeks. Are you okay?" I could hear that old panic back in his voice.

"Michael, something in here is making me sick. I feel like I'm losing it!"

"For God's sake Jillian! Fine time to be conking out . . ."

"Michael!" I seethed under my breath, "I don't need anger, I need understanding . . ."

He looked somewhat sheepish and was about to respond when the classroom door opened. Mrs. Allen greeted us and invited us in. As I brushed past her, I almost gagged! She reeked of perfume, as if she had bathed in the stuff! I could feel myself falling apart by the second. I could barely think straight! All I could mumble was that I wasn't feeling well, and that Michael would have to talk to her himself. Shaking, I excused myself, ran down the hall, and escaped out the front door into the fresh air.

Once outside, my head began to clear. I felt less agitated. My first thought was: *No wonder poor Nathaniel has problems! Maybe he's sensitive to these things, just like I am.* One thing I knew for sure - I couldn't function in that environment!

What amazed me was that I'd walked around feeling sick for years but I'd never known why. Now, bit by bit, I was beginning to piece things together - like a jigsaw puzzle - much like the fragmented figure on Dr. Rowland's chart.

By the time I made it home, I was feeling somewhat better. About an hour later, Michael arrived. He was rubbing his head and looked quite haggard.

"Look, I'm sorry I snapped at you at the school, but I was really looking forward to us doing something together - even if it was something as difficult as talking to a teacher about our kid's problems."

"Michael, I'm sorry . . ." Here I was once again apologizing for being sick. Guilt flooded over me in waves. Familiar feelings of shame and inadequacy as a wife and mother returned. Perhaps Eva was right - we could use some counselling.

"I'm just so tired of doing everything alone . . ." He looked away and I could feel his loneliness. I began to cry. The devastation of being sick with an unrecognized illness was bad enough, but its effect on those around me and the guilt associated with it was even worse.

"Michael, I'm sorry I'm sick! I'm sorry you're tired of it all! And I'm sorry you feel lonely . . . I just don't know what else I can do. I know I'm on the right track . . ."

"You probably are, Jilly. I'm sorry too, but it's the way I feel and I've felt this way for a long time. Every once in a while it just gets to me. Meanwhile, Nathaniel's behavior at school is getting worse. It seems that the kid Mrs. Allan describes is not quite the one we know at home . . ."

"In what way?"

"Well, we know he's always been a difficult kid, but she seems to be implying that he's totally disruptive."

"I can tell you one thing - the odors at that school are causing very serious problems. As far as I'm concerned, Mrs. Allan's perfume has got to go!"

"Jillian, I know you're gung-ho on all this environmental stuff, but it doesn't account for everything. It's too easy to point the finger at one thing. Besides, just because these things are a problem for you doesn't mean they're a problem for Nathaniel . . ."

"But if I have the problem, who's to say he doesn't have the same thing? He *is* my son, you know!"

"Okay, okay, I've heard enough. My head feels like it's going to blow apart! I can't talk about this anymore. I have to lie down."

"Maybe you're affected by these things too. Did you have a headache before you went into the school?"

"Well, no . . ."

"Then how do you know that her perfume didn't cause it?"

"Jillian, give it a rest!" he shouted as he stomped off to the bedroom.

I fed the kids. After putting Max and Emma to bed, I spoke with Nathaniel. I asked him if he noticed a difference between the way he felt when he woke up in morning and after being in the classroom. His response was most interesting.

"Well, I feel a bit cranky almost every morning but after being at school for a while, it feels like my body can't sit still - like it has to move all the time. Everything bugs me . . ." Then he looked up at me and said, "Mom, you wouldn't want to be in my head. I feel so mixed up. It's like I can't help myself. Then I feel mad."

"And what happens when you get mad?"

"Then I start bugging other kids . . ."

"And then Mrs. Allan gets upset with you?"

"Yeah. Then I get yelled at and usually end up out in the hall." He looked up at me, his beautiful dark eyes welling with tears, and said, "Mom, no one likes me this year. I hate school."

My heart ached for my son. Deep inside, he really was a loving child. I held him for a few moments, feeling his pain and wishing I could do something about it.

"Nathaniel, last year you were doing okay. Mr. Grant thought you were keen and your report cards were much better. Why the sudden change?"

"I don't know, Mom. All I know is I really hate school." Fighting tears, he asked in a whisper, "Do I have to go tomorrow?"

"Well, yes you do. But Nathaniel, we're going to have to figure out why you're having so many problems this year compared to last. Run off to bed now. You need a good night's rest."

I gave him another hug and reassured him that we were doing everything possible to try to help him. Something wasn't adding up. I decided then and there to call the clinic first thing in the morning and have them put us on the cancellation list for testing. I was suspicious of the perfume. I wanted Nathaniel tested for it as well as for other chemicals.

The next morning I told Michael that I planned to put the whole family on an elimination diet.

"Well, leave me out of the experiment. I don't have any of these problems."

"Oh yeah? What about those headaches? What about the antacids you practically live on?"

"Ah! That's nothing . . . at least they don't interfere with my life. . . or my work!" His words were full of anger and sarcasm.

I couldn't believe the pain they evoked - *as if I didn't work*!

"I still plan on having pizza on Fridays, but I'll tell you what, I'll eat it at the office instead of at home," he mumbled as he munched on a piece of toast and gulped his morning coffee.

"That's fine, just don't bring anything home for the next couple of weeks that's not on our diet. First I'm going to scrap sugar and dairy products. Later I'll do the wheat/yeast thing . . ."

Michael looked at me with suspicion. "Jilly, why are you doing this?"

"Because I'm sure Nathaniel's stuffiness and crankiness, as well as Emma's asthma and Max's ear infections, are all tied into this . . ."

"And what makes you think that?"

"It's in all the books you refuse to read, and on all the charts I saw at Dr. Rowland's office . . . Which reminds me, I have a couple of short videos we need to watch together. Can we do it tonight?"

"Maybe, after the kids go to bed . . . Anyway, gotta go! See you later." He grabbed his briefcase and shot out the door.

I realized there wasn't much I could do about Michael - his health was his own responsibility. My main concern was the children.

When I spoke to the kids about the diet, their first responses were, "No way! No treats? No milk? What do we put on our cereal? No more Frosted Frooties!" But as soon as we talked about a reward system - better known as bribery - they were game. After all, a new pair of jeans and a Barbie go a long way! Max was no problem - he was too young to fully understand what was happening.

That evening when the kids were tucked into bed, Michael and I popped some corn and put on the first of the Doris Rapp videos that I had brought back from the clinic. The tape showed children of various ages being tested for foods, chemicals and airborne irritants. In some cases, their noses would stuff up, in others their handwriting would change from neat and tidy to an illegible scrawl. Sometimes a child's behavior would become uncontrollable and defiant. They would run around, and in some instances, even yell vulgarities. Michael kept saying, "Boy! I'm glad our kids aren't like that!" Of course, he was thinking of the many other children we both knew - nieces, nephews and some of the neighborhood kids.

"Well," I began, "our kids might not be as bad as some of *them*, but they sure have a lot of the same signs . . ."

"Like what?" asked Michael, somewhat defensive.

"Pale faces with dark circles under their eyes, stuffy noses, Emma's asthma, Max's ear infections, not to mention Emma's bedwetting. According to the video, these are some of the symptoms."

"True. But I see it more in my sister's and your brother's kids than in ours, don't you?" said Michael.

"Well, that's true. But from what Mrs. Allan says about Nathaniel at school, it doesn't sound like we're too far off the mark."

"What bothered me the most was the kid who reacted to the poor air in the school, and the little boy who became so tired and clingy from the disinfectant they used to clean the desktops. And, Jilly, the sweet little kid who reacted to chlorine. He went from being this adorable little guy to resembling a vicious animal. Give that kid a few years and he'll be an inmate at a reformatory! It's a good thing Dr. Rapp is onto this and can help them. No wonder you're so upset. It's really frightening."

His words were like music to my ears!

"I know you think I'm becoming a fanatic about this environmental health stuff, but I really am convinced that if it can devastate my own health to the extent that it has, it must be a part of the children's problems as well. After all, they *are* my kids!"

"Hey! They're mine, too! Maybe along with your rotten genes they got some of my good ones!" teased Michael, pulling me closer to him.

I smiled, thinking about his head and stomach aches. At least he was open to some possibilities. It was a beginning.

The next few days were busy - shopping for new foods and scouring recipe books for interesting meals. I set up a reward system on the fridge, using wild and wonderful stickers for each day. When I cancelled the milk delivery, the milkman stared at me as if I were crazy. I did the same with the kids' milk program at school. The secretary made me feel like I was a criminal. I sent juice with the kids so they would have something to drink with the other children.

Little Max kept asking for his milk. I told him over and over that the milk was all gone. After a few moments of whining, he'd forget about it until the next time and then we'd go through the story again - that the milk was all gone, the store had run out. I didn't like to fib, but he was too young to understand the truth.

The foods they missed most were cheese, ice cream and milk on their cereal. Because they weren't allowed sugar either, they found it hard to get used to the unsweetened cereals or those sweetened with fruit juice. They stuck with oatmeal, toast and rice cakes, eating dry cereal only occasionally. After a few days, they even began trying rice and soy milk.

Within a week, I noticed that both Nathaniel and Max had stopped honking and snorting. Their noises used to drive me crazy! Finally, they could breathe through their nostrils without obstruction. Nathaniel was easier to wake up in the mornings and was less grouchy. Emma had better color and hadn't used her puffer in days. Little Max scratched less and was calmer. Needless to say, these changes made my life much easier.

After one of our Friday night family dinners, near the end of our second week on the diet, Michael made an interesting comment.

"Jilly, this is the first night I can remember that we've all sat, talked and eaten without any commotion. We all interacted calmly, and no one jumped up and down to get this and that. I'm impressed! Something's working. Whatever it is, keep it up! It's great!" He hugged me tightly.

He had no idea how much those words meant to me! "It's got to be the diet, Michael. Nothing else has changed."

"Well, maybe it is. Then let's keep them on it," he said, rubbing his forehead, "I have to lie down, my head hurts again."

"Michael, if we're all on this diet, why don't you try it too? I'll bet you fifty bucks your headaches and upset stomach will disappear after a few weeks. The only hitch is . . . you'll have to quit coffee too."

"No coffee? I'd die! I need that pick-me-up."

"But if you stop sugar and dairy, you might not need the jump start."

"You could be right," he mumbled holding his head. He squeezed out a sheepish grin and said with resignation, "All right, all right, for fifty bucks, you're on. I'll try it with you guys."

I squeezed him tightly and went to get an ice-pack from the fridge. With the exception of the incident at the school, I was amazed at how loving I felt towards him these days. The more support he gave, the more affection I felt. Of course, the fact that I was physically stronger was significant. A few weeks earlier, I couldn't even think straight, let alone feel loving toward anyone!

Now I felt like we were all working together. It was great! The results spoke for themselves. I felt so happy!

I spent a good part of the weekend creating new recipes. I reviewed rotation diets, studied food families in preparation for a more formal version down the road - just in case. Michael decided to start his elimination diet Monday morning. I could hardly wait!

On Sunday afternoon, we visited my parents. They lived in Newbury, half an hour from where we lived. We were all in good spirits.

Mom and Dad were excited to see us. I'd previously told them about our dietary restrictions, and unlike Michael's folks, they respected our wishes. They'd been on a health kick themselves ever since Dad's heart attack two years earlier. Part of their escape from the stress of urban life was to move to the outskirts of this sleepy little town. They had recently bought a sprawling old Victorian home on a picture-perfect street with huge rambling yards and gnarled old trees. The kids loved it.

Emma and Max raced up to the attic as soon as we arrived, looking for old dressup clothes. Nathaniel headed out to one of the outbuildings that still held antique farm machinery. Mom commented on how well we all looked - especially me.

"Darling, I'm so glad that doctor was able to help you. You've been through so much over the past while."

"Mom, since I've followed this diet, I haven't felt better in my entire life. I'm great as long as I stay away from malls and crowds . . ."

"Because of the perfumes?" she asked.

"How did you know? Did I tell you that?" I was trying to recollect phone conversations in which I might have mentioned it to her.

"No dear. But Mrs. Wilson down the road gets so sick from smells of any kind - perfumes being the worst. She can't go near malls at all. In fact she's had to stop going to church, and for her, that's crushing."

"Well, perfumes are only one of the things that set me off. I suspect there are lots of triggers I don't even know about yet. But Dr. Rowland will be able to test us for those . . ."

I had just started to tell her more about Dr. Rowland and the clinic, when Max ran down to tell us that Emma was sick. He pointed to the attic. We all rushed up and as we approached the door, we could hear her gasp for air. Michael ran out to the car to get her mask and pump. The moment I opened the attic door, I was assaulted by the musty smell. I felt myself becoming disoriented and irritable. By the time we got down to the main floor, I was totally spaced out. Michael gave Emma her mask. She responded more quickly than ever. Within moments, she was fine - a record recovery! I, on the other hand, felt awful.

"Jillian dear, you look terrible! Only minutes ago you looked great - better than you've looked in years. Now you're pale, almost grey. What is it?" asked Mom, very concerned.

"It's something in the attic . . . it smells like mold. I really feel sick. I need some water."

Mom helped me downstairs and filled a huge pitcher. I opened my vitamin C and poured some into a glass. Dr. Rowland had suggested I take high doses of C or a mixture of tri-salts whenever I was exposed to anything which set off a reaction. It was supposed to help the body to detoxify quickly. I drank three full glasses, and excused myself, saying I needed fresh air. She insisted on accompanying me.

After breathing the crisp air for a few minutes, I started to feel better. Mom could see the color come back to my face. "Jillian, you look better already. What a difference! But now . . . when I think about it, even as a child, you'd often go from having rosy cheeks to being washed out."

"You're probably right. I don't think I was ever well."

"I'd have to agree with you on that one. You'd be the sweetest child one minute and the next, we'd all wonder where you came from! You'd be totally unreasonable - unmanageable. Jilly, do you remember the picnics we used to go on?"

I nodded. "Do I remember! You'd spend most of the time yelling at me, telling me what a terrible child I was."

"But you were, dear." She stopped and looked at me. Her eyes brimmed with tears. "And don't think I didn't feel bad. I did. I just didn't know what to do. Your Aunt Maggie used to tell me you were a bad seed. Some days I didn't know who you were."

"Mom, I now know that some things in the air, chemicals and certain foods make me sick. Those picnics were loaded with sugary, sticky foods - cakes, pies, squares. You name it, we ate it. Then Uncle Harold would always run out and buy two big tubs of ice cream. Dr. Rowland says I've always been highly sensitive to these foods. I could kill after eating sugar; dairy leaves me totally stuffed up; and wheat exhausts me. Remember all those ear infections I had? The colic you always attributed to 'the baby from hell'? It was dairy products all along!"

"You really think these foods caused you to be so miserable?"

"I don't *think* so, I *know* so. Mom, I remember trying so hard to be good and then just wanting to scream, never knowing why I felt that way. I felt like a prisoner in my own body - like a little bird trapped in a cage, wanting so hard to get out, only not being able to find the way. I always felt sad, irritable. Anything would set me off. I felt as if I hated the world around me - at times, even myself. I'm lucky I didn't do something really stupid - maybe even kill myself, and don't think I didn't think about it because I did."

Mom winced, tears spilling down her cheeks as she listened.

"My private hell was probably worse on me than on you. I never understood why I was scolded all the time. I didn't even know why I would do the awful things I did. I was so highly reactive."

Mom held me close and whispered, "I had no idea. Jilly, can you forgive me for not knowing?"

"Of course I forgive you, Mom. I only wanted you to love me." I hugged her back. Tears flowed freely. I could feel her pain as a mother. I thought of Nathaniel, Emma and Max. In between sobs, I whispered, "How *could* you have helped me? We didn't have the information back then . . . but now, we do. And I've made a commitment to myself that my kids will never suffer the way I did."

She wiped my tears with her glove and gently pushed back a strand of hair that had fallen over my eye. "And they won't. At least my grandchildren will have a better chance at being happy. I have every confidence that you'll make sure they will. I'm so proud of you - that you kept on searching, even after we all gave up on you. The changes in you over the past few weeks have been remarkable. You're like a new person."

"Mom, I *feel* like a new person. And I want nothing but the best for my kids - and for you. Dr. Rowland says my sinus problems and mood swings may be showing up in you as arthritis."

"What do you mean?" she asked.

"It means that certain foods or chemicals may also be triggering *your* problems - that the sugar, dairy and wheat that cause my difficulties may be the triggers for your arthritis. Remember how you'd fall asleep right after every meal?"

"Well . . . yes . . . but . . ."

"Remember how cranky we'd both get when we shopped?"

"No wonder. You always wanted the most outrageous clothes - and the most expensive."

"Mom . . . it was far more than that! Even after five minutes of being in the store, you'd become highly irritable - long before we even got into any discussions. I admit, I wasn't much better, but you were part of the equation."

She appeared to be deep in thought. "Well . . . maybe you're right. Just the other day, I had the strangest experience. Every afternoon this past week I spent an hour to an hour and a half on the phone trying to form a bridge club. I noticed that after three calls, I felt irritable. Your dad made the mistake of poking his head in the den. I all but bit it off! Not only was I fit to be tied, but I became extremely tired. I lay down on the bed. After about an hour, I was fine. The next day, the same thing happened. Only this time, I became even more irritable. I thought I was becoming paranoid, having listened to you talk about environmental sensitivities."

"So did you ever figure out what was setting you off?"

"Well yes . . . Mrs. Wilson from down the street - you know, the one who gets sick from perfume - popped in for a cup of tea. I told her about my strange experience. She immediately asked me questions about whether or not I felt better in or out of the house, and whether I had purchased anything new in the den."

"And? What happened?"

"You won't believe this. It was the telephone! Your dad had exchanged the old phone for a brand new one - same color, same model. I didn't notice the difference - but my body sure did! Mrs. Wilson insisted I smell the receiver. It reeked of a strong chemical odor - I nearly gagged! I phoned the manufacturer and in the beginning, received the usual runaround. One rather rude employee thought I was crazy to suggest that I could be reacting to their phone. In the end, they put me in touch with one of their researchers. He suggested I put the phone out in the hot sun or in the oven at 125 degrees to help it outgas."

"That *is* an incredible story! And how many people would ever connect their daily irritability and fatigue to a new telephone! See? I'm convinced that identifying cause and effect is the key that unlocks so many chronic problems. There are thousands of people out in the world who react to all kinds of things - only they haven't made the connection. Sad, isn't it?"

Mom nodded.

As we walked, I told her about my experiment with the kids and that Michael was ready to join us. She was very interested since she had experienced unpleasant side effects from her arthritis and migraine medications. By the end of our walk, she was ready to make an appointment with Dr. Rowland for herself.

When we went inside, Michael was still talking about Emma's instantaneous response to the mask. Then it struck me! "Maybe her response was due more to getting her out of the attic than it was to the medication. Maybe she's sensitive to mold!"

Mom piped in, "You may be right, dear. You always said Emma gets much worse in the spring and fall . . ."

"That's it! It must be mold. I'll bet Dr. Rowland can test her for it at the clinic. I can't believe I never made that connection before."

The rest of the visit was one of the best we'd ever had. I was calm and relaxed. Dad couldn't believe how well behaved the kids were, especially Max and Nathaniel. It felt great to be complimented!

"If only your brother's kids were half as good as your three. Between you and me, they drive us crazy! Don't ever tell them, but your mother and I are exhausted by the time they leave here. It takes us almost a week to recover, doesn't it Helen?"

"Dear, they're just children . . . ," said Mom, playing her usual role as mediator, " . . . but they are a handful, I must say!"

All I could think of was my brother making fun of my health problems over the years. In the meantime, his kids were little demons - wired from morning till night. I wondered if he'd be open to hearing what I'd learned over the past few weeks. The Doris Rapp tapes were just what he needed to see!

The drive home was relaxed and enjoyable. Michael told the kids how proud we were of their behavior. I agreed. We talked about how giving up sugar and dairy products might be responsible. Their input was an education in itself.

Emma said that with the exception of the episode in Nanny's attic, her chest felt better - clearer with less tightness. Nathaniel told us it was great to be able to breathe so easily through both nostrils, and that he felt happier these days. He was also less irritable and had fewer detentions at school. Max, in his dear little way, said his skin didn't feel creepy-crawly anymore and that he hardly ever needed to blow his nose. In democratic fashion, we all agreed to continue the diet beyond the two week limit, with, of course, the lure of material rewards in the future.

I felt so positive! Our lives were definitely taking a turn for the better. We were on our way to wellness!

Then, overnight, my life fell apart.

*Each year people are exposed*

*to thousands of toxic chemicals*

*and pollutants in the earth's atmosphere,*

*water, food, and soil.*

*People now carry within their bodies*

*a modern-day chemical cocktail*

*derived from industrial chemicals,*

*pesticides, food additives,*

*heavy metals, anesthetics,*

*and the residues of*

*pharmaceutical, legal, and illegal drugs.*

**The Burton Goldberg Group**
**Alternative Medicine: The Definitive Guide**

# 13

# Will There Be a Morning?

*We should never forget that the brain is the most common allergic target organ and the one most frequently overlooked.*
Sherry A. Rogers, M.D.

*I* awoke feeling nauseated, cold and clammy. After Nathaniel and Emma left, I drove Max to pre-school. I was weak and so cold that my teeth chattered. By the time I got home, my heart was racing and pounding so hard I could feel it in my throat. Waves of paranoia washed over me. Had I left the stove on? I was afraid to get out of the car and go into the house. What if there was a burglar hidden inside? Or a murderer?

Exhausted, I collapsed on the living room sofa. My muscles ached. I could barely move. Life seemed dark and foreboding. I was gripped with fear. In my mind, all I could see was Michael lying dead in a ditch, the car a crumpled heap nearby. What was happening to me?

Everything seemed senseless, meaningless. Michael and the kids were better off without me. I was full of self-pity and self-doubt, questioning the value of my life, my very purpose for being. I was useless - a burden to everyone. Let them find a healthy woman who'd be able to live life fully with them. My eyes welled with tears. "Why doesn't he just leave?" I sobbed aloud. Where were these thoughts coming from?

The prospect of making lunch was too much. I felt overwhelmed. How would I ever cope? Even the thought of calling Michael for help was more than I could deal with.

I didn't want to live. God! What was happening? I had everything to live for. Yet, only negative, dark thoughts loomed in my mind. Lying curled up, my body was freezing cold, shivering. How would I ever manage to get up to the bedroom?

Sliding off the couch, I began the long climb up the stairs. Weak, numb and aching, I literally crawled on my hands and knees.

Finally, I dragged myself to the bedroom and into bed, pulled the blankets over my head, huddled under the covers and wept.

The phone rang but I didn't answer it. Then I thought of Max. Who was going to pick him up? I couldn't. I'd have to call Michael. Thank God the phone was beside the bed!

"I'm sorry, Jillian, he's on another line," replied Andrea, his secretary. "Could I get him to call you back?"

Teeth chattering, I stammered, "Y-y-yes, please," and hung up. Again, I began to sob. Terrifying thoughts arose and lingered, consuming me - Michael bleeding by the roadside, the children with terminal illnesses. I screamed and wailed from a place deep within. Thank God no one was home.

The phone rang. I fumbled for it but couldn't speak. Michael's voice seemed so far away. "Jilly?" Silence. "Jilly, what's wrong? Are you okay?"

I whispered, "M-m-michael, p-p-pick up Max. I c-c-can't do anything. I feel so s-s-sick . . . just want to d-d-die. I'm no g-g-good for anything, f-f-for anyone . . ."

There was dead silence on the other end. Then Michael said, "Jilly, I'm coming home. Get into bed, stay put, and don't do anything. I'll be right there!" He hung up and I retreated back under the covers.

The pounding! I could feel and hear my heartbeat throughout the room. I couldn't get warm. I curled tightly into a fetal position and tried to block it all out.

The sound of my heart gave way to that of footsteps racing up the stairs. The bedroom door flung open. It was Michael. He raced toward me, took one look and said, "Jilly, what happened? You look terrible! We've got to go to the hospital."

"No! I won't go! I c-c-can't go! Th-th-they'll drug me. They'll k-k-k-kill me! Call Dr. Rowland. M-m-m-maybe he c-c-c-can help." I could barely speak.

"Where's his number?"

"In m-m-m-my ad-d-dress book in m-m-my purse." My teeth chattered uncontrollably.

He piled more blankets on me, filled the hot water bottle and plugged in the heating pad. It helped. I stopped shaking.

"I'll be right back." I could hear him dial the phone in the den.

Moments later, he shouted, "Jilly, Dr. Rowland wants to speak with you. Pick up the phone."

As soon as I heard his voice, I began to sob, "Dr. Rowland, I'm s-s-so sick! I j-j-just want to die . . ."

"Jillian, it sounds like you're having a severe reaction to something - the question is, to what? What changed over the past day? Think very carefully . . . Michael tells me you were fine yesterday. It's got to be something you've been exposed to . . . think . . . try to think, Jillian. It's very important."

"I don't know, I d-d-don't know, I just feel so s-s-sick . . ."

"Are you nauseated? Chilled?"

"Yes. I'm so depressed . . . and s-s-scared . . ."

"Jillian, did you start the antifungal?"

"No, not yet . . . just the bacteria, the acidoph . . ."

"Just the acidophilus. Think carefully . . . did you eat anything unusual?"

"No . . ." It was so hard to concentrate.

"Were you someplace you usually don't go?"

"Only my parents' place."

"When were you there?"

"Yesterday afternoon and evening . . . I'm so s-s-sick . . . s-so sick . . ."

"Michael, are you still on the line?"

"Yes."

"Did anything happen at her parents' place?"

"She got pretty wiped out from their moldy attic, but she was fine after getting some air."

"Open her vitamin C powder and start giving her a thousand milligrams every half hour until she has loose stools, then cut back until the stools become normal."

"Vitamin C powder? Jilly where is it?"

"In my purse, I think . . ." Vitamin C powder . . . water . . . something started to connect. "Michael," I mumbled, barely coherent, "I think I know what happened . . ."

"What? What happened Jilly?"

"Michael . . . the water . . . the water at Mom's place . . . It was tap water . . ."

"Tap water? Yeah . . . so? How could . . ."

Dr. Rowland interjected, "Jillian, was that the first time since going on the diet that you drank tap water?"

"Yes . . . I totally forgot . . ."

"Does your mother live in the city?"

"No, but she lives in Newbury . . ."

"I bet that's what you're experiencing, Jillian. A very severe reaction to chlorine. Michael, wrap her up warmly, and take her outside. Breathe along with her until she starts to normalize. Keep pushing the vitamin C into her. Call me if she doesn't start to improve by lunchtime."

"Dr. Rowland, I really appreciate this. I'll definitely call you back to keep you posted." Michael hung up. I could hear him dial again.

He shouted, "Jillian, I'll be right there! I'm calling Beth . . ." I could barely hear what he was saying . . . something about picking Max up at the pre-school and looking after the kids . . .

He picked me up. I was still wrapped in blankets, hot water bottle and all. The winter cold felt like a slap. It was freezing! Michael acted like a birthing coach, breathing in and out with me and feeding me little sips of spring water with vitamin C. Gradually, the paranoia eased, the terrible suicidal feelings lifted. I felt like a wilted flower being brought back to life.

My head began to clear. I could now see some light at the end of what felt like a long, dark and dismal tunnel. It took me back to days not so long ago - except that this was far more extreme. Michael kept talking, reassuring me that it was only a chemical reaction that had made me so paranoid and depressed, and that I'd be better soon. After a while on the porch, he carried me back to bed.

I slept fitfully the rest of the day. It was as if I had been drugged. In my stupor, I was vaguely aware of Michael coming into the bedroom every now and then to check on me. At one point, he crawled into bed, held me and rocked me ever so gently. I reached up to touch his face, and could feel warm tears on his cheek. I was too weak to respond.

Sounds of the children's voices faded in and out of my consciousness as I drifted in and out of sleep.

I awoke to the sound of the alarm. Sunlight danced on my face. I was glad to be back in the world of the living. I felt almost normal! Could last night have been real? A bit of nausea and a slight headache were the only symptoms, the only remnants of my night of terror. It was frightening to think I had lost control, even if only for a short time. I rolled over and hugged Michael close to me. I was glad to be alive. He opened his eyes, squinting. "You're back! You're okay?"

I smiled, touched by his concern.

"Jilly, I was so worried about you! That was definitely the worst you've ever been!"

"Well, I can tell you now, I'll never drink tap water again! We must buy a filter for the whole house."

"Yes, we certainly will. Dr. Rowland recommended that when I called him back last night."

"What did he say?"

"He said you were probably reactive all along to tap water, but by eliminating it for the past few weeks, you unmasked the problem. It's likely one of your worst sensitivities. He says he'll test you for chlorine during your next appointment. You'll be able to get desensitization drops to reduce your reactivity in case you're ever accidentally exposed to it again."

"That would be a life-saver! You know, Michael, I had those same sorts of feelings when I was a teenager, only not as extreme."

"What sorts of feelings?"

"I was often depressed, full of anxiety, despair. As I got older, the feelings faded somewhat, but during the past three years, they've resurfaced. I always wondered why I felt depressed when there was nothing in my life that warranted it. I remember Mom and Dad sending me to a psychiatrist and I recall just sitting there with really nothing much to say."

"True, the last three years have been bad, but I don't remember you ever being quite that reactive before . . ."

"But you know, Michael, when I think back, I remember as a child, begging my parents not to put me in swimming lessons . . ."

"Afraid of the water, were you?" Michael teased.

"No, actually we spent our summers at the cottage swimming every day. It was indoor pools that turned me off. I didn't know why. I just knew I didn't want to be in or around them."

"Could it be that on some level you knew?"

"Maybe. In any case, I'm starting my anti-fungal tomorrow . . ."

"Dr. Rowland wants you to hold off for a few days until your system settles down . . ."

"Michael, I'm just so anxious to start feeling good again!"

"Well, I reserved Beth for today, so you can rest . . ."

"That's so sweet of you!" I leaned over to give him a kiss. Stretching, I let out a big yawn and said, "I'm so glad I feel better. You know, I still find it difficult to believe that one day I feel like I'm dying and the next morning I'm almost normal again. Don't you think that's weird?"

"It is strange, but then, when you think about it, you've been like that for quite some time. One day you're functional and the next, totally strung out. In fact, you've even gone from being sick one hour to being well the next."

"And I never knew why. Now at least I'm starting to see some links, some cause and effect . . ."

"I think that's also why no one believed you when you told them how sick you were . . ."

"What do you mean?" I started to bristle.

"Well, recall that incident at your parents' place the other day. You were fine one moment and within minutes of being in the attic, you felt awful. Then, after a short time in the fresh air, you were okay again."

"You never really believed I was that sick, did you?"

"Well . . ." Michael looked away.

"Am I right? You must have thought I was just lazy or that I wanted to get out of obligations, commitments . . ."

He smiled sheepishly, "Well . . . maybe some of the time I did . . . but Jilly, I guess I didn't understand it . . . or I was too focused on work . . . I don't know . . ."

"You believe me now, don't you?"

He drew me close and said, "Jilly, you scared the hell out of me yesterday. Quite frankly, there were moments when I wasn't sure if you'd see morning."

Later that day, while reading my health diary, I noted that Emma had kept the bed dry three days in a row, while Max's skin had become smooth and he hadn't yanked at his ears for two weeks - touch wood! Our family dinners had consistently remained calm over the past few weeks. Michael even commented that Emma was far less whiny these days. So, apart from my temporary setback with chlorine, I felt we were making progress.

Three days later, I started the enzymes and acidophilus. A few days after that, I began the antifungal, one capsule per meal. Immediately I noticed a decrease in my abdominal gas and bloating. At first, I was more fatigued and became a bit light-headed and irritable, but that too passed after a few days. I definitely didn't get the more severe die-off symptoms described in the books. I guess I was lucky. Or Dr. Rowland could have been right when he suggested my elimination diet helped starve the yeast. In other words, I'd done a lot of the work already.

After about two weeks on this regime, my bladder settled down and my vaginal symptoms disappeared. The most exciting part was that my joint pains, which had gotten much better from the elimination diet, became a thing of the past! My energy increased daily and my cerebral symptoms had all but vanished. My weight dropped even more! I then added flax seed oil to my regimen. I continued to lose weight, without effort. At this rate, I'd soon be back to my weight of twenty years ago! Even if I had to say so myself, I was starting to look pretty good! My skin, previously dry and flaky, was far softer and my hair took on a new lustre. I no longer needed all those creams on which I'd spent a small fortune over the years.

I actually looked and felt healthier than I had in my entire life - as long as I wasn't exposed to chemicals. Even perfumes at church set me back. Interestingly, though, the longer I was on the antifungal, the less sensitive I became. It was like a miracle!

In the meantime, Michael stuck religiously to his diet and I became fifty dollars richer!

Dr. Rowland and Eva had both told me that the journey toward wellness wasn't an even, steady climb. There would be setbacks, each one serving to teach us more about ourselves. I thought of all those who were locked away in mental institutions under various labels - paranoid, manic, or schizophrenic. How many of them were highly reactive to things they ate, drank and inhaled?

And how many of us waste precious time feeling unwell - mentally and physically - because of our daily habits?

My new mission was to unmask our problems and deal with them head on. No more hospitals and weekly doctors' appointments for us! Whatever it took, I was determined to find the road to wellness.

We were already on our way.

*As you continue*

*to become better acquainted*

*with your body*

*and become more adept at*

*influencing it in positive ways,*

*you can gradually assume*

*more responsibility*

*for your healing.*

*When you feel this happening,*

*introduce yourself to the new*

*health manager in your life.*

*Yourself.*

**O. Carl Simonton, M.D.**
**The Healing Journey**

# 14

# The Healer Within

*Ultimately, our best teacher is ourselves. When we are open, aware, and watchful, then we can guide ourselves properly.*
**Tarthang Tulka**

*L*eah Irwin turned and faced me head on. "Jillian, imagine you have only six months to live. Then a friend calls to ask a favor on a day that you'd planned to do something special for yourself. Would you grant the favor?"

"Well . . . yes . . . why wouldn't I?"

"Bernie Siegel, a surgeon and well-known author, posed this question at a lecture I attended. Almost every arm in the room shot up - including my own. His reply to this large show of hands shocked us all. He said, 'Chances are, you aren't going to make it!' This statement changed my entire approach to illness - and to life."

"How?" I was puzzled.

"I walked away from that lecture with the realization that most of us spend our lives doing for others and not for ourselves. Before you know it, life will be over! People will always have expectations of us, making demands on our time, energies and talents. But do you know what? We don't have to feel guilty if we say no."

"But isn't it wrong to put yourself first?"

"No. In fact, if we don't put ourselves first, especially when it comes to our health, we can develop illness, actually create it."

"What do you mean?" I started to become defensive.

"Illness gives us many messages. How, for instance, are you handling the everyday stresses in your life? Do you need help but never ask for it? What makes you angry? What makes you uncomfortable? What do you need? What does your body need? What resentments are you hanging on to? These basic issues are neglected when we constantly focus on others."

"But I grew up believing that one should always put others first."

"Your not the only one! The common belief is that to put yourself first is selfish."

"That's true. I remember reading a book called *The Art of Loving* when I was in my late teens . . ."

"Ah, yes, by Erich Fromm."

"That's the one. I was intrigued by his concept of self-love, but when I discussed it with my father, he thought it was the height of selfishness and narcissism."

"I'll bet your dad was gloomy and resentful a lot of the time, always appearing to be the 'good guy', pleasing and sacrificing for others . . ."

"He sure was! How did you know?"

"Because most of the people I see have similar mind-sets. You need to learn to love yourself first. Otherwise, it's impossible to nurture others in a healthy way - at least not without resentment and anger. It's time to take care of *you* - because if you don't, no one else will." Dr. Irwin paused for a moment. "Jillian - how's your relationship with your husband?"

I thought about it for a moment. "Well, he tries hard and acts as if everything's fine most of the time, but I know he's angry with me for being sick so much . . ." I felt a lump in my throat, tears beginning to form. Michael wanted to do so much with me, but couldn't because most of the time I was usually sick or just too tired.

"Perhaps a lot of his anger comes from whatever he experienced earlier in his life - long before you were even in the picture. Remember, you can't help *his* anger, only your own. What you *can* do to help create a supportive environment, is to come for counselling together. That way we can deal openly and honestly with your feelings as a couple."

"We definitely need to do that . . . we sure could use the help," I mumbled, blowing my nose.

Deep in thought, Dr. Irwin gazed out the window. After a few moments she began to speak in a hushed voice, "Jillian, you must feel very lonely, misunderstood . . . even victimized. If you had cancer, diabetes or some other disease we all recognize, you'd get proper acknowledgment for your suffering. Environmental Illness is, after all, considered by many as the 'disease of neurotics'. That must make you feel very angry."

As my tears began to flow, I blurted out, "It does! I'm never believed. My own brother looks at me as if I'm crazy. Even Michael thinks I'm a little weird. I've had so little support from him. A couple of weeks ago, I had a horrible reaction to chlorine - so bad we both thought it was game over. It took *that* to make him finally believe my illness was real." I was getting angry just thinking about the years of pain and isolation. "Dr. Irwin, how do I deal with all this anger and resentment?"

"Good question, Jillian. This is where the housecleaning begins. Woody Allen once said, 'I can't express anger. I internalize it and grow a tumor instead'."

I barely managed a smile.

"It's very important that you let your anger out. Perhaps a good first step you could take is to write a letter to all those you feel have let you down. Tell them how you *really* feel . . ."

"I'm not sure I could do that. They'd be so upset!"

She smiled. "Oh, you wouldn't have to send it to them. This exercise is for *you*. The important thing is that those feelings be released."

"Oh, I see . . ." I sighed with relief.

"Then, you might want to write one to Michael, telling him how you feel about his lack of support all these years."

"Do I give it to him?"

"Not right away, but you might want to bring it to the next session when, hopefully, both of you will be here. You could read it to him then."

"Although he's much better than he was, I still have a fair bit of resentment . . ."

"That's what we need to work on together. You see, resentment and anger usually result in blame, which is one of the surest recipes for staying stuck emotionally. After venting our anger, we need to move on - make room for understanding. One way we can get to that place is to picture the other person as a small child. After all, we're really nothing more than little children deep inside. Now, think of the environment in which that child grew up. It was probably filled with criticism and shame, causing pain and suffering. This pain and suffering gets transmitted from one generation to the next . . ."

"Along with sensitivities . . ." I thought of Eva's chart, *The Family Patterns of Hidden Sensitivities*.

"Yes, that's very true. Quite often, underlying this emotional baggage is a physical imbalance. The bottom line is that we're basically all victims of victims - whatever the cause. We need to end that pattern and rid ourselves of victim consciousness in order to heal. And yes, often it means working with the body first in order to become more balanced - more open to receiving the information necessary to heal our emotional wounds. For others, healing emotionally sets the stage for healing their physical selves."

"I think I've got the physical under control now. I'm ready to do the emotional healing."

"You don't mess around, do you Jillian? You really *are* ready to let go, to move on. It takes time and effort, but you're already well on your way to freeing yourself. Letting go is the first step. It happens when you acknowledge people as a product of their environment, and acknowledge that they're doing the best they can. Then, once you've reached that level of awareness, you apply it to yourself - and let go . . ."

"Let go of what?"

"Of all the things you feel guilty about; of all the things you feel inadequate about; of all the things you criticize yourself for. Do you know what I'm talking about?"

"You mean my feelings about my illness? That I'm an inadequate wife, an absent mother? Things like that?"

"Yes, but go even deeper. We may need to explore your childhood."

"Dr. Irwin, I try so hard to be positive."

"No, no, trying is to perform - to pretend - and that's hard work. Our goal here is letting go, to achieve self-acceptance and peace of mind - all of which facilitate your physical healing."

"How do I find peace of mind?"

"Begin by stopping long enough to reflect: close your eyes, go deep inside, and be still. What comes up? What do you feel? What do you see?

One way to get in touch with that part of yourself is by quieting the mind. Meditation certainly helps me do that by letting go of thoughts as they arise. I'm not talking about suppressing them, but simply acknowledging them, touching them lightly and letting them go."

"And how can I learn to do this?"

"We have classes every week here at the clinic. We also have an outreach program that enables our patients to learn right in their own communities."

"How will I ever have time for all this? As it is now, I spend most of it in the kitchen . . ."

"This is a perfect opportunity to let go of the mother/martyr syndrome and learn to ask for help." Dr. Irwin smiled.

"I can just see Michael making meals." I said somewhat cynically.

"Well, perhaps it's time for him to start."

"Actually, now that I think about it, he *has* been pretty good lately. He probably could take on some of the cooking without much difficulty. He was great when I had that reaction to chlorine and I couldn't do a thing for myself . . ."

"Do you need to wait for things to get that desperate? Maybe, just maybe, part of your illness is caused by overloading your system - your barrel - with non-physical stressors. Asking for and accepting help may be one of the lessons you need to learn in your recovery process. We can all benefit from opening ourselves to the love, help and support that are available to us."

I thought about what she said. Perhaps she was right. There might be more to my illness than just the physical. After all, Dr. Rowland emphasized the whole person, not just the body.

"Illness often forces us to make changes. One of my patients, a mother with three young children, developed ovarian cancer. In order for her to heal, she had to undergo a complete overhaul of her lifestyle, including giving the care of the children over to their father, so she could focus her energies on healing. Healing is a full-time job. A year later, her priorities are straight and she's doing fine. Her tumor is barely detectable. She may fully recover."

"What about her children?"

"She and her husband now share the raising of the children more equitably. This is one example where illness can bring about positive change. Now, let's talk about sickness and what it means . . . "

"What it means?"

"Yes. Quite often illness gives people permission to do things they would never otherwise allow themselves to do. Bernie Siegel says it can make it easier to say no to the demands of everyday life. It can free us to do what we've always wanted, but have been too busy to start. It can provide us with the opportunity to take time off to reflect and re-evaluate our lives."

"Boy! You, Dr. Rowland and this Bernie Siegel character make it sound like this is some kind of wonderful opportunity!" I said, with a touch of sarcasm.

"Jillian, it is! It's a *perfect* opportunity to learn and grow. Your illness is already teaching you so many things. The first lesson is how out of touch you were with your own body, ignoring your intuition. Did you have any inkling that all those medications you were taking might have been the wrong course of action?"

"Yes, many times. I often questioned my doctors about the antibiotics Max and I were on. But every time I did, I was met with resistance, coupled with annoyance, irritation, even criticism. Some doctors were even patronizing. You know, I had a hunch all along that Nathaniel was bothered by certain foods, but was told repeatedly that I was an overprotective, neurotic mother and that foods had absolutely nothing to do with his behavior."

"How did that make you feel?"

"Completely stupid. As if I were worthless and knew nothing . . ."

"At any time did you ever feel that your workplace or home renovations were making you sick?"

"Yes. I could feel it all happening, but I ignored the signals. Whenever I brought it up with my doctors, they'd tell me that one had nothing to do with the other. I convinced myself they were right - after all, they were 'the experts'. Now I know better."

"You know, Jillian, I once heard a famous toxicologist lecture on health and the environment. He made a statement that will stick with me forever: *No one is an expert in anything and everyone is an expert in everything.* No one on this earth is a better expert on you or your children than *you!* We're too quick to give our power away to others. Now it's time to reclaim it. Healing helps us to do just that. Sure, we can ask for outside help or guidance, but ultimately, the truth resides inside each and every one of us."

"But Dr. Irwin, I have a real problem with the concept that sickness gives us permission to do things we normally wouldn't do. It sounds to me like a cop-out, as if I created this illness in order to get out of my responsibilities . . ."

"Well . . . that may or may not be the case, at least on a conscious level. Let me ask you a very simple question - were you happy in nursing?"

"Quite honestly, no. Intuitively, I've always felt that our approach to healthcare is wrong. Medication is used far too often, numbing not only the body but the mind. Before working at the Children's Hospital, I had a part-time job at Stadona General. If someone was depressed, we medicated. If someone was grieving, we medicated. To treat their bodies was one thing, but to numb their feelings? Drugs became the answer to everything. Deep down, I knew it was wrong."

"Could you imagine going back to nursing, knowing what you now know?"

"Never. Not unless it changed dramatically. My whole life is different now. I'm not the same person I was back in September . . ."

"Ah-ha! So maybe the higher purpose of your illness was to help you grow and evolve to the point where you could be open to listening to your inner voice - to hear the message that nursing as you know it is no longer for you . . ."

"Right! In fact, with all the information I've learned over the past few months, my life is heading in an entirely different direction."

"Is that all right with you?"

"It is. It actually feels good. But I have one major concern - I'm afraid of leaving everyone behind. They all think I'm a little strange with my new lifestyle. They just don't understand."

"How could they? They have no concept of what you're going through or what you've gone through."

"Not yet, anyway!" I exclaimed, thinking of what Dr. Rowland had said about everyone eventually being affected by their lifestyles in one way or another.

"I'll bet they all care, but don't know how to give you what you need. Remember, they're doing the best they can but aren't yet ready to make a change. They're not in the same time and space as you."

"But I want to share everything I've learned . . ."

"Jillian, your enthusiasm and your willingness to help others is so refreshing! I hope that never changes. Close your eyes and relax for a moment. I have a great image that might help you deal with some of the isolation you're feeling right now.

I sank back in my seat, feeling quite drained.

"Imagine you're on a huge ship filled with people, all of them vibrant and happy. You've just pulled away from the dock into clear weather full of warmth and sunshine. The shore you've left behind is dark, foggy, and crowded with suffering people. You tried to convince them to take the trip with you. Some came while others stayed behind - everyone made their own choice."

"But I'd want to jump off the ship, swim to shore and rescue them - especially those closest to me."

"I understand. But it would be senseless. Everyone must make their own decision when *they* are ready. The choice is not ours to make. You can wave to them, cheer them on, and encourage them should they decide to attempt the journey, but if their time hasn't come, you can do no more. Jillian, you don't ever have to go back to shore where it's dark, foggy and people are sick. The best place for you is on that ship, sailing toward the light! Your example gives others hope that there's a better place for them as well."

I opened my eyes. "That image is so powerful! I guess I need to let go of all those who aren't yet on the journey."

"You do. Their time may or may not come. It's not up to you - it's up to them. You're right where *you* need to be and they're right where *they* need to be."

"It's a hard one to let go."

"The most difficult thing in life is to let go, and ultimately, to forgive. Jillian, let me ask you a simple question. Do you feel loved?"

"Of course I do!"

"Relax and sit with the question for a while."

I closed my eyes and let the question resonate deep inside. I began to squirm, feeling very uncomfortable. My chest tightened and my belly tensed. Tears spilled down my cheeks.

Leah leaned over and put her arm around my shoulders. "You're a very honest woman, Jillian," she whispered. "This is a brave first step toward healing the pain you feel. That pain resides deep inside many of us."

"I've never felt loved!" I sobbed, thinking back to my childhood. "I never felt wanted or loved for who I was, only for what I could do . . ."

"Ah yes. Jillian, look at me . . ."

I looked at her, my sobs subsiding somewhat.

"Do you *want* to be well?"

"Of course I do. It's just that at times, it all seems so hard . . . I feel so alone . . ."

"Jillian, this is where it all begins. Everything in life is a choice. And so too, is wellness. You must *choose* wellness. Close your eyes one more time. Take some deep breaths." She guided me through a relaxation technique. I felt my body lighten and relax as never before. I felt peaceful.

Dr. Irwin said quietly, "Let yourself be with your feelings." She paused. "Where are you right now?"

"I'm in my gut and I'm starting to feel tense and frightened."

"How old are you?"

"About eleven . . ."

"What color do you see?"

"Grey. Silvery-grey all around me."

"Where are you?"

"In my grandmother's hospital room." I could feel my throat tightening, tears starting. "Her beautiful silvery-grey curls pressed against the stark, white pillow . . ." My breathing felt labored.

"What's happening? Jillian . . . what are you seeing?"

"She's slipping away . . . Don't go . . . please don't go! I need you!"

"It's okay, Jillian . . . stay with it . . . don't push it away . . ."

Sobs wracked my body. "She's dying! She's the only person who ever loved me for being *me - who accepted me for who I was*. I need her here so badly . . . " I let out an anguished wail, a sound I'd never heard before. Leah held me, silent, stroking my hair.

A few minutes passed. Once I'd calmed down, she asked softly, "Have you ever felt unconditional love from anyone at all - other than your grandmother?"

I shook my head.

"Maybe now it's time to internalize that feeling so you can call it up whenever you need to."

"How can I do that?" I asked through my tears.

"One way is to imagine your grandmother living within you. She is warm, wise and all-loving. She wants only the best for you. Do you think you'll be able to visualize her as part of you?"

I loved the image. The very thought of her was so comforting. "Yes! I can feel her," I whispered.

"Keep her with you. You can even talk with her. Just take time each day to go inward and visit. We must learn to disconnect from the hectic pace of life - even if only for a few minutes a day to reconnect with our original being. You know, Jillian, peace and tranquility already reside within you - right *now*. All you have to do is peel off the layers to allow yourself access to that core of self-acceptance."

"I'm not sure I understand."

"When you were a tiny baby, did you have to do anything to prove yourself?"

"No . . ."

"Babies are the centre of the universe. They're free to be who they are. When they're upset, they cry. When they're hungry, they're fed. Their needs are met all the time - they're loved unconditionally. Then we get older and learn to live without this kind of love. We receive only conditional love . . ."

"You mean you're loved and accepted as long as you do well in school or are pretty or sweet?"

"Exactly. This type of love is what we internalize because it's what we're taught from a very young age. Later, the critical and unforgiving internal parent takes over where our real parents leave off. This results in our inability to love ourselves in the way we need to be loved - unconditionally."

"I always thought I liked myself . . ."

"As long as what? As long as you're healthy and vibrant? Did you love yourself when you were down and out - only a few weeks ago?"

"Well . . . no, not then."

Leah reached around to a small table and pulled out a mirror. She passed it to me. "Jillian, take a look. Can you tell that person in there that you love her?"

I began to squirm and blush. "Well, it's kind of a silly exercise . . ."

"But a very revealing one. You see, most of us don't know how to love ourselves. Once we learn how to do that, everything else becomes secondary. This will be the goal of our sessions over the next little while - to show you how to gain access to that love. Hopefully, by the end of our time together, you'll be able to embrace that person with compassion, understanding and forgiveness."

I passed the mirror back to her.

"As a first step, write a letter to your parents, expressing your true feelings about the way you felt as a child . . ."

"And give it to them?" I asked, horrified at the prospect.

"No, you wouldn't have to show it to them. As we discussed earlier, this exercise is for *you*. The important thing is to articulate and release those feelings."

I sighed with relief.

"But getting back to your comment about illness being an excuse for avoiding obligations and responsibilities, why not look at it as an opportunity to make changes? Jungian psychotherapist, Arnold Mindell, said: *I don't believe that a person actually creates disease, but that his soul is expressing an important message to him through the disease.* She paused for a moment, reflected and asked, "Jillian, what do you think your soul is expressing through this illness?"

I thought for a few moments. "That I take on far too much in life, and I leave nothing for myself. That I need to ask for help long before sickness forces me into a position where I have no choice . . ."

"That's a great start! Anything else?"

"That I need to change my vocation to something more in harmony with my nature as I have come to understand it. I'm now positive that nursing as we know it, is definitely not where it's at for me . . ."

"You're doing well. Anything else?"

"That I need to be more tolerant, kind and loving toward myself. I can look at myself as that little child that needs unconditional love. I think your idea of internalizing and talking with my grandmother is brilliant."

"Why, thank you," smiled Leah. "In *Peace, Love and Healing*, Bernie Siegel says: *Illness and death are not signs of failure; what is a failure, is not living.* We are, by nature, joyful, loving creatures. Illness often forces us to acknowledge those parts of ourselves . . ."

"By backing us into a corner?" I grimaced.

"Well, sort of - at least in the sense that we are forced into making decisions - similar to the story of my patient with ovarian cancer. You can choose mere existence or to live life fully - basking in life's richness."

"I could use some basking right about now. How do I do that?"

"Once again, through meditation. It can bring us into the present - into the moment. We tend to be very past and future oriented. Our minds are always somewhere else - everywhere but where we need to be - here, now."

"Do you mean we're always worrying about tomorrow?"

"Yes. Or reminiscing about the past . . ."

"Is exercise or listening to music a form of meditation?"

"Some people think so, but I look at it as yet another way of filling space. All types of relaxation or enjoyment are important, but nothing takes the place of meditation where there are no distractions whatsoever. You are with yourself, by yourself. A famous spiritual teacher once said it so beautifully: *Yesterday is gone, tomorrow is not yet born. All we have is today.* Meditation can help us be present, be in the moment."

I couldn't help but notice Dr. Irwin's intensity and beauty. She must have been in her late fifties or early sixties. Her hair was a snowy white, elegantly swept up in a French roll. She had fine facial features, like a porcelain doll, and the deepest twinkling blue eyes I'd ever seen. She, too, had that quality I'd observed earlier in Jane, Dr. Rowland and Eva. Maybe it wasn't just their great diets. Were they all able to live more in the moment than the rest of us? Whatever it was, I, too, wanted that same quality in my life.

"Dr. Irwin, is it meditation that gives you that youthful energy, that vibrance?"

She giggled with a schoolgirl shyness. "Well, it probably contributes. You know, Jillian, meditation is so effective in reducing stress and tension, that in 1984, the National Institutes of Health recommended meditation over prescription drugs as the treatment of choice for mild hypertension."

"So it's not just a spiritual practice . . ."

"Not at all. Its health benefits are enormous. But since each of us is one being - a whole total being - it's difficult to separate the physical from the mental and the emotional from the spiritual . . . Meditation addresses all levels. I guess what I'm trying to say is that wellness is really a total package. We need a good diet, exercise, clean air and pure water. Meditation would certainly expedite recovery."

"A total overhaul, right?" I grinned.

"That's about it! Jillian, we need to take the time to ask ourselves these questions: What do we want and need? What would help us feel better? What are our feelings trying to tell us? Our bodies? Our intuition? Then we must quiet the mind so we can listen carefully - the answers will come."

"It's like making a date with yourself, right?"

She smiled, "That's a good way of putting it!"

"But if we live in the present moment, how do we plan for the future?"

"This doesn't mean that you don't plan or have a vision of what you want your future to be like. But remember, even planning takes place in the present. You work on creating something, but then you let it go - you don't dwell on it. You then focus your attention on the *process* instead of the end result. You'll find life flows much smoother this way."

"I'm not sure I understand. Can you give me an example?"

"One of my patients is a perfect example. He's a lawyer who despises the prospect of wining and dining clients in order to increase his income. He feels he's prostituting himself. I asked him why he felt that way. He replied he felt he was using people in order to get their money. "But Jim," I said, "what about the *process* - getting to know your clients personally, listening to their stories - all those pleasurable things. Why focus only on the end result?"

"So are you saying the end result will happen regardless?"

"It likely will, yes. If it doesn't, at least you'll have relaxed, and spent time enjoying the moment. Focus on the *process*, the *now*. Then you'll be completely present and the other person will feel that presence. This, in turn, will probably get you what you want and need."

"Hmm. I suppose . . ."

"Another example is in this book, *Peace is Every Step* by Thich Nhat Hanh, an internationally renowned spiritual leader and Zen teacher." She held up a small, thin book. "In it he describes the simple act of washing dishes . . ."

"What's dishwashing got to do with being in the moment and peace?"

Dr. Irwin laughed. "You obviously must plan to wash them, but the important thing is to focus on the act of washing while you perform the task, instead of going off in your head to something that happened yesterday or something that might happen tomorrow. It's this jumping in, out and all over the place that causes tension. He talks about enjoying the act of holding the dish, feeling the water, and the movement of your hands as you wash the dish. If you want to finish the dishes quickly so you can have dessert, you'll likely not enjoy the dessert either. You'll be focused on the next activity and as a result, the texture and flavor of the dessert, together with the pleasure of eating it, will be lost. You will again be focused on what is *going* to happen as opposed to what *is* happening. You're always dragged into the future instead of living in the present. Understand?"

"From the sound of it, I'm hardly ever in the moment!"

"Take heart, Jillian, very few of us are. It takes effort. To empty the mind of all the chatter and to focus on what you're doing at the time is what helps create peace in your life. By the way, Thich Nhat Hanh does admit it takes him a bit longer to do the dishes, but he says he lives *fully in every moment* - very happily."

"Gee, does he need three kids to help him with the dishes?" I joked. "On a more serious note, along with all the other changes in my life, it looks like I'm going to be working on living in the moment as well."

"It's worth it. Peace, joy and happiness are present here and now, in everything we do and see - in ourselves. All we need to do is realize it. Meditation simply unlocks the door."

"You mentioned classes at the clinic, but didn't you also say something about outreach programs?"

"A schedule is posted in the main reception area for all the upcoming classes in various locations. Emily can also give you a comprehensive reading list on creative visualization, mind-body healing and meditation. My own personal favorite is *The Language of Letting Go* by Melody Beattie. It's a collection of daily tidbits of wisdom, each one ending with a strong affirmation. This book is profound and has empowered many people." Dr. Irwin glanced at her watch. "Goodness! Our time is almost up. But before we end the session, I have something I'd like to give you." She pulled a small, round object out of her desk drawer and handed it to me. It was a button that read: *Enjoy Life! This is not a dress rehearsal!* I chuckled.

"And this leads me to my final point. Over the next few weeks, I'd like you to laugh at least three times a day. Laughter is wonderful medicine!"

"And how do I incorporate that prescription into my life? Where do I find it?"

"Anywhere and everywhere. Just allow yourself *time* to find it. It's all around you. Seek it out. Play with your children - but be fully there. Forget about your to-do list for that time. Watch a funny movie. Seek out fun-loving friends. Give yourself permission to have a ball!"

I smiled. "What about support groups? Do you think they're helpful?" I asked.

"A good idea in general, but be careful. Some people choose to dwell exclusively on their pain and suffering, keeping themselves well entrenched as victims. Others can be a wealth of information, emphasizing what's positive - the healing process. The key is not to focus on what made you sick but rather on what can make you well. You know, Jillian, some people actually become addicted to support groups."

"Are you kidding?"

"Not at all. It's quite common. Oh yes, before we end our session . . ." She passed back the mirror she had handed me earlier. "You may feel uncomfortable about telling yourself you love yourself. That may come later. But how about 'I am well, I am vital, I am healthy'?"

"But I'm not there yet . . ."

"But you mustn't wait until then . . . You need to feed those positive messages to your body *now*. It's not, 'I'm going to be well' because that doesn't address the moment. 'I am well'! Try both out for size and you'll very quickly discover the difference. 'I am well' is a very powerful message. Try it right now. Just say it aloud - even without looking in the mirror."

"I'm going to be well. I *am* well . . . I *do* feel the difference. The latter is by far the more intense of the two."

"Good. So, Jillian Stowe, you are ultimately your own healer. All you need to do is stay in touch with yourself in order to receive guidance whenever you need it. By making changes in your diet and environment, you've already taken charge of a big chunk of your life. Now, all you need is some fine-tuning."

I could see that housecleaning meant more than a change in diet and physical environment. It meant I had to take a good look at the messages my thoughts and feelings were sending to my body. That short encounter with the memory of my grandmother demonstrated their power!

I knew that Leah Irwin was right - within each of us is the wisdom that is the source of all healing. We just need to slow down, stop, look and listen. I was now ready to go inward and trust my inner teacher.

Strontium 90, released through
nuclear explosions into the air,
comes to earth in rain
or drifts down as fallout,
lodges in soil,
enters into the grass or corn
or wheat grown there,
and in time
takes up its abode
in the bones of a human being,
there to remain until his death.

Similarly, chemicals sprayed
on croplands or forests or gardens
lie long in soil,
entering into living organisms,
passing from one to another
in a chain of
poisoning and death . . .

As Albert Schweitzer has said,
"Man can hardly even recognize
the devils of his own creation."

Rachel Carson
Silent Spring

# 15

# Garden of Eden, Revisited

*When it comes to pesticide use in Canada we are a human experiment*
*without records being kept. We have chemical warfare*
*going on in our neighbourhoods.*
**Dr. June Irwin**

*A*February thaw. It was spring and my heart was singing! I hadn't
felt this good in years. I was meditating, exercising regularly, and paying
close attention to everything I put into my body. Knowing which foods
triggered my symptoms was revolutionary. I could now take responsibility
for my own health! It gave me a newfound freedom - the freedom of choice.

I was about to meet Jane Harding. Not only had she been ill herself,
but she'd nursed her four children back to health. Apparently, she was an
expert on everything I would need to know in order to make our home a
safer place. Dr. Rowland had told me that she'd been bedridden after the
birth of her third child. Today she spent a great deal of her time on the
lecture circuit, talking about how to create healthy homes and work
environments. She was even in the process of writing a book on the subject.

I rounded the corner and turned onto Lakeside Terrace. There it was,
number thirty-six. Trees and shrubs surrounded the property, a huge
weeping willow embracing an entire corner. I parked the car and proceeded
up the walk. Everywhere I looked there were raised-bed gardens with
walkways in between instead of the usual front lawn. I could just imagine
how lush everything would look in the summer.

I rang the doorbell and heard a cheerful voice say, "Just a moment. I'll
be right there!"

The door swung open. I couldn't believe my eyes! *Jane*, the woman I
had met in the schoolyard way back in September, the woman who had
launched me on this incredible journey, stood before me. She was as vibrant
and beautiful as I remembered. And there was little Abby, peeking out
from behind her mother.

Jane grabbed my arms, and squealed with delight. "Oh my God, you
did it - you really did it! You went to Gabe! Look at you - you look terrific!

Come in! When Emily called with your name, I was so excited! I can hardly wait to hear the details!" She ushered me into the front hall. My attention was immediately drawn to the glistening hardwood floors and natural light that poured in from all directions.

"Gabe?" I asked, puzzled.

"Well, yes, Gabe - Gabriel Rowland. He's a dear friend of mine. We were sick about the same time, except that he was light-years ahead of me in terms of knowledge and information. We became close friends as we struggled to find the missing links needed to resolve our health problems. So . . . what did you think of him?"

"He's an incredible human being! I guess having been ill himself makes him that much more compassionate and understanding."

Jane hung my coat in the closet. "You know, I used to wonder whether one needs to have a disease in order to understand it. Now I believe that to *truly* understand it, you really do."

"I think you're right," I said, recalling the frustration and loneliness of my own illness.

She bent over to pick up Abby. "What did you think of Eva? Isn't she a hoot? She cracks me up - she's so passionate, so into her work!"

"I've never met anyone with so much knowledge and compassion - other than Dr. Rowland, of course. No one even comes close to what she knows about diet and nutrition."

"I couldn't agree more."

"I still can't believe how great I feel!"

"Jillian, I'm so happy for you. Doesn't it boggle your mind that common foods and chemicals can make you so sick?"

"What really frustrates me is that so many people are unable to find the help they need because most nutritionists and physicians refuse to acknowledge that what goes into our bodies can be so devastating."

"It's sad, isn't it?" Jane said softly. "Their usual solution is medication, much of which is unnecessary and often, potentially harmful."

"Or surgery," I added, reflecting on my nose operations and all those needless tonsillectomies, hysterectomies and ear surgeries. "I'm just so grateful to be off medication. Now my goal is to expand my knowledge base even further. I need to learn how to make my home a safer place to live and *you*, Jane Harding, have been recommended as the expert."

"You know," she laughed, "the more I learn, the more I realize how little I really know. Come, sit in here while I make some tea."

I followed her into the kitchen and sat at the table while she put on the kettle. "Dr. Rowland mentioned that you give lectures. I believe he said your workshops were called *Creating A Healthy Home*."

"Well, after years of learning about the subject, I suppose I have quite a bit of information to share."

"Jane, I owe my recovery to you. If it hadn't been for you that day at the playground, who knows where I'd be."

"But remember," Jane touched my arm gently, "all I did was give you Gabe's name and number. You were the one who made the call, went for the appointment and followed his instructions. You accepted the responsibility - and you made the changes. Give yourself some credit. You're quite a woman!"

Feeling embarrassed, I blushed. "Nevertheless, I'm forever indebted to you for putting the bug in my ear."

Tray in hand, Jane led me to the living room. Abby sat beside her on the floor playing with crayons and coloring books. Turning to me, Jane smiled and said, "So let's continue our journey. . ."

She was right. I was on a journey, whether I liked it or not. And I could tell it was time to fasten my seat belt for the next phase! I smiled inwardly, reflecting for a moment on the vast amount of information I'd digested over the past few months. It was far more intense than any course I'd ever taken. I thought of that day at the playground, watching Jane and Abby playing on the swings. "Jane, would you say that you're completely well?"

She laughed. "What is wellness? I've often asked myself that question. Over the years, I've come to understand that wellness is really a journey, not a destination."

"What do you mean?"

"Simply that we are evolving organisms, constantly interacting with an ever-changing environment, where nothing is static. We're always in a state of flux. We never really arrive. We only reach plateaus every once in a while and then move on. The minute we feel we've made it, everything changes and we need to adapt again."

"So are you suggesting we're always in process?"

"Yes, I believe we are - we never stop changing, adapting. At one time, I felt that if I did all the right things, I would reach a state of health and stay that way forever. Now I realize how naive that was. But you'll know what I mean once you've been on the path a bit longer . . . "

Just then, the doorbell rang. "I'll be right back. It's probably my sitter coming for Abby."

"Abby, Holly's here! Come on sweetie, time to go." Abby abandoned her crayons and raced out the door. After a few moments, Jane returned. Pouring the tea, she continued, "So, you're here to learn about how you, too, can have a healthy home. Today, we'll just be able to cover the basics. I hope you don't mind, but I invited a few people who missed my last workshop to join us in a little while."

"That's fine with me. A group always makes for a more stimulating discussion."

"That's what I always say."

The doorbell rang again. As Jane went to answer it, I leafed through a couple of books on the coffee table. The first one that caught my attention was *Your Home, Your Health, Your Wellbeing* by Rousseau, Rea and Enwright. The information appeared to be specific, practical and included great illustrations of healthy versus unhealthy indoor environments - a very user-friendly book. The other was *The Healthy House* by John Bower. A line near the beginning summed it up: *If there were more healthy houses there would be more healthy people.*

I was deeply engrossed in one of the chapters when I heard footsteps approach and the sound of voices. Jane appeared, followed by a rather handsome, bearded young man and a plump woman, closer to my age.

"Jillian, I'd like you to meet Martha Webster, a neighbor of mine, and Andrew Coughlin . . ."

As they introduced themselves, the doorbell rang once more. Jane excused herself again.

"You sick too?" asked Andrew, looking at me.

"Yes, but I'm much better than I was a few months ago. Once I discovered that foods were causing much of my grief and that the water I was drinking was toxic to my body, I began to mend."

"Doesn't it blow your mind that most doctors aren't onto this? I'm still amazed - no, not amazed - outraged would be a better word. They still want to medicate or write you off as a hypochondriac!"

I could relate to his anger. Martha quietly added, "I was depressed for years and never knew why. It got worse after my last child was born. All they offered me were drugs, drugs . . . and more drugs. One night, after hearing Eva speak at a conference, I discovered I had other options. I've never looked back. But, along the way, it cost me a great deal - my job and my marriage."

"Because of your sensitivities?"

"It sure had a lot to do with it. Most of the time I wasn't operating with a full deck. I'd fly off the handle at the slightest thing. I spent a good deal of time crying, my sex drive was at an all-time low, and I was sixty-five pounds heavier than I am now. You can only imagine what it was like!" I think she knew, by the look on everyone's faces that we'd all been there. "But the worst part was that my husband never believed me. He never believed I was physically sick because all the tests would come back negative. He'd accuse me of being lazy, unmotivated. Nothing could've been further from the truth."

"That's the worst," Andrew commiserated. "Being doubted and unsupported, especially by those you love. It makes you feel so alone." We all nodded, empathizing with every word he said. It was sad, yet I felt somewhat reassured to be with people who really understood.

"Jillian, Martha, Andrew, I'd like you to meet Samantha Webber . . ."

"Just call me Sam," smiled the pretty young woman standing in the doorway beside Jane.

"Sam, please find a seat and help yourself to a cup of tea."

Andrew turned to the newcomer. "And what brings you here, Sam? Poison in your food, water, or air?"

His bitterness and anger cut like a knife. Beneath it was real pain. I felt it. I knew it. I'd been there - and not so very long ago.

"Actually, I guess you could say it was the air. My two children and I were poisoned by pesticides."

"Pesticides?" asked Martha. She sounded surprised, and immediately stopped leafing through the book on her lap.

"You know, the kind you spray on your lawn year after year for that perfect turf - just like all your neighbours. You know, the stuff that's supposed to be perfectly safe . . ."

Andrew snorted, "Oh yeah, the same way carpeting, airtight buildings, additives, colorings and preservatives in our foods are safe!"

"While you're at it," added Martha, "don't forget breast implants and estrogen replacement therapy." She sounded almost as cynical as Andrew.

Sam continued in her quiet way. "They don't tell you that chemicals like 2,4-D, marketed under more than forty different trade names and commonly found in granular fertilizer and weed-killer mixtures, can be dangerous - and these pesticides are considered among the *least* harmful. In fact, one lawn care company told me it was safe enough to roll in it! I later learned that organophosphates can be potent neurotoxins."

"And then there are the so-called inert ingredients, "continued Jane, "that can comprise up to ninety-nine percent of a pesticide solution - and are usually a trade secret due to competition. They consist of substances as benign as water and as harmful as neurotoxic chemicals, which can damage the central nervous system and the brain. For example, xylene - an 'inert' used in almost 2,000 pesticide products - can cause impaired memory, organ damage, hearing loss and fetal death. Others are known carcinogens."

"Great!" Andrew exclaimed, "Agent Orange - right in your backyard!"

I shuddered at the analogy.

"And to make matters worse," added Sam, obviously up on the subject, "the EPA's evaluation of hazards is generally based only on the active ingredient, not the inerts. But what's really a shocker is that chemicals banned as actives can turn up as inerts!"

"All we really need to ask is a basic question," suggested Jane. "If a substance is lethal enough to kill weeds and insects, what does it do to our bodies?"

"And not only are pesticides on lawns," murmured Sam, "but they're in the very food we eat."

I recalled my session with Eva Sandor at Dr. Rowland's clinic. "When I first heard about these insidious chemicals on our food, I just sat there with my mouth open - in shock - at the number of allowable pesticides used on fruits and vegetables we eat every day."

"The reality is that we live in a pesticide smog and there's probably not a corner of this earth that hasn't been contaminated by pesticide residues. And North Americans seem to be the worst offenders. In 1984, the United States alone used 34 percent of the total volume of all pesticides applied; Western Europe used 19 percent; the Far East, 16 percent; Latin America, 10 percent; Eastern Europe and Russia, another 8 percent; with the balance of the world using the remaining 13 percent. . ."

"We're really leading the way to self-destruction," mumbled Andrew, "and for what?"

Jane continued to rhyme off statistics,". . . and 43 percent of all pesticides used were herbicides; fungicides accounted for 18 percent; while other pesticides accounted for the rest. So given these figures, it shouldn't come as a surprise that the primary source of toxic pollution from upper income urban homes is lawn pesticides."

"It sure isn't a surprise to my family." Sam looked as if she was about to cry. Her voice then took on a sharper tone. "I still find it hard to believe I live a culture where having a perfect lawn takes precedence over health!"

"What happened to you and your family, Sam, only confirms that the suburban dream of a well-manicured lawn is fast becoming a suburban nightmare. North Americans are overdosing their lawns with chemicals they know nothing about . . ."

"And I'll have you know, these products are far from safe!" Sam's indignation was obvious. "Not only are pesticides linked to neurotoxicity, declining male fertility rates and birth defects, but they are cancer-causing as well. And these are the same chemicals with which we regularly douse our lawns - just to get rid of a few little bugs and weeds!"

The poor woman! I wondered how I would have handled a similar situation had it been my children who had become ill from such a needless practice.

"And are you aware that in the U.S., lawncare companies are legally prohibited from claiming their products as safe, but that no such protection exists for Canadian consumers?"

"I believe it," replied Andrew. "Years ago, long before becoming ill, I asked the head greenskeeper at one of the golf clubs about the pesticides that were used on the course. His reply was that the chemicals they used were government-approved and practically non-toxic. In fact, he actually went on to state that my child would have to eat several cupfuls of treated grass before he'd experience any side effects!"

"Had we taken him up on his suggestion, we'd likely all be dead!" retorted Sam.

"I'd also suggest he take a look at this," said Jane, retrieving a chart from her folder. "These figures are based on EPA documents, standard toxicology references and extensive files from the National Coalition Against the Misuse of Pesticides (NCAMP)(fig. 14). As you can see, it's not a pretty picture."

We studied the chart for a few minutes. Out of thirty-six pesticides, 30 were sensitizers; 21 neurotoxic; 15 caused kidney/liver damage; 14 were linked to birth defects; and 13 were carcinogenic. How ignorant we were of the harm these chemicals caused! I wondered if everyone needed to become sick, like us, before heeding the warnings. What was it about human nature that required a catastrophe to bring the point home?

"2,4-D has an X in every category!" exclaimed Sam.

"Jane, I get all mixed up with the terms pesticide, insecticide and herbicide. Could you explain the differences?"

"Pesticide is a broad term that encompasses all pest-killing substances, including insecticides, which kill insects; fungicides, which kill fungi and molds; herbicides, which kill weeds; rodenticides, which kill rodents; and nematicides, which kill worms."

"And if I refer back to my high school Latin classes," interrupted Andrew, "cidium or cida means to kill."

"So we can safely deduce that by definition alone, pesticides are toxic. They're designed to kill various forms of life. There are two commonly used groups of pesticides - insecticides and herbicides. The insecticide agents most commonly used on lawns and gardens are diazinon, malathion, propoxur, chlorpyrifos and carbaryl . . ."

# Most Commonly Used Lawn Pesticides and their Health Effects

## (fig. 14)

| | Cancer | Birth Defects | Reproductive Effects | Neurotoxicity | Kidney/Liver Damage | Sensitizer |
|---|---|---|---|---|---|---|
| **INSECTICIDES** | | | | | | |
| Acephate | C | | | X | | X |
| Bendiocarb | | | | X | | X |
| Carbaryl | | X | X | X | X | X |
| Chlorpyrifos | | | X | X | X | X |
| DDVP | C | | | X | | |
| Diazinon | | | | X | X | X |
| Isazophos | | | | X | | X |
| Isofenphos | | | | X | | X |
| Malathion | | X | | X | | X |
| Methoxychlor | | | X | | | X |
| Trichlorfon | | X | | X | | X |
| **HERBICIDES** | | | | | | |
| Atrazine | C | X | | X | X | X |
| Benefin | | | | | | X |
| Bensulide | | | | X | X | X |
| 2,4-D | X1 | X | X | X | X | X |
| DSMA | | | | X | | X |
| Dacthal | X2 | | | | X | X |
| Dicamba | | X | | | X | X |
| Diphenamid | | | | | | |
| Endothall | | X | | | | |
| Glyphosate | | | X | | | X |
| Isoxaben | C | | | | X | |
| MCPA | | X | X | X | | X |
| MCPP | | X | X | X | X | X |
| MSMA | | | | X | | X |
| Pendimethalin | X3 | X3 | | X | X | |
| Pronamide | C | | | | X | X |
| Siduron | | | | | | X |
| Trifluralin | C | | X | | X | X |
| **FUNGICIDES** | | | | | | |
| Benomyl | C | X | X | X | | X |
| Chlorothalonil | B2 | | | | X | X |
| Maneb | B2 | X | | X | X | X |
| PCNB | | X | | | | X |
| Sulfur | | | | | | X |
| Triadimefon | | X | | | | |
| Ziram | X4 | X | X | X | | X |
| **TOTALS** | **13** | **14** | **11** | **21** | **15** | **30** |

### Source documents: EPA, Standard Toxicology and NCAMP files

B2 = EPA probable human carcinogen   X2 = contamination by Dioxin & HCB
C  = EPA possible human carcinogen   X3 = contamination by chlorobenzene
X  = demonstrated adverse effects   X4 = National Toxicology Program studies
X1 = NCI epidemiological evidence

Information supplied by: **Ecology Action Centre**, Halifax, N.S., Canada

"I've only heard of the first two . . ."

"No wonder. The 600 or so basic pesticides are marketed in 45,000 to 50,000 different commercial formulations and under a wide variety of trade names. They're found in wasp and hornet killers, ant traps, grub killers, soil insecticides, and fruit and garden pesticide solutions. For instance, propoxur is commercially known as Baygon, chlorpyrifos as Dursban, and carbaryl is known as Sevin . . ."

"The neighbor behind me sprays diazinon in every corner of his yard," said Andrew with disgust. "Between that and his lawn chemicals, we have to keep our windows closed most of the growing season."

"A wise move," commented Jane. "Since all living creatures are biochemically similar, we can assume that given certain conditions, pesticides can harm humans as well. According to NCAP - the Northwest Coalition for Alternatives to Pesticides - diazinon can produce abnormal chromosomes in human cells. Farmers who are exposed to it have an increased frequency of lymphoma . . ."

"And I know that golf courses have banned its use . . ." interjected Andrew. "

"Carbaryl isn't much better. Exposure can cause abnormal sperm in workers and an increase in brain cancer in children living in houses where it's used."

"Children are especially susceptible to these chemicals," observed Sam.

"Certainly studies in animals have indicated that the young are more vulnerable to pesticides than adults. It's true for any chemical, since the breathing rates of children are more rapid than those of adults. In fact, just a few days ago, the *American Journal of Public Health* published a study that adds to the growing concern that pesticide use in and around the home may be associated with cancer in children. Although the study doesn't prove that any of these chemicals are carcinogenic, children whose yards were treated with herbicides and insecticides had four times the risk of cancer."

"And of course they haven't proven that certain chemicals are carcinogenic since none of the more commonly used pesticides have ever been completely evaluated!"

"This conversation reminds me of a grotesque scene at my friend's place last summer," began Martha. "Her newborn son was napping in his carriage on the back deck. Esther glanced out the window only to notice a figure dressed in protective gear from head to toe - gas mask and all - spraying the lawn next door. She ran out, grabbed the baby, and immediately began screaming at the guy to stop. These companies can spray without giving any warning to anyone!"

Jane nodded, "And pesticides are the second most frequent cause of poisoning in young children . . . after medication. Sixty percent of the pesticide cases reported to poison control centers in 1988 involved children under the age of six."

"But acute, as well as chronic symptoms of pesticide poisoning, such as headaches, nausea, diarrhea," Sam pointed out, "are often chalked up to other illnesses, like the flu.

Jane nodded in agreement. "That's right. No one makes the connection." She then explained, "Then, you have the second group - the herbicides, such as 2,4-D, MCPP or mecoprop, and glyphosate - the three most common pesticides applied to North American properties. While not as acutely toxic as the commonly-used insecticides, their chronic hazards can be serious."

"My favorite sport for years was golf," began Andrew. "I took up the game because it was an activity where I could relax in the midst of an outdoor paradise - you know, green grass, trees, beautiful skies, water. I've since learned that golf courses are among the highest users of chemicals in the world. According to Dr. Melvin Reuber, formerly with the Washington, D.C. based National Coalition Against the Misuse of Pesticides (NCAMP), ten of the pesticides used on fairways are known carcinogens."

"A study sponsored by the Golf Course Superintendents Association of America (GCSAA) revealed that superintendents have a higher rate of mortality from several different cancers, two of which have been linked to pesticide exposure - non-Hodgkin's lymphoma and brain cancer."

"God only knows what I'll end up with!" exclaimed Andrew. "All I know is that when my illness was at its worst, I couldn't even go near the course. I had to stop playing."

"What would happen?" I was dying to know.

"For starters, my legs would ache and my throat would burn. But far worse, my brain would fog up to the point where I couldn't think clearly or articulate words. Can you imagine me - speechless?"

Somehow, I had a difficult time conjuring up an image of a subdued Andrew.

"If that wasn't bad enough, I'd be highly agitated one minute, then deeply depressed the next - so depressed I wanted to end it all - yes, even kill myself. It was *months* before I made the connection. I tell you, treated golf courses have to be one of the biggest hoaxes of bringing nature to urban life . . ."

"If any of you hear about a golf course that doesn't use pesticides, be sure to let me know . . ."

"I read recently that Eagle's Nest is experimenting with integrated turf management. You might want to look into it further."

"You seem to be up on golf courses, Jillian. Do you play?"

"No, but my husband does. I just happened to come across that article during my own research into pesticides."

"In 1991, a survey involving Japanese doctors," Jane stated, "indicated that of 500 patients with suspected poisoning from agricultural chemicals, 125 were associated with golf courses, 97 of them being employees. Symptoms included skin rashes, respiratory illnesses, asthma, allergic rhinitis, disorders of the eye, ear and throat, and damage to the central nervous system. In response, a Japanese company announced plans to build fifteen chemical-free courses."

"I think I'll move to Japan!"

"You may not have to go that far," smiled Jane. "As Jillian mentioned, there are courses that are aiming to reduce, even eliminate, these chemicals, primarily due to public pressure."

"Hallelujah! We should compile a list."

Sam piped up, "You might also be interested to know that the average homeowner who applies pesticides to his lawn uses ten times more per acre than most farmers."

"And did you know that Environment Canada states that 2,4-D can remain on the lawn for up to *six weeks*, even though requirements for signs posted on those same lawns are mandatory for only forty-eight hours?"

"Oh, do you mean those skimpy little signs that are barely noticeable?" Andrew never missed an opening.

"They are a bit of a joke, aren't they?" scoffed Martha.

"How old are your children?" I asked Sam.

"Naomi's six. Malcolm's only two."

"How did you know that it was pesticides and not something else that made you sick?" questioned Andrew.

"Because right after the lawn care company sprayed the neighborhood, Malcolm developed skin rashes and breathing difficulties. Naomi and I got sore throats we couldn't shake, and we all suffered from chronic diarrhea. At first, we thought we had a bad case of the flu. Before long, I realized what had happened. I could taste chemicals in my mouth. My memory was shot. I still have problems recalling simple things like my post box number. Ever since that day we haven't been able to fight any bugs and we get every virus that's on the go. It seems that we're always sick. We begin to react immediately if we go near areas that have been sprayed. One of my responses is instant, uncontrollable crying. It's become a nightmare . . ."

You could have heard a pin drop. Her story was akin to a twenty-first century horror movie.

" . . . My children can't play outdoors in spring and summer because they've become hypersensitive to pesticides - especially to those applied to lawns. And now we're all sensitive to just about everything - foods, perfumes, dust - things that were never problems before."

"What Sam has just described is known in environmental medicine as 'the spreading phenomenon'," Jane explained. "A massive exposure to one chemical can lead to sensitivities to other substances that had previously never posed a problem. The difficulty lies in being able to unravel the mechanism that would prove cause and effect."

"Right!" scoffed Andrew. "If you can't prove it, it doesn't exist."

"I'm just curious, Sam," began Martha, "did you ever have any tests done?"

"Yes, we did. Our urine and blood were sent to a toxicology lab where they found high concentrations of several chemicals . . . 2-4,D was just one. Besides detecting high levels of chemicals classified as inerts, they also found high levels of mecoprop and chlorpyrifos, the latter being one of the most widely used insecticides in the U.S. today."

"No one ever offered me tests like that when I was trying to find out what was happening to me," mumbled Andrew.

"Are you seeing Dr. Rowland?" I asked.

"Not yet. He's so heavily booked, but I have an appointment in six weeks."

"You might want to ask him to check for pesticides," suggested Sam. "But if you're checking for 2,4-D, the specimen has to be sent within seventy-two hours of exposure, since it's rapidly eliminated from the body . . ."

"That's very true," added Jane, "but its effects can persist for years."

"It certainly can!" exclaimed Sam. "And it can sensitize you to many other substances." She directed her gaze towards Andrew. "The lab that did our urine and blood also analyzes a wide range of chemicals, many of which are found in the workplace. Mind you, your family doctor may not know about these tests. You have to ask specifically for them and there's a charge - one I gladly paid."

"I wonder if I should get it done," I said, thinking aloud.

"Hey, you're looking so great you probably don't need it."

"Why, thank you, Andrew." I could feel myself blush. As good as I looked and felt, I did want to know what was floating around in my body. "Being informed is the name of the game."

Sam continued, "We're presently undergoing detoxification therapy to rid our bodies of this stuff . . ."

"Detoxification therapy?" Martha looked puzzled.

"We have to take frequent saunas and huge amounts of supplements. The only foods we can tolerate are those free of pesticides. In addition, we have to use neutralizing drops twice a day so we can at least function. That's why I'm here today - to learn how to reduce our total load even more - by making our home cleaner and safer. As far as our outdoor environment is concerned, I'm afraid we'll have no choice but to move, since so many of our neighbors still continue to spray chemicals."

"Where's it safe to move these days?" asked Martha.

"We're thinking about a place in the country where we can own a larger piece of land. That way, we'll at least be able to have more control over our immediate environment . . ."

"Good luck!" grunted Andrew disdainfully. "Then you run into farming areas that are commercially sprayed - nowadays, even Christmas tree farms!"

"Well . . . you might be right about that . . . But do you know what grosses me out the most? Even after informing my neighbors that several studies have shown that children from homes where pesticides are used are more likely to develop cancer, they still continue to spray. Information that links breast, prostate, liver and brain cancers to pesticides doesn't deter them either. I just don't get it!"

"But remember, it's a multi-billion dollar industry. Their employees are well-coached to respond to consumers' questions and concerns. The latest words they like to use are 'green industry' or 'enviro-something', but don't be fooled. Their main business is selling toxic chemicals that make them bundles of money. Dr. Phillip Szmedra, of the U.S. Department of Agriculture's Economic Research Service said there would be a two billion dollar economic impact on industry if 2,4-D were banned. And that's just *one* chemical! So you can bet it'll be around to stay - as long as we continue to buy."

"And don't forget that grass is only one item in the yard that's routinely sprayed. What about trees, shrubs, flower and vegetable gardens? The average homeowner can walk into any hardware store or plant nursery, purchase these pesticides, and indiscriminately spritz these chemicals to his heart's content - without a clue as to what's in those containers, or how they interact with one another . . ."

"Or, how all these chemicals used in combination affect human beings!" remarked Sam."

"That's right," nodded Jane. "Once again, we're looking at the chemical soup phenomenon - which brings to mind something Rachel Carson wrote in *Silent Spring*." She fumbled through a pile of books on the chair next to her. "Ah! Here it is." Opening it to a dog-eared page, she read: *The piling up of chemicals from so many different sources creates a total exposure that cannot be measured. It is meaningless, therefore, to talk about safety of any specific amount of residue.*"

"Nothing could be closer to the truth," proclaimed Martha. "I have a dear friend who has to move out of her house a couple of weeks every spring and fall while her neighborhood is saturated with these so-called 'safe' chemicals."

"What happens to her when she's exposed?"

"Symptoms similar to those you and Andrew described. Within moments, she's reduced from a happy, positive, self-confident person to a candidate for the psychiatric unit. Her self-esteem vanishes right before your eyes. She goes from despair, to hysteria, to being suicidal. If that's not bad enough, she also gets physical symptoms. She writhes on the floor in agony from stomach pain. Her diarrhea and headaches can last days. It's heartbreaking to watch."

"You see, it's these types of reactions," said Jane, "that no one ever connects to the culprit. Yet, these symptoms are on the rise. Most people have no idea of the damage these chemicals can cause. And just like your family, there are increasing numbers of people who can't go outdoors in the warm weather because of their high levels of reactivity. In this neighborhood alone, there are several people who have to wear masks in order to go for a stroll! It truly is reminiscent of science fiction . . . And I'll bet there are many more who don't connect their everyday symptoms to the lawn spraying."

"I used to think people who wore masks were whacked out - totally weird - until I got sick."

Jane acknowledged Andrew's honesty and continued to speak. "Dr. David Collison, in *Why Do I Feel So Awful?*, states that by 1980, 400 synthetic chemicals had been identified in human tissue, mainly in blood, breast milk, liver and nerve tissue. By 1986, there was not a single known species of animal on this earth, humans included, from Antarctica to the most extreme reaches of the North, that was free of traces of DDT, a pesticide that's stored in fatty tissue. Although many of us have lived to tell this tale, others haven't been quite so lucky. This particular pesticide was considered at one time to be our salvation - it rang in the Green Revolution. Just look at the horror stories now."

"I've read studies that indicate that pesticides have the ability to mimic estrogen."

"If that's true, then we must be swimming in a *sea* of estrogen," Sam said scornfully. "At least it's true where I live!"

"Women in specific areas of Long Island, New York, that were constantly sprayed with DDT, have one of the highest rates of breast cancer in the U.S.," said Jane. "In fact, in early 1993, a study showed that women with a high concentation of DDT residues were four times as likely to develop breast cancer as other women. A recent article by Dr. Carolyn DeMarco, author of *Take Charge of Your Body*, states that another study, of 229 New York women, showed that those who developed breast cancer had higher levels of PCBs, DDE, and other pesticides in their fatty tissues than those who didn't develop cancer. She goes on to say that when levels of the pesticides DDT, lindane and BHC in Israeli dairy products (previously 100 to 800 per cent greater than in U.S. dairy products) were reduced, the breast cancer death rate fell dramatically - by approximately 20 per cent."

"Even though it's been off the market for two decades now, DDT continues to haunt us," murmured Sam.

"What more proof do we need!" Now it was my turn to be angry. "I've lost two close friends to breast cancer over the past year. Something's definitely wrong! What's it going to take? More statistics - more deaths?"

"Well, from reading the report entitled *Measures of Progress Against Cancer*, put out by the National Cancer Institute - yes. With the exception of colorectal, breast and lung cancers, all of the prevention trials are either pharmaceutically-based or non-existent. When I read that pesticides were at the top of the list as a prime epidemiological or etiological factor in brain cancer, I expected to see at least *some* indication that attempts at reducing pesticide use would be one of the main strategies recommended. No such luck! I was appalled."

"No wonder," sighed Andrew. "It *is* appalling! I would think that stopping organochlorine pollution of the environment should be one of the priorities in cancer prevention strategies."

"I agree wholeheartedly, Andrew. Nevertheless, we must put everything into proper perspective," suggested Jane. "I really believe that it's the *combination* of exposures to many different sources of estrogen that creates the monster."

"What do you mean?" No sooner had I asked than I began to answer my own question. "Oh, I get it." I was thinking aloud. "You mean like the constant exposure to lawn pesticides, oral contraceptives, residues in our food, and estrogen replacement after menopause . . ."

"Yes," replied Jane, "although to trigger responses such as what Sam and her children experienced, a one-time exposure could be sufficient. These chemicals are potent sensitizers. Everyone has a particular level of tolerance and no one knows what that level is. That's what's frightening about all this. By the way, did you know that the use of 2,4-D and other lawn pesticides has been linked to malignant lymphoma in dogs? That study is right out of the *Journal of the National Cancer Institute*. Often, a health threat to pets brings the message home faster than a threat to ourselves or our children."

"Or our cars," said Andrew cuttingly. "I remember a meeting last year where we were discussing a proposed garbage incinerator. Some of those who attended were from an area near a group of smokestacks. Their biggest concern was that the emissions were damaging their cars! My question to them was, 'Hey guys, if it's doing that to your cars, what's it doing to your lungs? What's it doing to your overall health'?"

"The lesson in all this," Martha said quietly, "is that we just can't assume anything to be safe until we've thoroughly researched everything connected with it."

"Our entire existence would be spent checking everything out!" exclaimed Andrew. "We'd be too busy to do anything else. You know the old saying 'get a life'? We wouldn't have a life!"

"That's true," said Martha, "But another option is to try to avoid anything about which we're unsure. That which we believe to be safe is often harmful. Why just the other day, my neighbor two doors down inadvertently poisoned her cat . . ."

"Who's that?" asked Jane.

"Sylvia Murphy. You know, the one who bought Harrison's old house?"

"Ah yes . . . The woman with the three kids."

"Well, last summer her cat had fleas. So like any good pet owner, Sylvia went to the local grocery store to buy flea powder and a flea collar - you know, those white ones you see on so many animals. She dusted the cat lightly with the powder, put the collar on its neck and went about her business. A couple of hours later, she went upstairs to get ready for bed. There was the cat - unable to move, barely breathing."

"It wasn't the flea powder, was it?" Sam's eyes widened in disbelief. She shrugged her shoulders. "Why do I continue to be surprised?"

Martha continued her story. "She called the vet right away. He told her to immediately cut the collar off and immerse the cat in a bath - to wet it down to the skin, so the flea powder would wash off. It wasn't until much later that Sylvia read in a cat book that flea collars should be stretched and left outside to offgas for at least three days. Apparently, when they're first purchased, the concentration is far too high. Other sources suggest that these products should never be used. Both carbaryl and dichlorvos, two common active ingredients in these collars are toxic organophosphates."

"That's awful!" I cried. "What happened to the cat?"

"The cat was fine by the next afternoon, but it really was touch and go all night."

"An environmentally ill cat! So what else is new?" commented Andrew.

"I can't believe manufacturers are allowed to sell such dangerous products!" I was outraged.

"Especially when there are alternatives to flea control that are far less harmful," said Martha.

"Using pesticides, whether on a lawn, a bush, or on an animal, is like having a time bomb ticking away. It may never go off, but there are no guarantees. In fact, using any of these products as a preventive is about as ridiculous as using chemotherapy on a healthy person - 'just in case they get cancer'."

"Or giving an antibiotic to a child with a cold 'in case it develops into something more serious'!" I couldn't help but bring it up, considering how common the practice was - and what I'd learned about its side effects.

"And next to these 'safe' flea collars for our pets," added Andrew, "are tins of fly sprays, roach powders and pest strips - all of which contain dangerous chemicals."

"And right alongside our foods - in the grocery store!"

"It seems we have to be experts in everything these days or else suffer potentially catastrophic consequences," commented Martha.

"Life in the nineties, folks!" Andrew was right on the mark.

"I must read to you an excerpt from *Why Do I Feel So Awful?*:

> One of the most senior Australian public servants charged with overseeing the use of pesticides and herbicides said publicly not long ago that critics of 2,4,5-T and 2,4-D spraying programs were quite wrong in linking these herbicides with the high rate of birth abnormalities in people frequently exposed to them, even though both had long been known to be teratogens. 'Such abnormalities,' he said, 'could equally well occur in a group living in the vicinity of a pizza parlour or a telephone box.'
>
> Earlier, he had declared that the whole herbicide controversy had been drummed up by the marijuana growers, afraid that their crops would be wiped out by spraying.
>
> I think we still have a long, long way to go.

As extreme as this attitude may sound, it's far too often true when speaking with government officials - although, there are some agencies that are looking towards reducing the amount of pesticides used - especially in lawns and gardens. In fact, Environment Canada has a fact sheet called *Alternatives to Pesticides in Yards and Gardens*. It's full of statements such as: *Pesticides are poisons, otherwise they wouldn't work; Like any poisons around the home, pesticides should be used as a last resort and with extreme caution; Using a pesticide can be compared to taking a prescription drug, in that the benefits must be weighed against the side effects. Pesticides alleviate symptoms, but do not provide a cure.* It encourages homeowners to look at non-chemical pest control alternatives."

"So what do you do if you have a huge lawn and want it to look as good as everyone else's?" asked Martha.

"There are many options," replied Jane. "The first possibility is to do what I did - do away with the lawn altogether. As you probably noticed, my entire front yard is landscaped with raised gardens. In summer it becomes a paradise - in which I grow herbs, vegetables and annual flowers. Surrounding the beds are flowering shrubs, interlocking stones and perennials. More and more people are adopting this style of landscaping."

"It's certainly popular in England and Europe." I remembered being impressed with their gardens and the way they made the most of them.

"If you do decide to go with a lawn, your first step would be to have the earth tested for fertility and pH levels. You can have that done for a nominal fee. Essential nutrients include nitrogen, phosphorus and potassium. Then make sure you plant the type of grass that's appropriate for the conditions in which it's meant to grow. In other words, you wouldn't plant the same variety for a dry, sunny spot as you would in a damper, shadier part of the yard. Ground cover is another option."

"What about weeds?" asked Martha.

"I dig them out, but each year I have fewer of them because the healthier the soil, the less prone it is to weeds and pests. Just as your body needs good nourishment, so too, does your lawn. I encourage clover because it adds nitrogen. Feeding it natural fertilizers like compost, manure and seaweed is like feeding your body the best of food. Using synthetic fertilizers and pesticides leaves it more prone to disease. Then, it becomes drug-dependent. These chemicals disrupt the natural balance, repelling or killing earthworms and microbes that are the essence of healthy soils."

"It reminds me of the effect that overuse of antibiotics has on our bodies."

"A great analogy, Martha!" exclaimed Jane. "Next, de-thatching regularly with a brisk raking, and aerating the lawn in spring and fall, both help to keep the lawn healthy, thereby keeping weeds down to a minimum."

"What do you mean by aerate?" I asked.

"Aerating is a process where holes are punched in the soil to reduce compaction. This practice enables the water, nutrients and organic matter to penetrate the soil, thereby encouraging deeper rooting of the grass. Some people use aerators; others use pitchforks. Last year, I bought a pair of aerating shoes which are similar to golf shoes, except the prongs are much longer and you strap them on your regular walking shoes."

"I remember watching you walk around with those on!" laughed Martha.

"And as I recall, you want to borrow them this spring. Then there'll be *two* 'weirdos' walking around this neighborhood!" laughed Jane, turning back to face us. "But the most important rule of thumb is to keep your mower blades sharp and keep the grass fairly long, since taller grass will help to shade the soil, grow longer roots, and crowd out weeds."

"And don't rake up the grass clippings," suggested Sam. "Once free of chemicals, they act as a natural fertilizer for your lawn."

"That's right. Also, don't forget to water slowly and deeply in dry spells. Never water in strong sun or heat as the grass will burn, and don't water at night. Cool moisture can shock the grass, while dampness encourages disease. A tip when watering, is to place cups at different distances from the sprinkler. Irrigate until one inch of water has accumulated in the cups."

"So, essentially, the deal is to get to know your lawn in the same way you should know your body," commented Andrew.

"Exactly! It's the only way you can practice true prevention."

"Just recently," said Sam, "I came across an elderly gentleman who shared his secret to having a picture-perfect lawn, without synthetic fertilizers or pesticides. He told me that besides using fishmeal and pulling weeds by hand, he overseeded his entire yard every fall. And guess what? The total cost of that was one bag of good quality grass seed. This guy had the best lawn on the block. So it *can* be done!"

"It sure can," agreed Jane. "My backyard is also living proof that one can have an exquisite lawn without using one ounce of synthetic fertilizers or pesticides. No lawn is worth the very serious health risks created from routinely using harmful chemicals. Always remember, finding information about chemical-free management strategies is harder than finding information about pesticide products. In fact, if you're shopping around for a lawn care company, be sure to ask if their staff has been trained in Integrated Pest Management. The second question to ask is if they have a strong organic lawn care program."

"What's Integrated Pest Management?" asked Martha.

"It's an approach that focuses on prevention by considering the ecosystem as a whole. In terms of yard care, this includes ideas such as selecting the proper variety of plants and grasses for your location, monitoring potential problems, and recognizing that pests are part of the natural ecosystem whose presence should be expected and tolerated to a certain extent. In the beginning, organic lawn care is somewhat more expensive and more labor-intensive, but after a couple of years, it actually becomes far less expensive as the natural synergy is restored."

"So if I wanted to educate my neighborhood in this area, how would I go about it?" asked Andrew.

"You can start with one of these." Jane picked an object out of her bag of props and held it up for all to see. It was a pink wooden tulip. On it were the words: SUPPORT A CHEMICAL FREE LAWN. "It's from a no-pesticide campaign modelled after one created in Halifax, Nova Scotia. We commission their manufacture from a sheltered workshop. Each neighborhood sets up an environmental committee that sells them door-to-door for a nominal fee. They also distribute a brochure titled *Get Your Lawn Off Drugs*. It's always accompanied by a letter explaining the rationale for the program - that they want to make their community a safer place in which to live."

"What a great idea!" exclaimed Sam. "There may be hope yet!"

"How successful has the program been?" asked Andrew.

"If you take a drive around," said Jane, "you'll notice quite a few of these hot pink tulips popping up on lawns. All in all, I'd say the program has been quite effective. For example, if we know a particular homeowner is an avid user of pesticides, we try to educate the neighbors. Once they all have these pink tulips on their lawns, it puts pressure on the offending homeowner to follow suit."

"Great idea!" exclaimed Martha, "And done in a direct, but relatively subtle way. Sam, it might be a way you could remain in your home . . ."

"I think it's too late for us. But what a wonderful way to get the message across."

"What if you're an avid gardener, and are into flower and vegetable gardens?"

"Tolerate small numbers of unwanted pests. Control them only when the damage they cause begins to reach intolerable levels. Use biological pest controls before resorting to chemicals. A first step would be to douse infested leaves with a solution of soap flakes and water. Cutting off infected areas where possible also helps. Any of the Safer's products would be the next reasonable step. Pyrethrum is a natural substance derived from flowers of the chrysanthemum family, while *Bacillus thuringiensis* or thuricide would be two fairly benign alternatives as well. But keep in mind, even natural pesticides are designed to kill, so using them sparingly is the key."

"What about crop rotation and companion planting?" asked Sam.

"What's *that*?" asked Andrew, obviously not a gardener.

"Rotation of crops each year prevents the soil from being depleted of nutrients and controls soil-borne disease. For instance, if you planted tomatoes in one bed, cabbage in another, switch them the following year, since each takes different nutrients from the soil. An example of companion planting would be to plant marigolds or chrysanthemums throughout the garden to protect tomatoes, beans and other plants from a variety of insects."

"How does that help?" asked Andrew.

"Vegetables and flowers have different odors and root secretions that are believed to affect the activity of insects and the growth of nearby plants. For instance, basil seems to keep tomatoes free of infestation while savory seems to protect beans . . ."

"Who would ever have guessed!"

"In a nutshell, consulting magazines such as *Organic Gardening Harrowsmith* and similar books or publications would be a great start."

"How can we get more information about pesticides?" asked Martha.

"There are several excellent resources. One is the *Rachel Carson Council* and the other two are those we mentioned earlier - the *National Coalition Against the Misuse of Pesticides* (NCAMP) and the *Northwest Coalition for Alternatives to Pesticides* (NCAP). The latter maintains an extensive library of over 8,000 articles, studies, books, government documents, videos and other reference materials. This group is prompt and thorough in replyng to any requests for information. Their addresses and telephone numbers are all on the resource list I'll hand out at the end of our session. Jane stood up and stretched. "I suggest we all take a break. How does that sound?"

"Sounds great to me!" yawned Andrew. "Could you point the way to the washroom?"

She motioned, "Top of the stairs and to your left. Let's get our jackets on and get some fresh air."

"A great idea!" exclaimed Sam. "Coming, Jillian?"

"I'll be there in a minute. I just want to finish writing a couple of items in my book."

After the others left the room, I reflected on the morning. When I first arrived, I assumed I was going to discover how to maintain a healthy home. Well, I'd already learned a great deal, but we hadn't even made it to the front door! I'd never even considered my outdoor environment - right from my yard to the golf course down the street!

There was so much to learn, but I was determined to stick with it - to continue on the journey I'd begun. And I no longer felt alone. Not only was Michael more supportive, but I'd just spent the past hour with others who had begun to walk their own paths toward wellness.

I was ready for more.

*It is a difficult concept*

*for many people*

*to come to terms with,*

*but air pollution in their own homes*

*often poses a greater threat to*

*their health*

*than the pollution*

*outside their front doors,*

*serious enough as that is.*

David R. Collison, MB, BS,
Why Do I Feel So Awful?

# 16

# Sleeping With the Enemy

*Healthy people are those who live in healthy homes, on a healthy diet;*
*in an environment equally fit for birth, growth,*
*work, healing and dying.*
**Ivan Illich**

*T*he break seemed to revive everyone. Jane clicked the last leg of her lecture board in place. "There, now we can begin." A familiar chart faced us - the barrel filled with all those stressors. "Is everyone familiar with the *Total Load Theory?*"

We nodded in unison. It was obvious we had read the same books.

"Good! We're all on the same track. If we reduce the total load, through cleaning up our diet and our immediate environment, we can begin the healing process. I'm aware that each of you has already begun to work on one aspect or another, but today, we're going to focus specifically on sources of environmental contaminants and how we can keep our homes clean and healthy. It's a vital part of beginning to empty the barrel. For instance, did you know that the air inside the average North American home is more polluted than the air outdoors? In fact, an EPA study found that toxic chemicals are frequently more concentrated indoors than out. Typically, it's 10 - 20 times higher but has been known to reach as high as 500."

"Yeah, don't I know it!" exclaimed Andrew. "I'm living proof - just call me exhibit A." Laughter rippled around the room. As bitter as he was, he still had a great sense of humor. "Seriously, I was healthy all my life - until I renovated my house and began working in a sealed office tower that was re-carpeted a year ago. My life hasn't been the same since."

Jane's face looked grim. "The sad part is that no one is immune. One day you're fine. Then, you get hit with a heavy dose of a toxic substance which could sensitize you for years - not only to that specific chemical, but to many others."

"Like me and my two kids," whispered Sam.

"Or you're exposed to low levels over a long period, but never make the connection between the constant exposure and chronic symptoms - symptoms which are often written off as stress or the flu." It was apparent that Andrew had read quite a bit on this subject.

"And some of the more specific symptoms," added Jane, "can be misdiagnosed as sinusitis, bronchitis or digestive problems. Then the endless rounds of tests and medication begin."

"How can indoor air be more hazardous than the air outdoors?" asked Martha.

"Outdoor pollution comes and goes, depending on weather patterns. Our contact with it can vary greatly as we move about. Pollution in the home, office or school is always there - our contact with it is relatively constant, ongoing. Most of us spend about ninety percent of the time indoors, breathing in substances that continually outgas - only most people don't realize it. Products we consider the homeowner's dream - furniture built from more affordable materials such as pressboard and upholstered with stain-proof polyester fabric; mold-inhibiting wallpaper; and stain-resistant carpeting, fill our homes with dangerous, and often odorless vapors."

"So our homes which we think of as safe havens," summarized Andrew, "may be one of our worst health hazards."

"That's right," replied Jane. "The EPA estimates that as many as 31,400 premature deaths occur annually as a result of indoor air pollution. Other studies attribute 7,000 to 30,000 deaths to radon alone. So, given the latter figures, that EPA estimate is probably conservative. The greatest tragedy is that the medical profession, on the whole, is virtually uninformed with respect to the adverse effects of environmental contamination on our health. And as Andrew pointed out, this is especially true of our homes where we spend so much time."

"And our workplace . . ." observed Andrew, "but we don't realize we're affected until it's too late - until our conditions become chronic."

"If only I had known then what I know now," remarked Martha, "I could have prevented a lot of this."

"Easy to say in hindsight," commented Sam. "What I'm learning is that often it's our life experiences that bring us to a higher level of knowledge and understanding . . ."

"I would have to agree with that one!" I exclaimed. We all turned our attention back to Jane.

"There are two major sources of contaminants in a home - biological and chemical. The former includes molds, bacteria, dust mites, pollen and animal dander. Chemical contaminants include combustion gases, radon, pesticides, asbestos, formaldehyde and volatile organic compounds (VOC's). The latter is commonly released from paints and household products."

"What's radon?" asked Sam.

"Radon is a colorless, odorless radioactive gas emitted from the natural decay of uranium in certain rock formations. It's a serious threat in some areas. It's a known carcinogen. In fact exposure increases the risk of developing lung or throat cancer. The acceptable standard in the United States is 4 picocuries per litre of air, while in Canada it's 21.6 - five times higher. Obviously, the Americans are more concerned about this lethal gas than Canadians."

"Canadians are either a hardy bunch or they wear lead shorts!" I joked.

"Actually, more recent Canadian studies have shown that radon isn't as serious a hazard as we once thought - especially when compared to mold contamination."

"How does it get into the house?" asked Sam.

"Through unsealed or cracked foundations, unfinished crawl spaces, drains, sump pumps . . ."

"Can you test for it?"

"Yes, radon tests are available and are relatively inexpensive," replied Jane, "but I'd like to shift our attention to molds because they're often the source of many other problems commonly found in homes. Keep in mind, as you look for cracks in basement walls and floors, possible sources of moisture which can lead to mold, you're also finding potential sources of radon infiltration. In other words, you're really killing two birds with one stone."

"How can we detect whether or not mold is a problem?" asked Martha.

"One step that would help identify whether or not your home has an indoor air quality problem, is to ask yourself some of the following questions: Do you feel better when you're away from home than you do when you're in it? Do you notice any odors as you enter the house? Are your symptoms better at a particular time of day or year? Have you renovated lately? The next step is to conduct a simple sniff test."

"A sniff test?" We exclaimed in unison.

"Yes. Close all the windows and doors. Then spend the day outside. When you walk back into the house, follow the odors. If you smell a musty smell - an 'old' smell - chances are, your house has a moisture problem. A recent survey by Health Canada found that thirty-five percent of Canadian homes had indications of excessive dampness or mold. Obviously, if you are highly sensitive to molds, you would *not* be the best candidate for this job."

"What if the damp smell is in the bathroom?"

"You can clean the mold from the tile grout and from around windows, and get rid of any carpet, but these are only band-aid measures. Installing a high-powered fan is wise, and certainly replacing carpet with floor tile would be a good move. But always remember - you must remove the *source* of the problem. Are there leaks in the foundation? Leaks in the roof? Is there a downspout that's pouring water into the foundation? Do you have a feeling of unwellness when you spend time in a family room that's below grade? Any unexplainable aversion to going downstairs?" One visible sign would be mold growth on a basement wall."

"Are there times when the problem goes unnoticed?"

"Yes, even if there are no visible signs, and no smells can be detected, contaminants can still be present. For instance, mold can grow inside walls. Just last week, I gave an in-service in one of the local schools where many teachers and students had become ill. The walls were literally bulging with moisture. One teacher put a bit of pressure on one of those spots, and black mold literally burst through!"

"Did they resolve the problem?"

"The school board says it doesn't have the funds. Can you imagine? How can they afford *not* to fix the problem! One should never underestimate the health hazards that accompany indoor molds. Many of them produce mycotoxins which can have a very serious impact on our health - in extreme cases, they can even cause death. They're certainly a common factor in respiratory problems in children. I could also cite many examples of office buildings where employees have become extremely ill due to molds. The last building I visited was contaminated with three types - *Aspergillus Alternaria, Stachybotyrs Atra,* and *Penicillium Fellatanum.* The workers were continually sick. Andrew, did you have a question?"

"I understand that even dust, dust mites, and animal dander can be detrimental to our health. They can cause not only stuffy and itchy noses, but severe behavioral changes in some people, especially small children. What's your take on all this?"

"Are any of you familiar with Dr. Doris Rapp?"

"Only from the references in some of the literature I've read," replied Martha.

I piped up, "I've read both *The Impossible Child* and *Is This Your Child.* They were great, full of vital information. But her videotapes are what's truly remarkable. They show children reacting adversely to a wide range of environmental irritants, dust being only one of them. And I mean *extreme* behavioral swings." I could tell Andrew was impressed. I was beginning to feel more like one of the team!

"And keep in mind," declared Jane, "that dust is a complex particulate, comprised of dander, soil, fiber, hair, dust mites, and even scales from the human body - all of which can hold moisture, a perfect medium for mold growth. And dust itself can act as a chemical sponge. In one study alone, a sample contained *twenty-four* different hydrocarbons, half of which were heavy semi-volatile organic compounds (SVOC's), several of them suspected carcinogens. Combine this with the chemicals emitted by new carpets and you could be in trouble."

"I can just see all this dust entrapped in a brand new, thick, plush wall-to-wall carpet with a baby crawling around on it!" exclaimed Martha.

"Not a very pretty picture, is it?" Jane commented. "Then, when the house is heated, these contaminants are re-circulated into the air we breathe. The problem of fried dust has been known to cause problems for sensitive individuals. And let's not forget dust mites . . . they thrive in moist environments, so the best solution once again, is to search out the *source* of excess moisture in the house. And if you can't find it yourself, call in the experts. Always remember," Jane wagged her index finger in the air, "if you don't remove the problem, you can't cure it."

"So really what you're saying is that moisture is the primary source, the breeding ground, for major biological contamination in buildings."

"Absolutely. So again, as important as it is to remove carpets and musty furniture from basement areas, these are only stop-gap measures. Even if you check for leaky windows and floor drains, regularly operate the rangehood fan in the kitchen, remove plants, and adequately vent the bathroom, you may not completely resolve the problem - as long as all other sources of moisture have not been identified."

"Are you suggesting," said Andrew, "that even if you scrub down that green and black stuff growing around your windows and shower stall, it's really of little use because it'll only grow back?"

"Exactly. The entire house has to be checked out if the problem persists. You know, it's not much different than looking at the body - the *cause* of the problem must be addressed, not merely the symptoms. And when removing mold, it's extremely important to wear protective clothing, especially a face mask. A five percent solution of chlorine bleach, or for those chemically sensitive, baking soda or vinegar in water should do the trick. It goes without saying that you should keep the area well ventilated."

"Should the area be vacuumed first?" queried Sam.

"Absolutely not. Scrape it, bag it, and get it out as quickly and carefully as possible. Vacuuming would only make a bad situation worse because the molds would be blown out through the exhaust into the indoor air."

"So you'd be recycling mold. What a thought!" moaned Sam.

"What about carbon monoxide from heating sources such as gas appliances, kerosene heaters and wood stoves?" asked Martha. "I understand it's another potential hazard in homes, especially where there's inadequate ventilation or if the appliance is not operating properly."

"Portable kerosene heaters are one of the most toxic devices you could use for heat. The odor permeates and contaminates the air . . ."

Sam piped up, "I read somewhere that now you can get a plug-in device that can detect carbon monoxide."

"That's true," Jane replied, "but the detectors are set to go off at 90 - 100 parts per million. This is adequate to avert death, but not to forewarn of the potential ill effects which humans can suffer from concentrations as low as 5 - 35 ppm. And often, the early symptoms of carbon monoxide poisoning mimic flu symptoms such as sleepiness, headache, dizziness, blurred vision, irritability and the inability to concentrate. Remember, there's no taste or smell to carbon monoxide. Thinking it's a virus, the poisoning can be left to progress into nausea, vomiting, shortness of breath and convulsions. In severe cases, carbon monoxide poisoning can result in death. Ultimately, appliances and heating systems should be checked regularly for defects and leaks."

"I'll say! What we don't know could kill us!" proclaimed Martha.

"One thing for sure," declared Jane emphatically, "is that the heating system is another key to healthy air in the home. If, for example, there's a problem with backdrafting or the fuel supply to the furnace, serious health consequences can result. Upgrading to a sealed combustion furnace with an external source of oxygen is an option. They're also more cost- effective."

"What about humidifiers?"

"They generally create more dampness and mold. Unless you live in an unusually dry climate, I would rather see you invest in a good set of filters for your furnace. A high-efficiency particulate arrestance (HEPA) air filter is great, but requires a powerful fan to force the air throughout the house. They do, however, work well on single room air cleaners or air exchangers. Keeping the ducts clean is another important preventive measure."

"Is there one heating system that's better than another?" asked Andrew.

"They each have their good points and drawbacks. It's almost the same as asking, what's the best diet for everyone? And we already know how difficult that is to answer!"

"We sure do!" We exclaimed emphatically, then laughed at the immediacy of our response.

"The problem is that there is no one perfect system. You end up compromising somewhere. However, I think it reasonable to say that a safe heating system would include many or all of the following features: a heating source that is sealed off from the rest of the house; fuel that doesn't add pollutants to the indoor air or spread them around; low temperature heat to avoid the problem of fried dust; and heating elements that are cleaned and serviced regularly."

"What about radiant heat?" asked Andrew.

"For those sensitive to electromagnetic fields, electric radiant and electric baseboards could pose a problem. Hot water radiant heat may be more appropriate. The most important thing to keep in mind is to never - I repeat - *never* use radiant in-floor heating with wall-to-wall carpeting. The chemicals from the carpeting, underlay, and glues can outgas into the air for even longer periods than normal and at higher concentrations."

"Tell me about it!" snorted Andrew.

"Ideally, ceramic floors are the safest surface when using radiant heat."

"What about hardwood floors?" asked Sam.

"Well, that would be a good second choice, but it's critical to make sure the finish is as harmless as possible and that it outgasses for an adequate period of time before anyone moves in."

"I've read that making sure the house has a good ventilation system is also very important," stated Andrew.

"What about opening windows?" asked Martha.

"Open windows bring in air from outside, but it's certainly not the most economical way of ventilating."

"I hear from some of my friends," interjected Sam, "that a central exhaust system is helpful."

"It is," replied Jane, "but it still only exhausts air from the building. It doesn't provide a source of incoming air. The ideal system is a heat recovery ventilation system (HRV), which not only exhausts stale air from the house, but also supplies fresh air from outside. I often call these systems 'the lungs of the building' - they allow the house to breathe on its own. The air can be almost as fresh indoors as out. Although initially somewhat more expensive to install, especially in an existing home, it's the way to go. And during allergy season, it can clean the incoming air. Many newer building codes now require builders to install ventilation systems in new housing. My own motto is: *If you build it tight, do it right.*"

"Mind you, an HRV is little good in neighborhoods where everyone has a woodstove. It draws the smoke into the house."

"Oh no," groaned Martha, "I can't imagine living without my woodstove. Are they all that bad?"

"It's virtually impossible to have either a fireplace or woodstove without some risk of combustion spillage, so for someone with sensitivities, they're probably not a great idea. In fact, there are those who can't even walk in their own neighborhoods because of wood smoke. But certainly, if and when used, only woodstoves upgraded to high-efficiency or a catalytic converter type should be used. Fireplaces should always be fitted tightly with glass doors and the wood should be stored in a place separate from the house."

"Because of molds?"

"Yes. It's also important to burn only clean, dry wood. It helps keep creosote buildup to a minimum."

"What about the dust factor?"

"Well, there's definitely an increase in dust with these heating systems."

"Just what we need," moaned Martha, "more work!"

"Speaking of housecleaning, many people don't realize how hazardous everyday cleaning products can be." Jane looked at me and asked, "For instance, Jillian, what's in your bathroom, your laundry room? What's under your kitchen sink?"

"Under my kitchen sink?" I asked rather naively.

"Yes, what cleaning products do you use?"

"Do you mean things like detergents and sprays?" asked Sam.

"I mean furniture polish, scouring powder, oven cleaner. Are you using stuff that contains ammonia? What kind of disinfectant are you using?"

"Well I'm slowly changing over, but I must admit, I'm still using most of the same products I've always used, only less of them. I know . . . I know . . ." Sam responded somewhat defensively. "It's time to get rid of them."

"You see, not only do the cleaners themselves provoke symptoms in many people, but their use in combination can result in additional adverse effects. Used alone, a few may be acceptable, but they were never intended nor tested for use together as a chemical cocktail. Or, as Dr. Rowland suggests, the total load must be considered at all times because in real life, nothing is used in isolation." Jane looked at Martha. "Would this be a good time to share your Black Friday story?"

"Sure," said Martha, clearing her throat. "When my oldest daughter, Sarah, was nine, I noticed that every Friday she was impossible to live with. She was tearful, belligerent, and would do her best to push me to my limits. In fact, most Fridays, I felt like throttling her . . ."

"I can relate to that," I commiserated. "I used to feel that way almost daily with my oldest son, Nathaniel. He still isn't quite where I think he could be, but I must say, since we changed his diet, he's much improved."

"Well, it just so happened," continued Martha, "that every Friday I had a cleaning lady come in from 8:00 in the morning until 4:30 in the afternoon. At first I thought Sarah didn't like Zelda. Then one day, I came across a story in a women's magazine about the hazards of common, household cleaning products. The article explained that many of them can be toxic, especially if used over long periods of time. I decided to eliminate as many as possible. As soon as we were rid of them, Sarah no longer had the problem on Fridays. The biggest surprise was that I, too, felt better! It really was that simple. Since then, we've learned that not only does Sarah have difficulties with many chemicals - but so do I."

"What other chemicals do you mean?" For every answer, Sam had another question.

"We're both very sensitive to formaldehyde, phenols, perfumes and auto exhaust. These accounted for her feeling sick on long car trips, and for our dreadful shopping episodes. I always thought we argued in malls simply because of the usual differences between mothers and teenage daughters."

"See?"commented Jane, "we're forever trying to find deep psychological reasons for every negative behavior."

I quickly recalled the many aborted shopping sprees caused by my irritability, brain fog and fatigue which would start not long after being in the stores.

Martha went on. "And I recall that fabric shops and the cheaper department stores were the worst. I now call them hazardous wastelands."

"Sizing in fabrics and new clothes, rubber from shoes, plastics, cosmetics, cleaning agents, poor lighting and lack of proper ventilation all add up to a very toxic environment. For many, indeed most of us in this room," Jane glanced at each of us, "shopping trips become very unpleasant."

Suddenly it clicked. Could this be why my kids flipped out whenever we were in crowds? Church functions, weddings, movies - places where there were lots of people in a small space were always problems. The kids would be great at home. Then, suddenly, their behavior would change - for no obvious reason - at least not one that I could pinpoint.

Jane was still speaking. ". . . perfumes, colognes, and other scented personal care products can trigger horrendous reactions in some children."

"And not only in children!" I exclaimed, thinking back to the day I had to leave the parent-teacher interview with Mrs. Allen. "*I* can't be around them anymore. In fact, I wonder if Nathaniel's poor behavior in school might be caused by his teacher's perfume."

"It's certainly worth checking into," Jane suggested. "Aberrant behavior is a common manifestation of chemical sensitivity. Did you know, there are over 4,000 chemicals used to make fragrances, several hundred of which can be used in a single product alone? And not only are people with environmental sensitivities affected. Some perfumes contain products *known* to be toxic to humans. Many have been implicated as the cause of sore throats, runny noses, sinus congestion, muscle pain and asthma. They've also been known to affect the ability to concentrate and can cause severe irritability, nausea and seizures."

"Why wasn't perfume such a problem years ago?"

"I think the answer to that is at least two-fold. Today's perfumes are made from less refined and cheaper synthetics; and our bodies are unable to withstand the onslaught of these chemicals, especially if our internal ecology is imbalanced, causing our gastrointestinal tracts to be more permeable."

"Banning scents from public places will be commonplace in a few years' time," declared Martha.

"Yeah, just like *no smoking* campaigns," added Andrew. "It takes time to raise awareness, but I think more people are becoming aware that it's a real health hazard."

"It's already happening," said Jane. "In fact, my health club and church have instituted *no scents* policies . . ."

"And we can only guess why!" laughed Andrew.

Jane, with a lopsided grin, responded, "Well, I suppose it does help that they know I do this kind of work . . ." She stood up abruptly and walked into the middle of the room. Her eyes flashed as she looked at each of us in turn. "And don't ever forget that *everyone* in this room has the power to make profound changes. One example is the pink tulip program that started with one concerned citizen. Even if it seems like you're taking baby steps, they're at least steps in the right direction." Her enthusiasm was contagious. She made me feel as if I could make a real difference.

Martha looked up from her notepad. "Speaking of perfume, let me tell you a quick story about my friend's fifteen year old daughter. You wouldn't believe what happens to her when she's exposed to scented products."

"What?" we chorused.

"She becomes amorous and behaves like someone who's had too much to drink. She gets kissy, huggy and slightly delirious. Now, just imagine her on a date with a young guy plastered with aftershave!"

"I can well imagine!" remarked Jane.

Andrew snapped his fingers. "Instant pregnancy!"

Jane's tone took on a more serious note. "And the pregnancy would likely be blamed on her lack of morality, poor judgement, or lack of parental guidance - you name it. While in a few instances this may be true, more often than not, we underestimate - even dismiss - the effect our *physical* environment can have on our lives."

"So we institute *no-scent* policies at home, in church and in other public places, but what about magazines? They invade our homes, saturated with unwelcome fragrances, advertising the latest and the smelliest," said Martha disdainfully. "I actually hang them on the line to air them out. I pray that it doesn't rain before I get a chance to read them."

"They *are* intrusive," replied Jane. "You need to notify the publishers immediately. Tell them you don't want scented pages in the copies delivered to your home. You could cancel your subscription, but if you write to most magazines, they'll supply you with unscented issues. That's what our local school library does. It's been my experience that companies respond favorably to these requests - after all, it's business and they need yours as much as the next."

"What about kids' birthdays? Their friends love to give them perfumed soaps, lotions and shampoos."

"I simply put at the bottom of the invitations, 'no scented products please'. Since then, I've rarely had the problem. Would anyone like more tea?" offered Jane.

"I would. It tastes great. What kind is it?" inquired Sam.

"It's an herbal one called Morning Mist - it has mint, chamomile, and a few other herbs I can't remember right off. Glad you like it." She poured while we held out our cups. "Looks like we're on empty! Martha, you know where everything is. Would you be kind enough to put the kettle on?"

"My pleasure." She got up to go to the kitchen. "You know, I've had quite a time trying to find unscented shampoos, gels and hairsprays. When I finally located a few, I couldn't test them in the drugstore because just about everything there was scented. Then, when I tested them at home, I realized that almost every one had an odor! I ended up phoning the companies that manufactured them. The standard line was that 'a little smell has to be added to mask the odor of the alcohol'. I gave up."

"And although unscented is a vast improvement," commented Jane, "it may not be the ultimate solution. Although some portions of these products are made from natural ingredients such as lanolin, beeswax and other oils, dangerous chemicals are often added to prolong shelf life as well as to add color and attractive scents. Gary Null, in *The 90's Healthy Body Book,* calls personal care products 'pretty poisons', pointing out that the skin is our largest organ, key to the detoxification of the body, and that some of the chemicals added to these products are toxic."

"Oh, I read that book!" exclaimed Martha, on her way back in. "He talks about the hazards of anti-perspirants that stop perspiration flow with aluminum salt . . . and moisturizing creams with . . . with . . . oh, I can't remember . . ."

Jane helped her out. "With parabens to kill bacteria; mascara with 'lash extenders' containing nylon fiber that's been known to scratch the cornea; lipsticks made with coal-tar dyes; hair colorings and perms that contain chemicals such as ammonium thioglycolate which has been implicated in serious burns to the scalp and face, as well as permanent loss of hair. In fact, Debra Lynn Dadd, author of *The Nontoxic Home & Office,* cites an investigation done by *Consumer Reports* magazine, revealing about twenty different chemicals used regularly in hair-coloring products that are potential human carcinogens. And where the scalp is very porous, these chemicals can be easily absorbed."

"And we use these products regularly, without a second thought!" exclaimed Martha, running her fingers through her hair. "I'm as guilty as the next person."

"I got to the point where I couldn't tolerate the smell of any of them," declared Sam.

"Your hair is so shiny, you probably never needed them in the first place!" remarked Martha.

"Actually, I've been using henna, a coloring derived from plants. But when I was at my worst, I couldn't even use that."

"What price, vanity!" exclaimed Andrew. "I'm not quite at the point where this has become an issue, but several of my friends use dyes regularly. I'll be sure to point this out."

"Hopefully by the time you need it, there'll be a larger choice of naturally-derived products . . . Even better, go *au naturel*! I must tell you this little anecdote about a good friend who thought I was being far too stringent with my new lifestyle. She used to wear the most pungent perfumes - you know, those heavy, sweet, nauseating, designer ones."

We all nodded, knowing exactly where she was coming from. Some of these scents were so sickening that even people without sensitivities complained bitterly about them.

"Well, she suffered from headaches constantly - at least three times a week, if not more. I suggested she stop wearing her perfume for several days - just as an experiment. Lo and behold, her headaches disappeared. But the biggest shock was that she experienced withdrawal symptoms from not wearing it!"

"What kinds of symptoms?" I asked.

"Irritability, inability to concentrate and severe headaches for the first few days after she stopped using it. She was so hooked, she would soak a cotton ball with her perfume, wrap it up in a plastic baggie, and go outside to sniff it during her breaks. It was the only thing that relieved her pain. In the end, I urged her to give it up completely. She eventually ended up being treated at the clinic for her sensitivity. Her headaches became history, and for the first time in years, she felt calm, focused and productive. And not only did *her* health improve, but so did that of those around her!"

"So you can be addicted to perfumes just as to food?"

"Absolutely. The adaptation and masking phases often leave people quite oblivious to the fact that their own scents cause them to function at less than optimal efficiency, often making them feel headachy or tired before they've even finished breakfast."

"You really do crave that to which you are sensitive," commented Martha. "The books I've read all say that."

"Yes," nodded Jane, "you either crave it or have an aversion to it - the same as with food sensitivities. One group that adopted a scent-free policy pointed out that they've now become far more aware of other scented products in their environment. The reality is that by going scent-free, they unmasked a sensitivity they'd had all along, but had managed to live in the adaptive stage for a much longer time than many others."

"What do you mean by 'adaptive'?" Andrew appeared to be stumped. I couldn't believe there was something he didn't know!

"In order to understand the adaptive stage, let me explain the three stages of sensitization. First, there is an acute reaction - your initial response to an odor. This may take the form of an intense like or dislike. This may be followed by an adaptive stage in which there is a *suppression* of the initial symptoms. This is usually the point at which you no longer smell the substance. Finally, you may become maladapted and produce acute responses you may not connect to the initial sensitization."

"So is it like walking into a carpet store, for instance, and initially hating the smell, and then a few minutes later, no longer being able to smell anything - but by the time you leave, you feel light-headed and disoriented?"

"Sort of. It's the phase where it appears that the offensive substance is well-tolerated, when in fact, it's producing a host of seemingly unrelated symptoms."

"What about 'natural' or 'naturally scented'?" inquired Sam.

"Natural is not necessarily safer when one has sensitivities. You see, it depends upon the particular substance to which you're sensitive. I might be fine with pine furniture and feel totally sick with vinyl. You, on the other hand, might be reactive to the resins in pine and feel better with something else."

"So are you suggesting that sensitivities are very individual?" asked Martha.

"You can quote me on that," replied Jane. "Also, beware of products claiming to be 'hypoallergenic'. Because sensitivities are so individual, no one product can be truly hypoallergenic for everyone. It simply means that the most common allergens have been removed, but they may still contain ingredients to which you are sensitive."

"Sometimes it must be just trial and error . . ."

"Yes. Often there's no other way of really knowing before the fact. But I do know one thing for sure - chemicals can be absolutely *devastating*. I know a fifteen year old girl who told her mother every morning that she hated her. Can you imagine living with that daily ritual of hostility? The puzzling thing was, that by the time her mother dropped her off at school on the other side of town, she'd be quite pleasant again, occasionally even giving her a hug before she got out of the car."

"I thought Jesse was bad!" exclaimed Martha.

"Well, you may find this hard to believe," said Jane, "but that fifteen year old was me."

You could have heard a pin drop.

"Every morning Dad would have his hot bath; Mom, her fifteen minute shower; and guess who walked in last? Me. The clouds of chlorinated steam destroyed me, reducing me to a hostile, very bitchy teenager."

I was riveted to my seat. "I can't believe you're telling this story! Only a few weeks ago, *I* went off the deep end after drinking chlorinated water. I've since learned that it's one of my worst sensitivities, too!"

"And how many more are out there," remarked Andrew, "who are just as sensitive, but who don't have a clue?"

"That's right. How many just haven't made the connection?" whispered Sam.

"And that's not the only problem with chlorinated water," declared Jane. "It's a suspected carcinogen. *The American Journal of Public Health* published a study in 1994 that examined fifty-six Finnish municipalities - the largest long-term study of its kind. They found a statistically significant relationship between exposure to chlorinated water and the incidence of stomach, kidney and bladder cancers."

"I know one thing," I declared, "I'll never drink city tap water again; nor will my kids. Now that my whole house is dechlorinated, I can smell it everywhere - from drinking fountains to public toilets!"

"A great example of unmasking!" Jane pointed out.

"You know," began Martha, "I always wondered whether it was a safe practice to give young children swimming lessons in indoor pools. And some of them are babies, only a few months old."

"I don't imagine it's very wise when you consider that the skin is our largest organ." Jane became subdued, reflective. "I remember poor Mom in the bathroom, doing her hair and make-up, and invariably, a huge fight would erupt - all due to my reactivity to chlorine. Just imagine the years of stress we could have avoided had we known about my sensitivity."

"How'd you finally figure it out?"

"About eight years ago, my husband and I went on a southern vacation. We spent a good part of our days immersed in a chlorinated pool. By the end of our holiday, I was a basket case - and didn't have a clue as to why. From that point on, anytime I was near a chlorinated pool, I'd become irritable and tearful. When Dr. Rowland tested me for chemical sensitivities, chlorine showed up as my worst. What I regret most is how it ruined the relationship with my mother during that time - all those wasted years - when it could have been very different."

"I know this is really none of my business, but I'm curious. Did you ever go to therapy for those outbursts?"

"I sure did. In fact, I even invented stories for the therapist so I wouldn't feel silly sitting in her office with nothing to say."

"I thought I was the only one who did that!" I blurted out. "When my family doctor suggested I see a psychiatrist - an appointment I never did keep - I, too, began to dream up reasons for my outbursts."

"Once again, it goes back to the same old point," sighed Andrew. "We need to look at basic things first - such as our physical environment. Unfortunately, the traditional medical establishment isn't too quick to embrace this approach."

"No, it certainly isn't, although, hopefully, the tide will turn someday soon. I can honestly say that before I met Dr. Rowland, my life was the pits. I was tired, irritable, stressed - just generally unwell."

"Perhaps we need to backtrack and re-evaluate our lifestyles," said Martha.

Andrew, jumping right into the thick of the conversation, declared, "Hear! Hear! Right on! We need to focus less on acquiring material possessions - many of which are harmful anyway - and focus more on improving the *quality* of our lives."

"In the meantime, on a more practical note, what do we do about cleaning?" You could always count on Sam to ask a good question. She was so intense.

"Aw, take a break! Forget about cleaning!" teased Andrew.

"Actually, there are many safe products you can use," responded Jane. "Old-fashioned stand-bys include vinegar, lemon juice and baking soda. Homes were kept clean long before chemical companies were around. There are also many safe, non-toxic cleaning products on the market. Health food stores carry several lines, as do more enlightened grocers. I'll give you a list of these products before you leave today. One of the best guides to environmentally safe housekeeping products is a book called *Clean & Green* by Annie Berthold-Bond."

"Is that on the list you're handing out?" asked Sam.

"Definitely. Another good one is by Debra Lynn Dadd, called *The Nontoxic Home & Office*. It's also on the list. Most commercial cleaners and detergents contain potentially dangerous chemicals. They can cause headaches, confusion, lack of concentration, and can even mimic symptoms of mental illness. Many of them can lead to respiratory, as well as liver and kidney disorders. These chemicals enter our systems via the lungs or by absorption through the skin."

"How ironic," groaned Andrew, gazing out the window, "we risk our health - our very lives - to live in what we are brainwashed into believing is a squeaky-clean environment, when in fact, all we've done is create a worse situation - one that's even more toxic." All at once, his expression changed to alarm. He bolted out of his chair and beckoned for all of us to come to the window. A truck with huge print, 'Pesky Pest Control' was pulling up into the neighbor's driveway.

Martha rolled her eyes. "At least they stopped using chemicals on their lawn last summer . . . but they haven't gotten the whole picture yet ."

"Martha, you've hit the nail on the head!" exclaimed Jane, still watching the truck across the street. People just don't get it. This is a clear indication that those connections are not as obvious to everyone as they are to us. It's not until we become directly affected that change becomes automatic. This brings to mind the trial attorney who just finished a book called *A Canary's Tale, Environmental Pollution and Environmental Illness.*"

"Sounds like a book we all should have," commented Sam.

"It's just been submitted for publication. In any case, the author wrote it as a result of his own poisoning from pesticides commonly used to treat termites. Within hours after the treatment, he became ill with a headache, burning eyes and nose, and nausea. He had to move out of the home he'd lived in for the past twenty-five years, and was subsequently diagnosed by a toxicologist as having organophosphate poisoning. He became intolerant of common chemicals, including such ubiquitous items as tobacco smoke, auto exhaust and new carpets . . ."

"That's a familiar story!" grumbled Andrew out of the side of his mouth.

"When it comes to these products, what we need are tougher regulations and better still, to refrain from using them at all. There are better ways to deal with many of these unwanted pests. Again, any of the books and organizations we mentioned earlier would be able to offer alternatives. One of the most complete consumer guides I've come across is another of Debra Lynn Dadd's, entitled *Nontoxic, Natural, & Earthwise*, which lists over 2,000 brand-name products as well as over 400 do-it-yourself formulas. She also includes a huge mail-order listing. And, in the rare instances where pesticides must be used, extreme caution should be exercised, starting with the least harmful first."

"It's my understanding that the State of New York has some of the most comprehensive regulations in the country regarding pesticide notifications. Notification must be posted forty-eight hours prior to the application of the pesticide, and must list the name of the applicator, the symptoms of pesticide poisoning, and the phone numbers of poison control centers and the regional office for the New York State Department of Environmental Conservation. Signs have to be posted at building entrances on the day of the application. Apparently, fines can be up to $5000 for first-time offenders."

"Hmph!" growled Martha. "Signs should be posted at least a week in advance!"

"You're probably right," replied Jane, "and don't forget those insect repellents we spray on our skin - and on our children - are pesticides as well."

"And who ever thinks of them in those terms!" shuddered Sam. "I never did - at least not until we became sick."

"That's right. Most people have no idea that DEET is the most commonly used pesticide in these repellents. According to the British medical journal, the *Lancet*, exposure to this substance has caused brain disorders, slurred speech, difficulty walking, tremors and even death. Of course, while most people won't suffer to this degree, it does make you think twice."

"So what can you use?" I asked.

"Dadd's suggestions include wearing protective clothing, eating lots of garlic, splashing a little vinegar on exposed skin, and preparing a concoction using citronella and vodka or vegetable oil. There's a safer solution for just about everything - if we look for one. Now, let's take a quick look at a typical day in the life of . . . the way I used to live and how too many people on this continent still live. It may sound somewhat extreme, but it depicts a typical nineties' lifestyle. And what's wrong with a bit of embellishment if it helps make the point, right?"

We all nodded, waiting to hear the story.

Jane began. "Every morning I wake up on a polyurethane foam mattress, treated with fire-retardant chemicals and covered with polyester fabric. If there's particleboard, it's likely outgassing formaldehyde from the urea-formaldehyde resins in the glues. For the past eight hours, I've been surrounded by synthetics - from my nightie to the pillowcases, sheets and comforter wrapped around me - polyester everywhere. The bedding has been washed and dried with scented products and sometimes even spray-starched to make it look and smell fresh. My bedroom is carpeted, panelled, or wallpapered, all of which offgas chemicals, one of which is formaldehyde, a suspected carcinogen. Potpourri lines every drawer, so my clothes will smell nice. Hanging in the closet are my newly dry-cleaned clothes, offgassing perchloroethylene. According to Dadd, this chemical is the most commonly used dry-cleaning solvent. Inhaling its fumes can cause nausea, dizziness, depression of the central nervous system, and eventually liver damage and cancer."

"No more dry cleaning for me!" I exclaimed.

"Hanging these newly cleaned clothes outdoors or in a well-vented room would be wise. And don't take everything that's marked 'dry-clean only' too seriously. Hand washing works well in many instances."

"Hey," interrupted Andrew. "I just read in *Health Naturally* about a guy who became extremely ill from his dry-cleaned sleeping bag. He's had a breathing problem ever since and has developed a wide range of chemical sensitivities as a result of that single exposure."

"That's the whole point! You never know when it's *your* turn. Sam, would you ever have believed that you and your kids would end up as sick as you did?"

"Never," sighed Sam. "Life is very unpredictable. That's why it's better to be safe than sorry - especially with things you *can* control."

"With all the reading I've done," Andrew mused, "and now listening to Jane list the hazards lurking in our bedroom alone . . . when you really think about it, every night we're sleeping with the enemy!"

"Quite literally, we are - and we don't even know it."

"I meant to ask you earlier," interrupted Martha, "what do you mean by offgas? We've been bandying that word around all afternoon."

"Offgassing is the emission of gases from any material during drying, aging or decomposition," Jane explained. "Many synthetics manufactured in the last fifty years are major sources of indoor pollution. If you want a clear demonstration of what offgassing is all about, just take a small piece of rubberized underlay and new carpet - especially one containing significant proportions of cheaper fibers such as polypropylene - and put the samples in a jar. Keep it sealed for a few hours, then open it up and take a whiff. But be careful. It's pretty strong stuff! What you smell is what you'd be inhaling daily, only somewhat more concentrated. Another method is to put the product out into direct sunlight. You'll get a clear idea of its potency."

"Most synthetic carpeting is lethal!" Andrew retorted. "Take it from one who knows first-hand. It's *full* of volatile organic compounds . . ."

"Toluene, xylene, benzene are only a few," interrupted Jane.

"Then there are the chemicals in the pesticides, fungicides and stain-resistant treatments often added after the carpet has been manufactured - a great way to get pickled! Not only did we find all the fish in our aquarium belly up, but almost every plant in our office keeled over within *days* of installing the new carpet - I kid you not!"

We giggled like schoolchildren at the thought of a bunch of poor limp, toxed-out plants being put up as sacrificial lambs! But the dead fish were no laughing matter. In fact it was gruesome.

He continued, "On a more serious note, just talk about toxic effects to any one of the 125 EPA employees. They became ill after their offices were carpeted - ten were even hospitalized! Or ask any of the thousands who have been exposed to newly carpeted, poorly ventilated workplaces. As far as I'm concerned, the big lesson in all of this is that the human body can be far more sensitive than any instrument used to detect these chemicals."

"That's often the case. It's reminiscent of the canaries that were taken into the mines to detect methane - there were many cases of miners being gassed while the birds went on chirping. Some of us are just better detectors than others. But it's not to say that what we're able to sense more easily or sooner won't have a cumulative, harmful effect on others."

"It's happening all around us. Co-workers are dropping like flies, but they continue to live in denial."

"Synthetic carpeting alone can produce up to one hundred potentially harmful gases," Jane pointed out, "many of which can easily be detected in the blood."

"Where can you have your blood checked for these sorts of chemicals?" asked Martha.

"The same labs that do pesticide analyses will check for these as well." She dug a book out of her pile and opened it to a flagged page. "Take a look at this - compounds found in human tissue samples out of more than one hundred tested chemicals." (fig. 15)

"Can anyone have these tests done?" asked Andrew.

"Yes. But you need to have your family physician request it."

"That could be a problem," mumbled Sam, "unless you happen to be seeing someone who believes in all this . . ."

"Good luck! They're few and far between," said Martha wryly.

"The best thing," suggested Jane, "is to shop around until you find one

# Compounds Found in Human Tissue Samples *

## (fig. 15)

| COMPOUND | PERCENT WITH TOXIN IN BODY FAT | SOURCE |
|---|---|---|
| Benzene | 96 | combustion |
| Butylbenzyl phthalate | 69 | VOC |
| Chlorobenzene | 96 | water |
| Chloroform | 76 | water |
| DDE | 93 | pesticide |
| DDT | 55 | pesticide |
| 1,4-Dichlorobenzene | 100 | VOC |
| Dioxin | 100 | pesticide |
| Ethylbenzene | 96 | combustion |
| Ethylphenol | 100 | water |
| Heptachlor | 67 | pesticide |
| Styrene | 100 | VOC |
| Toluene | 91 | VOC |
| Xylene | 100 | VOC |

Compiled by the EPA. National Adipose Tissue Survey of the Public Health Service.

**Source:   Your Health & Your House**
Nina Anderson and Albert Benoist
Keats Publishing, New Caanan
Connecticut, USA

*∗ more than 100 chemicals tested*

who'll be sympathetic. Of course, ideally, these chemicals shouldn't be found in our homes or workplace to begin with, but as luck would have it, we don't live in an ideal world."

She continued the story. "Throughout the house, there's wall-to-wall carpeting which, when new, can be extremely toxic, and when old, harbors dust, molds and chemicals - somewhat in the way a sponge absorbs water. In fact, one can often tell the history of all the chemicals used in a house, as well as the pesticides sprayed in the neighborhood, from a carpet or underlay sample."

"And you think it's a problem in homes!" Sam asserted herself. "I can't begin to tell you how many schools have closed down due to mold-related health problems, most of which improved significantly once the old carpeting was removed and when the source of the moisture was found and corrected."

"Rates of asthma and other respiratory problems certainly improve markedly with carpet removal," affirmed Jane. "Just listen to stories from pre-school and kindergarten teachers. Not only is mold a problem, but carpets are breeding grounds for viruses and bacteria. Kids at that age sit or play on carpets for a good portion of their day. If a washroom happens to be attached to the main classroom, urine can be tracked in daily!"

"Oh gag! Spare me!" moaned Andrew. "And don't forget what we said earlier about dust absorbing carcinogenic VOC's and SVOC's."

"Carpet absorbs all that stuff?"

"All the more reason to take off your shoes any time you enter the house," reminded Jane. "You track in not only dust with all its hazards, but other toxins such as lead, cadmium, PCB's, dioxins and as we said earlier, a wide range of pesticides." She threw up her hands. "And folks, we're only at the beginning of our journey! Shall we continue?"

We nodded, knowing there was no turning back. "Next, I enter the fragrance capital of the house - the bathroom. I turn on the chlorinated, fluoridated water, inhaling those hot, wonderful vapors for a good ten minutes. At the same time, the shower curtain outgasses vinyl chloride, which has been linked to liver dysfunction, birth defects, genetic mutation and even cancer. I saturate my hair and body with perfumed soap and shampoo. Out of the shower, I gel or mousse my hair, then douse it with hairspray - the more strongly scented, the better. An aerosol deodorizer is optional, but certainly not my antiperspirant! Heaven forbid that one should have any natural odor left and smell like a real human being!"

We cracked up at the thought of our North American obsession with cleanliness. Sam quietly asked, "But then, what do you use? I don't really want to walk around with body odor."

"First, if your diet is appropriate for you, odors should be minimal. Second, the health food stores, and even some of the more progressive pharmacies, carry safe, alternative deodorants. Many of my friends swear by plain old baking soda, patted on once the body is dried off. As you'll soon discover, there are less-toxic solutions for virtually everything we use or do. Standard, commercial anti-perspirants may contain aerosol propellants, ammonia, alcohol, formaldehyde, fragrances and aluminum chlorohydrate. Excess aluminum is a real health concern, as high concentrations of it have been found in the brains of those who die from Alzheimer's disease."

"I read in one book," said Andrew, "that more than eight different ingredients used in commercial deodorants were banned by the FDA or voluntarily removed by the manufacturer because they posed a health risk to users."

"I'm not a bit surprised," answered Jane, as she resumed her story. "Then . . . I slather myself with perfume so I'll smell nice at work. I dress in undergarments which reek of potpourri, and put on clothes that have either been laundered with scented detergent and fabric softener, or that still outgas dry cleaning fluids - not only into the environment, but into my body as well."

"It all sounds so ridiculous when you really stop and think about it!" remarked Sam.

"But so few of us ever do. We just go about our business every day without giving it a second thought."

"Fabric softeners are a pet peeve of mine," I said. "I smell that stuff coming out of dryer vents whenever I go for walks - trying to get fresh air. It's disgusting!"

"I agree. If only people realized they were such victims of advertising. We really don't need most of these things. One safer and much less expensive way of getting static out of clothes is by rolling up a ball of aluminum foil and putting it in the dryer. . . An even better way is to wear as few synthetics as possible. Natural fibers tend not to cling."

"What do you use for detergent?" wondered Andrew.

"There are many low-toxic, unscented brands available. Again, health food and some grocery stores carry them. But do you know what I recommend?"

We all shook our heads.

"Reusable laundry discs."

"Laundry discs?" We said aloud. It was obvious that none of us had any idea what Jane meant.

"Instead of worrying about detergents and soaps that may or may not work, I bought these reusable Tri-Clean laundry discs that replace the need for soap. They last at least two years, sometimes more, and are extremely cost-effective, averaging about three dollars a month. At the same time, it's great for those with sensitivities and the environment in general."

"What exactly are they?" asked Sam.

"They're special ceramic beads enclosed in three small discs with a hard casing. The beads are electrostatically active, making the water super soft - exactly what soap and detergents are supposed to do. And they've just come out with something similar for dishwashers."

"Do they actually get the clothes clean?" I couldn't imagine doing a wash without adding anything besides three discs!

"The feedback from people who use them has been very positive. My sister-in-law, who happens to be pretty fussy about laundry, introduced them to me. She's been using hers for the past year and swears by them -

and that's with three young children. She recommends pre-soaking stains and adding a bit of Borax to whites. Now, where was I?"

"You haven't even left the top floor yet, and I feel tired already," sighed Martha, bringing another pot of tea from the kitchen.

"Next, I go downstairs to join the kids in a bowl full of Choco Puffs, Sugar Bears, or perhaps, instant waffles full of processed flour and sugar, additives and preservatives. Orange juice with its lingering pesticide residues, eggs, and milk on my cereal - two potential sources of hormonal and antibiotic residues - round out my breakfast."

"Mmmmm . . . yummy!" Andrew groaned mockingly. We couldn't help but scoff at the absurdity of the situation.

My mind immediately leaped to the reactions that milk had provoked with my kids, but I decided not to interrupt Jane. I was just grateful to have finally made the connection.

"Then there's my caffeine fix - my lifeline until mid-morning break," continued Jane. "After all, *something* has to pick me up from the breakfast I just had. Time to leave the house for work. Sometimes I take the car - other times, the bus. If I take the car, I leave the engine running to warm it up and enjoy the new car smell . . ."

"Believe it or not," said Martha, "my neighbour told me the other day that she uses a spray that gives her car that 'new' smell."

"No!" I couldn't believe it.

"You've got to be joking!" Andrew looked aghast.

"No, I'm serious. Her sister bought some just the other day. She adores that new car smell."

Jane burst into laughter. "It's probably a bottle of vinyl chloride!"

"Is that what makes a new car smell?" asked Sam.

"Well, it's one of the main chemicals. But things are looking up. Volkswagen recently announced that it's conducting research on upholstery and carpet emissions in its cars. Let's hope others follow suit. . ."

"Getting back for a moment to warming up the car . . . what about garages that are built beneath living quarters? This is very common in my neighborhood."

"I live in one of those," mumbled Sam.

"That's about the poorest design one could have," commented Jane. "In fact, the safest place for a garage is separate from the house. Not only is it dangerous to live atop a place where cars are started up, it's also not wise to have a living space above a garage that's full of stored chemicals. They slowly outgas into the rest of the house - especially to an upstairs room." She looked at Sam. "If you happen to live in this type of arrangement, it's best to store chemicals in a shed apart from the house and to keep the car outside."

"Just another reason to make a move!" declared Sam.

"If I don't take the car," resumed Jane, "I'd probably take the bus. Inhaling diesel fumes from an idling bus is a great way to start the day! Then just think - forty or fifty people, crammed into a small space, all wearing different scented products, some with smoke all over their clothes. Imagine the quality of *that* air!"

Andrew feigned a choking sound. As funny as it appeared, I was beginning to get a clear picture - that living in the nineties was a scarier prospect than I had ever imagined. We needed to look well beyond our contaminated food chain - if that wasn't bad enough!

"Finally, I arrive at work. If I've driven my car, I'll park in the underground garage. There, I breathe in the fumes of hundreds of cars as I find my way to my office. On the elevator, of course, I'm inundated once again with everyone's personal scents. And of course, there's always someone who's just put out a cigarette . . ."

Andrew cut in. "Speaking of tobacco smoke, *nothing* upsets me more than seeing adults smoking in cars with small children inside - strapped in their car seats - especially when the windows are shut tight - like on a cold winter's day or when it's raining. It's nothing short of abuse!"

"I agree with you Andrew. According to the Lung Association, aside from the damage caused by the smoke itself, tobacco is a source of over 4000 chemicals, fifty-two of which are known carcinogens. And *thirty-five percent* of all cancers are linked to tobacco use!"

"Those are astounding figures!" exclaimed Sam.

"*Four thousand* chemicals! Are you sure about that?" I had a hard time believing this figure.

"I had the same reaction when I first learned about it," replied Jane. "In fact, I have the information right here." She pulled a sheet from her file folder. "Included in the list of these chemicals are the following poisons: acetone, commonly used as a paint stripper; hydrogen cyanide, used in gas chambers; mercury, lead and cadmium - all toxic heavy metals; carbon monoxide - the deadly, colorless, odorless gas in car exhaust; DDT; arsenic, used as poison for pest control; formaldehyde; and nicotine, a drug as addictive as heroin that causes blood vessels to constrict and blood pressure to rise."

"If smokers only knew . . . Do you think they'd be more apt to quit?"

"Good question. In fact, if there are smokers in a house, you may as well forget about many of the precautions we've discussed here today, because that alone outweighs all the rest. Smoking constitutes our number one health hazard. Nothing is quite as damaging - especially to young children."

"This has become a very sensitive subject with my husband and me," remarked Sam. "We've recently lost a long-standing friendship over this very issue. But we simply couldn't bear to watch our neighbour hold a mask over his asthmatic child's face while holding a lit cigarette in his other hand."

Andrew's face contorted. "I tell you, there's no excuse! It's a form of slow poisoning!"

"Given what we know about cigarettes and all the publicity about second-hand smoke," said Jane, "I'd have to agree - there is no excuse. These parents are killing their children!"

"You're right," mumbled Martha. "The key might be to increase awareness, but more often than not, it takes legislation - especially when it comes to the common air supply we all have to share. And by God, we have a right to clean food, water and air. It's our birthright!"

"Right on , Martha!" proclaimed Andrew. "Jane, I'm sorry for diverting you away from your story and getting everyone all riled up. I just had to make that point. It pushes all my buttons."

"It's quite all right. What you said makes sense." She grinned, noting his somewhat obsessive nature. "Meanwhile, back at the office . . . a mid-morning coffee and danish would give me that second kick-start while I struggle to stay awake in my sealed building among my scented co-workers. Add to this the odors from synthetic furniture; carpets, of course; emissions from photocopiers and computers; poor quality artificial lighting; correction fluids and cleaning products - including those great air 'fresheners' used in washrooms - and what have you got? I'll tell you - a *toxic brew!*"

"And we haven't even made it to lunchtime!" Andrew said with his usual disdain.

"That's right. Now I realize that all this may seem somewhat exaggerated, but in fact, this is the way too many people live today. I was one of them - getting sicker by the day and never connecting my symptoms to my daily routine."

"Is that how you became ill?" asked Sam.

"It was a combination of things," replied Jane. "But as we speak, many of my former co-workers are experiencing similar symptoms. Denial is the operative word when it comes to Environmental Illness. They tell me how their chests tighten when they're at work, how their eyes water and throats hurt all day. They tell me about their headaches and nausea after sitting in idling traffic, and that their concentration and ability to retain information is deteriorating. They list all the tests they've had and the medications they're on. They're also very quick to tell me that they have a handle on it, often ending the conversation with, 'But thank God I don't have what you have'."

"Right," scowled Andrew with bitterness in his voice. "I've heard that a few times before."

"Oh, so have I," Sam concurred. "My colleagues are afraid to admit it, partly because of their own denial, but also because they're terrified of losing their jobs."

"I know all about that," said Martha. "The teachers at the school were petrified of making waves with the administration. They were afraid that if they spoke up, they'd be penalized for years to come - you know, promotions withheld, transfers to less popular schools - or even the fear of being replaced. And we taught in absolutely shameful conditions!"

"No one wants to admit that our quick-fix, comfortable, affluent way of life is making us sick - neither physicians, nor government, nor labor organizations, and last but not least, not even we, the consumers. Perish the thought that we should have to give up our creature comforts! We prefer to chalk up our chronic health problems to some mysterious force outside ourselves. To admit that we may have created this monster is an admission that we must take responsibility for it."

"Sort of like my Uncle Gene being told by one bowel specialist that there was absolutely no connection between his Crohn's disease and diet. Another told him as long as he watched his intake of roughage, he'd be fine. So he continues to eat junk, and continues to lose yards of bowel.

He's well on his way to a colostomy. But because his doctors endorse the belief that his bowel condition is essentially unrelated to his poor eating habits, he continues to take drugs, to undergo surgery, and to refuse to look at anything that may truly help him."

"The very notion that an illness may be tied into our way of life is very threatening," said Jane. "Change is a scary prospect for most of us. It can make us feel frustrated, angry. Then we begin to rationalize, even deny the obvious. I recall when I first became ill, I'd have a sore throat, dry eyes and fatigue throughout the week. Halfway through the weekend, I would begin to feel better, but by Tuesday or Wednesday, I'd be unwell again. Rather than try to figure out the problem, I went into major denial - to my detriment, of course, because the longer I stayed there, the sicker I became."

"God, Jane, I can empathize with everything you're saying," confessed Andrew. "How long was it before you finally made the connection?"

"It took quite a while. I recall times when I wanted to throw a rock through the sealed windows because I wasn't getting enough air. Those feelings were far more extreme on Monday - often in the mornings - but without fail, by late afternoon. Now I realize why."

"Why?" asked Martha.

"They used to shut the air exchange system down at four o'clock sharp every day and keep it turned off all weekend. By Monday the air would be dead, and the molds rampant."

"What should they have done?" I wondered aloud.

"First, they needed to address the mold problem in the building, and second, they should have kept the air exchange running on low all night, cranking it up at least several hours before people arrived in the morning."

"Why don't they do that?" queried Martha.

"Because they don't want to spend the money," shrugged Andrew, rolling his eyes. "We could smell the paint from renovations being done on the second floor all the way up to the eleventh. How good could that ventilation system have been? It really doesn't make sense! In the long run, they actually lose money, due to decreased productivity, higher absenteeism, and long-term disability payouts. These substantially outweigh any savings they could have enjoyed had they operated the air exchanger properly."

"So Andrew, do you think it was the poor air quality alone that did you in?" asked Sam in her quiet way.

"That certainly was a significant factor. In retrospect, however, I can clearly see that it was right after those renovations that I started to feel fatigued, catching one cold after another. Then, slowly, both my digestion and ability to think clearly was affected. But even then it was difficult to pinpoint cause and effect. Like Jane, I kept making excuses, blaming my overall state of health on other things - independent of what was happening around me."

"Did others complain?" inquired Jane.

"A few did. We had several teams of air quality experts in and they told us repeatedly that everything was 'well within acceptable limits'."

Martha scoffed, "And we all know how accurate they are!"

"What they don't often tell us," explained Jane "is that there are several different so-called acceptable limits for chemical emissions. The 'standard' chosen is often based on a single exposure to the contaminant for a healthy adult male working in an industrial setting. What's not considered is the effect of long-term, low-level exposure - especially for children; nor does it address the chemical soup phenomenon - that the office, school or home air is only one of many chemical exposures experienced in the run of a day, week or month. In other words, it doesn't take into account the total load."

"At least governments are now developing Indoor Air Quality (IAQ) standards for non-industrial settings," offered Andrew. "Things are starting to change, but it's very slow."

"Too slow for my liking!" retorted Martha. "In the meantime, our children - the next generation - are directly affected."

"And not in some distant future, but this very minute," replied Jane. "Children who sit in polluted classrooms certainly bear the brunt of environmental assaults. That which is acceptable today often gets re-evaluated tomorrow as we discover that some chemicals are more hazardous than we knew at the time. And what's acceptable for one person - the so-called 'average' person - may be quite toxic for another, depending upon their immune status."

"Jane, just how sick were you?" Sam queried.

"My dear, when I was pregnant with Lara, my third, I was bedridden. I suspect it was the mold in my office building that pushed me over the edge. By then I was sensitive to just about everything - to life itself, only I didn't know it. I was sick more often than I was well throughout that entire pregnancy. People would comment on how awful I looked."

"As bad as I looked that day we met in the playground?" I asked.

"Even worse. But Jillian, that's how I knew you were sick. I could see it in your face. You were so pale, your eyes so puffy - you looked wiped out. I could also see it on your little one's face - his runny nose, dark eye circles . . . You have to have been there to recognize it, to *know* it."

"And thank God you saw it," I murmured to myself.

"What was frustrating in my case," commented Sam, "was that I looked as good as ever, yet I was feeling so sick inside. I often felt like I was dying."

"Yes, I know all about it. No one believed how sick I was. In fact, everyone would comment on how great I looked. My colleagues thought I was faking . . . and I've already mentioned what my family thought . . ." Martha's voice faltered as she fought back the tears.

Andrew tried to change the subject, directing his question to Jane. "So what happened after Lara was born?"

"I had to go on long-term disability under the guise of a stress-related disorder. I've never gone back to that job and now understand that I never could.   Nor would I want to work in that kind of environment again - knowing what I now know."

"I can't believe how we just accept everything, never questioning the status quo - but worse, never stopping long enough to look at what we're really doing to ourselves."

"At least not until we become very sick," replied Jane, shaking her head.  "And unfortunately, that may be too late.  But really, if we think about it . . . who gets enough fresh air and exercise?  Who gets natural daylight?  Who drinks clean water?  Who eats foods that aren't processed or full of pesticides?"

"Is it any wonder so many people walk around feeling unwell?" Martha pointed out.

Andrew added, "Yes, today, everyone's got a complaint.  When I was growing up, maybe one or two kids in the entire school had asthma. . ."

"Today, it's normal to find at least one or two children in *every class* ," suggested Sam.  "And in some schools, teachers have drawers full of puffers."

"And do any of you recall running to the doctor each time you had the sniffles?  Or running to the local emergency department with earaches?"

"I sure don't," replied Martha.  "Something is wrong somewhere."

"I agree.  And more often than not, our ill health has to do with . . . with what?  In the now famous words of Dr. Gabriel Rowland . . ." Jane prompted me to finish.

"With what we eat, drink and breathe on a daily basis!" I smiled.

"You've got it!" Jane and I had a good laugh.

She then asked Andrew to pass around the papers on the table next to him.  "I hand these out in my workshops.  Most of the recommendations we went over today are represented by these two simple drawings - an unhealthy house (fig. 16), and a healthy house (fig. 17).

We studied them intently.  Andrew broke the silence.  "Jane, could we touch for a moment on building materials such as flooring, wall coverings and plumbing . . ."

"Sure.  Two important issues come to mind - the use of low emission materials and the timing of renovations, especially in colder climates.  Spring and summer are preferable to fall or winter."

"Because of access to fresh air?"

"Precisely.  Also, it's preferable to renovate one room at a time and isolate it as best as possible from the rest of the house.  Ideally, to vacate the house during the renovation period is even better.  Unfortunately, most people either can't afford it, or don't want to impose upon their relatives or friends."

"What about the materials themselves?" asked Andrew.

"Let's talk about good versus poor choices.  Using particleboard for construction material instead of an exterior grade plywood or tongue and groove construction is definitely an undesirable choice."

"Isn't particleboard often used in kitchen cabinets and shelves?"

"Yes - all too often.  Ideally, it shouldn't be used at all.  The best solution is to use solid wood.  Even exterior grade plywood would be an improvement. . ."

"Why?" asked Andrew.

"Because it uses phenol-formaldehyde which is quite a bit less toxic than the urea-formaldehyde glues used in particleboard and interior grade plywood.  If using either of the latter products, at the very least they should be well sealed with a low emission sealant - prior to installation where at all possible."

# The Unhealthy House
### (fig. 16)

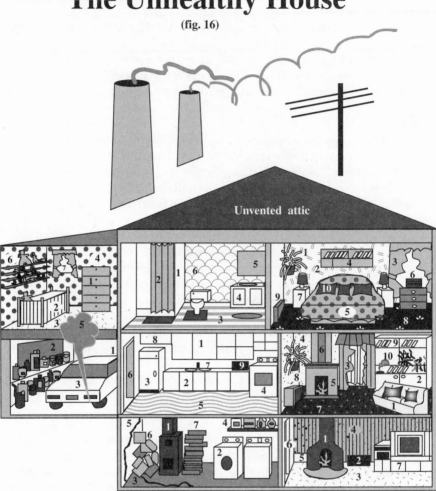

Unvented attic

## Laundry/Heating Area

1. Poorly maintained, unfiltered forced air system
2. Unvented dryer
3. Cracks in foundation allowing
   moisture & radon infiltration
4. Toxic, scented laundry cleaning agents, pesticides
5. No windows or ventilation
6. Storage of boxes, unused things
7. Storage of wood for fuel

## Family Room

1. Low-efficiency, poorly maintained
   woodstove
2. Kerosene heater
3. Wall-to-wall carpet on damp concrete
4. No windows/ventilation to outside
5. Dirty de-humidifier
6. Open doorway - toxic laundry/heating
7. Presswood entertainment unit

---

**NB: problems indicated in one room apply to all rooms**

# The Unhealthy House

## Kitchen

1. Cabinets made from pressboard
2. Toxic, scented cleaning compounds
3. Dirty refrigerator drip pan, stagnant water
4. Unvented stove
5. Vinyl sheet flooring or carpeting
6. Door leading directly to garage with car and toxic chemicals
7. Lead in plumbing of older homes
8. No windows/ventilation
9. Leaky microwave oven

## Living Room

1. Overstuffed furnishings made from synthetics
2. Entertainment units, furniture made from pressboard
3. Heavy drapes made of synthetic material
4. Walls covered in panelling, wallpaper or other unsafe materials
5. Fireplace without doors
6. Cracked, improperly maintained chimney
7. Wall-to-wall carpeting
8. Plants promoting mold growth
9. Books and lots of knick-knacks on open shelves (dust)
10. Cigarette smoke

## Bedroom

1. Plants
2. Wallpaper (esp. vinyl), or panelling
3. Draperies made from synthetics
4. Open bookcase headboard (dust)
5. Electric blanket, synthetic bedding
6. Dirty air conditioner
7. Furniture made from pressboard
8. Wall-to-wall, synthetic carpeting
9. Dirty humidifier, stagnant water
10. Excess pillows, stuffed animals

## Bathroom

1. Plaster, vinyl, gyproc tub/shower enclosure
2. Plastic shower curtain
3. Vinyl sheet flooring or wall-to-wall carpet
4. Cabinets made from pressboard
5. Cabinets full of toxic, scented personal care and cleaning products
6. No window or ventilation to the outside

## Room above Garage (especially if nursery!)

1. Furnishings and crib made from pressboard, plastics
2. Bedding made from synthetics (e.g. polyester)
3. Wall-to-wall carpeting
4. Wallpaper, panelling, toxic paints
5. Fumes from everything in garage, below
6. Clutter

## Garage

1. Attached, door to house often ajar
2. Open storage for toxic paint supplies, pesticides and other chemicals
3. Car exhaust permeates rest of house, especially room above

## Surrounding Environment

Close to:
1. industrial sites
2. high traffic areas
3. high-tension wires
4. heavily forested area, if mold-sensitive

# The Healthy House

(fig. 17)

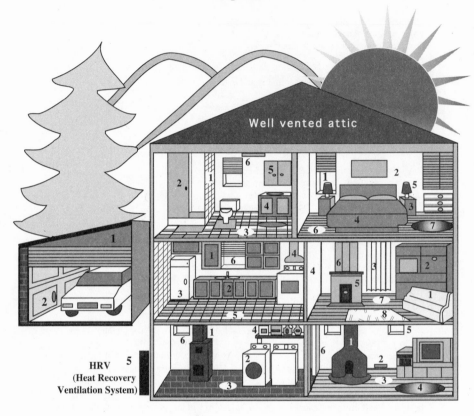

Well vented attic

HRV
(Heat Recovery
Ventilation System)

## Bathroom

1. Ceramic tile tub/shower enclosure
2. Glass doors
3. Ceramic tile/linoleum floor
4. Cabinets made from solid wood, metal or other safe materials
5. Cabinets containing safe, scent-free personal care & cleaning products
6. Window and powerful fan exhausted to outside

## Bedroom

1. Lots of windows with simple aluminum/wood shades - natural fiber curtains
2. Walls painted with VOC-free paints
3. Furniture made from solid wood, metal or other safe materials
4. Bedding made from natural fibers, as simple as possible
5. Lampshades made from natural materials (esp. important due to heat)
6. Hardwood, ceramic tile or linoleum flooring
7. Area rug made from natural fibers

---

**NB: factors affecting one room apply to all rooms**

# The Healthy House

## Kitchen
1. Cabinets made from solid wood, metal or other safe materials
2. Safe, unscented cleaning compounds
3. Clean refrigerator drip pan
4. Vented stove
5. Ceramic tile/linoleum/hardwood floors
6. Lots of windows - fresh air and light

## Living Room
1. Simple furnishings made from hardwood and natural fibers
2. Entertainment unit made from hardwood or metal with glass doors
3. Lots of windows, covered in metal or wooden shades, natural fabric curtains
4. Walls painted with VOC-free paint
5. Fireplace with tightly-fitted doors
6. Chimney that's tight and regularly maintained
7. Hardwood or ceramic floors
8. Area rugs made from natural fibers

## Laundry/Heating Area
1. Well-filtered forced hot air system, HWBB, electric, or solar heat
2. Vented dryer
3. Well-sealed foundation
4. Unscented, 'safe' laundry and cleaning agents
5. Heat recovery ventilation system (HRV)
6. Windows and/or ventilation system or both

## Family Room
1. High efficiency, catalytic type woodstove, properly maintained, or no woodstove at all
2. Electric baseboard, hot water baseboard or filtered forced hot air
3. Ceramic tile, linoleum or hardwood flooring
4. Natural fiber area rug
5. Well vented to outside, natural light
6. Doorway to 'safe' laundry/heating area

## Garage
1. Ideally, separate from the house - if not, seal off access
2. Low toxic-chemicals stored in closed cabinets

## Surrounding Environment
Far from:
1. industrial sites
2. high traffic areas
3. high-tension wires
4. heavily forested area, if mold sensitive

"I often wonder about those houses and apartment buildings built with pressboard - especially in damp, seacoast climates. It seems they're put up almost overnight. How safe can they be?"

"Good question. Since the material is affected by moisture, it's just about the worst choice one could make."

"I think we all know the answer to that," remarked Sam. "Just look at the list of chronic diseases that weren't in existence until the past decade or so. . ."

"Andrew, you had a question?"

"I realize we won't have time to go over this subject in any great detail," said Andrew, "and I don't know if anyone here is even interested as much as I am, but where can we learn more about construction materials?"

"A good place to begin would be to read this." Jane picked up a booklet from the table and held it up. "Put out by CMHC, it's called *Building Materials for the Environmentally Hypersensitive*, a resource I've included on the list you'll be getting at the end of our session."

"What's CMHC?" asked Sam.

"It stands for Canada Mortgage and Housing Corporation, a federal government agency that develops guidelines for quality housing. They've come out with several excellent brochures that deal with indoor air quality."

Martha inquired, "What about paints?"

"The paint industry has come a long way in recent years. VOC-free paints are now available, although the color selection is somewhat limited. By spring, some of the deeper shades will be on the market. Acrylics are a reasonable alternative to oil paints. For those extremely sensitive to latex and acrylic, old-fashioned milk paints that have recently made a comeback, are always an option."

"At least milk is good for some things!" mumbled Sam. A ripple of laughter went around the room.

Andrew piped up, "I'd heard that to help cure materials, it may be useful to conduct what is known as a 'bake out'. Can you comment on this procedure?"

"This is done by turning up the heat while simultaneously supplying adequate ventilation. Some say it offers only superficial curing while others seem to think it works well. The purpose is to prevent chemicals from migrating from one area to another and prevent absorption into porous surfaces such as rugs and furniture. Obviously, you don't want to be breathing in what's been outgassed."

"Speaking of furniture," I interrupted, "someone at the clinic mentioned that foam and synthetics can be a problem. Aren't most upholstered furnishings made from these materials?"

"And I read in one of the books," added Martha, "that some of these materials are made from plastic resins which not only irritate the skin, but can cause other health problems as well."

"They most certainly can," replied Jane. "And if that's not enough, they're almost always treated with chemicals for fire, mildew and stain resistance, which contribute to the outgassing process."

"And these additional processes can be detrimental to our health," Sam remarked. "Just a few weeks ago, my niece who's had asthma most of her life, made an interesting connection. She hadn't had an attack in months - especially since she modified her diet. This past January, she spent every Thursday at my sister's place. On each of those nights she ended up at the emergency department of the Children's Hospital. They finally tracked it down to a new, plush lazyboy chair that my sister had given to her husband for Christmas. That's precisely where Ellie would sit every Thursday night, watching her favorite program. As soon as the chair was removed, her asthma attacks became a thing of the past."

"Who would ever have guessed!" exclaimed Andrew, shaking his head. "A chair!"

"And that wasn't the end of the story," continued Sam. "My sister decided to pursue it even further. She took Ellie to a specialist in environmental medicine for testing. It turned out she was extremely sensitive to several chemicals, especially formaldehyde."

"I understand that one person in five is sensitive to formaldehyde," began Andrew, "but what alarms me most is that I've read that chronic exposure to this particular chemical plays a major role in the onset of chemical hypersensitivity - Environmental Illness." He looked around the room, "You know, the disease we all have?"

We acknowledged his comments, allowing Jane to address them.

"It's little wonder, since formaldehyde is found in virtually everything in our homes, office buildings, even hospitals - from our furniture, carpeting and construction materials, to fabrics and personal care products. According to experts in environmental health, the whole idea of 'acceptable limits' for formaldehyde should be discarded because of its sensitizing nature. In fact, I recently read that in West Germany, formaldehyde has been equated with dioxin as a health hazard. In March 1980, the American National Academy of Sciences added its formidable weight to the controversy when it concluded that formaldehyde, even at low levels, posed a serious health threat. Dr. Rowland tells me that there isn't a doctor in environmental medicine who hasn't encountered a whole host of complaints that result from this one chemical. And you can't avoid it - it's everywhere, from diesel engines to personal care products we use every day."

"It's one of the main reasons why so many employees complain of eye, nose and throat irritation, sneezing, coughing, chronic headaches and brain fog . . ."

"Which, of course, are common symptoms of flu viruses. No wonder people don't get the connection."

"And those are only a few of the many symptoms," Jane pointed out. "Others that no one ever connects to this type of exposure include memory loss, mood swings, apathy and depression. . . you'd probably chalk it all up to 'stress' or a natural part of the aging process."

"So if even our furniture is contaminated, what does one sit on?" asked Martha, her eyes darting about the room.

"Look around. Everything here is hardwood and untreated natural fiber. How do you feel sitting in this room?"

"Great."

"Fine."

"Feels wonderful. Feels clean."

"Dust is always a problem in my house," continued Martha, "especially since we took up all the carpets and now have the hardwood floors."

"Perhaps you need a better filter for your heating system," Jane suggested. "The one consolation is that at least now you can *see* the dust and dirt." She looked at the rest of us. "Have any of you ever ripped up old carpeting?"

"I have," replied Andrew, "and let me tell you, the amount of dirt that's under wall-to-wall carpeting would be appalling to anyone!"

"So you see, Martha," Jane explained, "the only difference is that you can now at least *see* it - which means you can do something about it. All I use is a damp mop on the floors and a damp cloth on the furniture. And it works! We really don't need all those smelly, expensive, toxic cleaners to keep our homes clean."

"I don't mean to change the subject," interrupted Andrew. "but I'd heard that the best age for a house is anywhere between thirty and fifty years old, since it would be built primarily from wood instead of synthetics or pressboard. I'd also imagine that a house that age might be rough on the old heating bill, but great for overall health - at least it breathes. Any merit in this?"

Only a few short months ago, I never would have believed that I'd be interested in this topic - now, I couldn't get information fast enough!

"The truth of the matter is that there's no ideal age for a house because each age has its problems. Obviously, top quality building materials are important criteria - whether new or old. Older homes can have lead paint, mold and asbestos problems. In fact, in Massachusetts, homes on the marketplace must be warranted free of lead. What I found interesting during my research, is that lead paint was banned in Germany just after the turn of the century, while Canada only banned it as recently as 1967."

"We really are far behind when it comes to our health," Martha commented.

"I agree. Maybe we should be looking at some of our European counterparts for precedents. And as we discussed earlier, newer homes should be checked for chemical contamination. Everything depends upon the materials used and the efficiency of the ventilation system. One of the most significant things you can do to help your health is to transform your bedroom into a sanctuary. . ."

"A sanctuary?"

"Yes . . . a place to heal. Because you spend about a third of your life in the bedroom, it's the most logical place to transform into a safe space . . ."

"A safe space?" I asked. I was beginning to sound like Sam.

"I mean a special location where you can get relief from everyday environmental assaults - a way of reducing your total load. It should be isolated from the rest of the house, infused with nothing but clean air and include furnishings made from non-toxic materials. An air filtration system also helps. This diagram gives more detail about how to create a healthy bedroom." (fig. 18)

As we examined the drawing closely, Sam shared more of her story. "I was so sick from that pesticide exposure, that I had to take drastic steps immediately to help myself. Creating a safe bedroom was crucial. I stripped

# Unhealthy & Healthy Bedrooms

### (fig. 18)

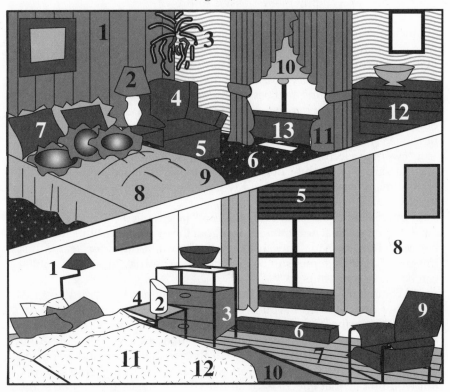

## Unhealthy Bedroom

1. Panelling/wallpaper/toxic paint
2. Plastic shade and base
3. Plant
4. Foam-stuffed chair
5. Synthetic cover
6. Carpet with rubber underlay
7. Foam-filled cushions
8. Synthetic bedspread
9. Foam mattress
10. Vinyl shade
11. Synthetic fiber curtains
12. Chest with particle board
13. Hot air duct

## Healthy Bedroom

1. Metal and glass lamp
2. Air purifier
3. Solid wood chest
4. Glass and steel table
5. Metal blinds
6. Electric or hot water baseboard heater
7. Hardwood floor
8. Non-petroleum, VOC-free paint
9. Steel and cotton chair
10. Natural cotton rug
11. Natural fiber cotton-covered bedding
12. Futon or cotton mattress
13. Natural fiber pillows

everything down to bare bones. What a difference it made! So, I can vouch for what Jane is suggesting, and I would highly recommend it."

"Thanks for the testimonial, Sam. There's nothing quite like personal experience. And let me tell you, if you've never slept on a cotton futon or mattress, you've missed something really special. I've never had such great sleep! But you have to make sure they haven't been sprayed with anything, especially fire-retardant finishes on the cover."

"Where can you buy them?" asked Andrew.

"Addresses and phone numbers for everything we've covered today are included in the resource list I'll give you before you leave. For those who want a regular bed, with boxspring and mattress, one can be custom-made from cotton and hardwoods. They're quite expensive, but it's often the only solution for very sensitive individuals. Another solution would be to cover the existing mattress with layers of cotton, flannel sheets or even quilts to create a barrier. A third option for those less sensitive, is to obtain one that's outgassed. Often, a display model is preferable to a brand new one. Andrew, do you have another question?"

"I went to a lecture given by a builder who specializes in healthy homes and he said that mobile homes were among the most contaminated environments one could live in. My girlfriend lives in one and she's not exactly a picture of health."

"Interesting you should bring that up," Jane replied. "I've often heard Dr. Rowland say that new mobiles are about the most unsafe living quarters around. They're made entirely of synthetics and outgas for years. Just imagine that hot summer sun beating down on one day in and day out. It can become a toxic inferno."

"What about apartments?" I inquired. "You have very little control over your environment if you're surrounded by neighbors who smoke, wear heavy perfumes or who clean with lots of chemicals."

"It could be a somewhat more difficult situation, but manageable. Your own unit could be outfitted with a small air exchanger - the kind that fits in a window. It would screen out most odors and outdoor airborne irritants, but wouldn't be that effective for smoke. To some extent, you'd be at the mercy of whoever owned or managed the building. You'd have to form a tenant group to ensure that cleaning and maintenance were done with non-toxic products. A couple more questions and we'll have to call it quits. Martha?"

"I've been reading a bit here and there about electromagnetic radiation and its potentially adverse health effects. Can you talk about that for a minute?" This topic was way beyond my scope.

Jane explained, "Electric blankets and waterbeds, space heaters, televisions, computers, and cellular phones, are all sources of electromagnetic fields. Video display terminals have been linked to increased levels of miscarriages, and even to cancer. Research is presently being conducted into a possible connection between cellular phones and brain cancer. As you can well imagine, living close to high voltage lines is definitely not recommended . . . "

"Why?" asked Martha with a puzzled expression on her face.

"Fatigue, flu-like symptoms, muscular weakness, memory impairment, mood swings, depression and irritability are only some of the symptoms that have been attributed to living near high tension wires. Even more significant is the relationship between childhood leukemia and proximity to sources of high voltage."

"So how do we protect ourselves from all these modern conveniences? We're not going to do away with T.V.'s and computers."

"That's very true, but we can take measures by limiting our exposure. For example, we can sit at least four to six feet from the television and reduce the amount of time we watch it. . ."

"Better for overall mental health and family life in general!" grinned Sam. "The best thing I ever did was cut off our cable T.V. We now spend our time chatting, reading and playing music. The quality of our lives has drastically improved."

"Did the kids go into withdrawal?" teased Martha.

"Only for a couple of days. Now it's almost as if they're relieved the option isn't there." Sam looked toward Jane, covering her mouth with her hand. "Oops! Sorry! I've interrupted you."

"That's quite all right. It's anecdotes such as these that bring home some very important points. Now, back to electromagnetic fields . . . we can either avoid electric blankets and waterbeds altogether, or at the very least, turn them off when in bed. It's also wise to reduce our time around microwaves. Microwave ovens should be regularly inspected for leakage. Using low radiation monitors or placing filters on older VDT's is critical. These are important precautions. Dr. Rowland told me of a patient whose cure was simply to stop sleeping on a heated waterbed. From that day forward, his chronic fatigue cleared up."

"*Harrowsmith* had an excellent article on reducing EMF exposure a few years ago," offered Andrew.

"Oh, if only *our* problems could be solved so simply!" lamented Sam.

"Before I forget, Jane," said Andrew, "can you recommend a good book on creating a more healthy home?"

Jane passed him *The Healthy House*, by John Bower. "Aside from being well-written, what I like best is its great index." She held up another book, *Your Health & Your House* by Nina Anderson and Albert Benoist. "It's hot off the press and clearly makes the connection between symptoms and health hazards around the house. It also contains a list of pollutants and their effects. Every home should have this book. And then," she held up a video, "Canada Mortgage and Housing recently produced a half hour video called *This Clean House*. It's full of very simple, easy-to-follow suggestions, and full of information that's helpful in tracking down the primary culprits. CMHC also has several exceptionally user-friendly booklets available at low cost: *The Clean Air Guide* is one; *Housing for the Environmentally Hypersensitive* is another; *Research House for the Environmentally Hypersensitive* is a third." She then held up two small booklets. One dealt with moisture and the other with procedures for cleaning up mold.

"Are those on the list as well?" asked Martha.

"Absolutely! They're an invaluable resource. All homeowners and institutions should consider getting them - they're life-savers. When I asked one of the authors whether there were equivalents to these publications in the U.S., she said they didn't believe there were any quite like these. I've included a toll-free number in the resource list.

"Jane," asked Andrew, "where can I learn more about electromagnetic radiation?"

"One of the best books I know is *The Zapping of America* by Paul Brodeur."

"I hate to say it again," said Martha, deep in thought, "but we really must become more aware - knowledgeable. Then we can make intelligent choices. Is that not true?"

"Yes, it is," replied Jane. "Information is critical and the more unbiased, the better. Take heart, though. There *is* an increasing awareness about the toxic world in which we live. These publications are good examples of the changes we've been seeing lately. A public opinion poll, conducted as far back as 1988, suggested that nine out of ten Canadians believed their health had deteriorated due to environmental pollution, and *ninety-three per cent* feared they were being poisoned by toxins that had not, as yet, been identified. So I think it would be safe to say that the public *is* more aware than ever before."

"Let's face it," summarized Andrew, "We're all becoming allergic to the 21st century."

"That's it in a nutshell!" declared Jane. "I couldn't have said it better myself. This is why books on this subject are popping out all around us, and why the media is providing greater coverage than ever before."

"But the real question is, are we ready to give up our perception of that perfect world for one that includes a few wormholes in our apples and some weeds on our lawns?" Andrew, as always, was very direct.

"I tend to be the eternal optimist and believe that someday we will be ready to change. Unfortunately, it may take much illness and many deaths before that occurs." Jane peeked at Martha's watch. "Is it really three o'clock already? Gosh! We haven't even discussed lighting. Are any of you scheduled to visit Lake of the Woods School in the the near future?"

"I'm going in a few weeks," I piped up.

"Is that the school that was renovated with environmental safety in mind?"

"That's the one. They're totally scent-free; have a state-of-the-art ventilation system; and use skylights and broad-spectrum lighting throughout. You really should check it out, especially if you're interested in making your schools safer places for your children. You wouldn't believe the difference. Even the school menu would knock your socks off!"

"How on earth did such a dream school ever come into existence?" asked Sam.

"Some very persistent parents, a few courageous teachers and a group of open-minded administrators made it happen," replied Jane. "It shows that we *can* make a difference."

"That's encouraging." Andrew stretched and yawned. "So Jane, do you think we'll ever be normal again?"

"The real question is, what's normal? If normal is going back to the lifestyle you lead prior to becoming sick, perhaps not. But is that what you really want, knowing what you now know?"

That was food for thought! I knew that if normal meant going back to eating the standard North American diet, full of additives, preservatives and colorings which caused much of our illnesses - mental as well as physical - the answer was no. Did I want our precious time spent in doctors' offices and emergency departments as a result of guzzling milk and eating ice cream every day? No way. Did I want to go back to cleaning with products I now knew to be toxic? Not a chance. Did I need a perfect lawn if it meant risking our health? Never!

I knew I could never go back. I knew I'd never *want* to go back. I made a decision to leave my old way of life behind in exchange for a whole new way of being. In that moment I knew my future would be one filled with hope, good health and happiness.

*Provocation-Neutralization*
*helps parents pinpoint*
*specific cause-and-effect relationships.*
*It often enables parents dramatically*
*to see exactly which allergenic substances*
*are causing each of their child's*
*individual medical complaints.*
*One item might cause*
*obvious hay fever during testing,*
*another asthma, a third depression,*
*and a fourth a rash.*

*Some patients improve immediately*
*during their first office visit,*
*others within a few days or months.*
*If this method is helpful, it is not unusual*
*for many children to improve*
*50 to 85 percent*
*within a few weeks or months.*

**Doris Rapp, M.D.**
**Is This Your Child?**

# 17

# Testing

*Flipping a coin in deciding on a food sensitivity is just as reliable for food allergy diagnosis as a scratch test.*
**Zoltan P. Rona, M.D., M.Sc.**

*T*esting day came a bit sooner than anticipated. Another family had cancelled and we were bumped up on the list. For four consecutive days, we would be poked and prodded to determine our sensitivities. Finally, we'd know exactly what effect specific foods, chemicals and airborne irritants had on us.

As we drove to the clinic, I thought of how pleasant our family outings had become. Looking back, it was difficult to imagine that I had accepted the constant whining and bickering as a normal way of life - as so many people did. Of course, when you're right in the thick of it and don't realize there's any other way, you come to accept it.

Michael was amazed by our progress, especially since my chlorine incident. He was impressed with the children's behavior over the past few weeks. But I think what really did it was losing his fifty bucks! I smiled to myself. Gone were his headaches and heartburn. Now whenever the subject of diet or environmental health arose, no one praised the clinic more than Michael. He had become a true believer. Today he'd finally get to meet Dr. Rowland.

I'd packed a knapsack for each child, filled with supplies to keep them quietly occupied - books, pencils, scent-free markers and paper. After explaining the procedure to Nathaniel and Emma, I promised them each a reward at the end of testing. I wasn't quite sure how well they would take to intradermal injections. Max, too young for this method, would be tested sublingually.

As we entered the reception area, Emily greeted us as if we were long-lost friends. "Jillian, your children are beautiful! They look just like you - especially this young lady," she said, placing her hand on Emma's shoulder. "And you must be Michael," she said reaching out to shake his hand.

She escorted us to the testing area. It was empty but for one person - an older woman quietly knitting with one sleeve rolled up. We were taken into an inner office and introduced to two young women wearing brightly colored lab coats. The room was sunny and decorated with pictures drawn by children of all ages. Two entire walls were devoted to shelf after shelf of tiny bottles. Gesturing to the young woman with curly red hair, Emily said, "Jillian, this is Jaime and she'll be testing you and Max." Then, nodding to the taller woman sitting at the desk beside the window, she said, "And this is Lori. She'll be working with Nathaniel and Emma."

Lori smiled at the children and said cheerfully, "Hi, kids! Are you ready for your first day of testing?"

"Does it hurt?" asked Emma, in a near whisper.

"Nah . . . feels like a mosquito bite. There's really nothing to it." At that moment, the woman from the waiting area walked in, sat down in front of Lori, and placed her bared arm on the desk. Lori then took a ruler and measured a raised bump on her arm, asked how she was feeling, what her pulse rate was, and then gave her another intradermal injection. Lori caught a glimpse of Emma out of the corner of her eye and could see she looked worried.

"See. Nothing to it . . . right, Mrs. Hilchie?"

"Right." She winked at Nathaniel and Emma. "And you wouldn't believe what I've learned from these tests! Why, in no time at all you'll find out what sorts of things get you into trouble! Really, there's not much to it. And Lori's an expert at this - she makes it so easy."

Lori laughed, drawing Emma close to her. Emma looked at Nathaniel and said, "You go first! You're older."

"No way! You're closer. *You* go first!"

Lori, obviously used to young children, took a coin out of her desk drawer. "Okay you two, let's flip. Heads go first." Emma won the honor.

Just then, Lori looked in our file and exclaimed, "Emma, Nathaniel, this must be your lucky day! Dr. Rowland wants me to start with chemicals." Looking at them both, she said, "And guess what?" Chemicals are tested sublingually - drops under your tongue. No need for needles today, so you can relax."

They were both quite relieved!

She selected a dropper bottle from one of the shelves and said, "Emma, honey, I'm going to put a tiny drop of this stuff under your tongue. Then, your Dad will time you and take your pulse. After seven minutes, he'll take your pulse again, and we'll give you another drop. How does that sound?"

"All right," mumbled Emma, not at all sure what was happening.

Lori turned to us and said, "I'm not going to tell you what you're being tested for until we're finished each substance . . . to avoid any power of suggestion. Mr. Stowe . . ."

"You can call me Michael . . ."

"Michael, I'm giving you this stopwatch. I'd like you to take the children's pulses and get them to write their names on a piece of paper. Or, they could draw a picture if they wish. Then, I'll give them a drop and you'll repeat the same procedure after seven minutes. Do you know how to take a pulse?"

Michael nodded.

"Good." She reached into her drawer and pulled out two pads and some pencils. Nathaniel wrote his name and Emma drew a sweet picture of a girl smiling with a sun over her head. "What a beautiful picture!" Lori had a wonderful way with children. She smiled. "So Emma, are you ready? Open your mouth and curl your tongue back, like this." She demonstrated it for her. She placed a single drop under her tongue and repeated it with Nathaniel. In the meantime, Jaime did the same with Max and me. I was in charge of monitoring my own pulse as well as Max's. We all trooped out to the outer room to wait our seven minutes. Michael pulled a newspaper from his briefcase to pass the time while the children played.

Suddenly, Mrs. Hilchie turned to Michael and said, "Excuse me, but the smell of newsprint really makes me sick. I'd appreciate it if you would remove it." I could tell that Michael was a bit put out. He mumbled, "Sure, no problem," and left the room. As he passed me, he leaned over, rolled his eyes, and whispered, "Now, this is a bit much, don't you think? I'll be back in a few minutes."

It reminded me of all the people and places I had to leave over the years because of smells that made me sick, whether it was perfume, aftershave, fabric softener, smoke or even unidentifiable odors. I admired Mrs. Hilchie for speaking up. It was certainly better than quietly slinking away and later apologizing - to someone who had polluted my space! I made a commitment right then and there to be more assertive in the future. We had a right to clean air.

A moment later, a bizarre thing happened.

Nathaniel went over to Emma and kicked her. Emma shrieked, burst into tears, and began to sob uncontrollably. Feeling increasingly unfocused and irritable, I snapped at both of them. Max, who had been playing with some building blocks, got up and started tearing around, yelling at the top of his lungs, collapsing into a sobbing heap on the floor. I was mortified! I gave Mrs. Hilchie an apologetic look. She looked at us with pity, yet with understanding. By the time Michael returned, we were completely out of control. He couldn't believe it. Ordering Nathaniel back to his seat, Michael vacillated between anger and embarrassment.

Refusing to listen, Nathaniel continued to badger Emma. He was becoming more fidgety, hyperactive, and louder by the minute. When Michael tried to calm him, he yelled,"No! Why should I? Who do you think you are, anyway?"

"Sit down, young man! Right now! Do you hear me?" hissed Michael under his breath.

"No I won't! I hate you!" Nathaniel stood up and staggered like a drunk. The entire scene reminded me of Martha's Black Friday story.

Emma continued to whine and yawn, constantly rubbing her eyes. She said repeatedly, "Mommy, I'm tired. I'm so sleepy." Max, completely out of control, climbed all over the furniture, making car and truck sounds. He was drooling from the corners of his mouth. It was a sad sight indeed. It brought back memories of some of our worst days at home.

Michael could see we were all reacting and that disciplining the children was hopeless. "God, Jilly! This is what it used to be like. I don't think I could handle that again. Look at your face!" He led me to a mirror near his chair. I was aghast! My face was as white as a sheet.

Mrs. Hilchie came over to us and said quietly, "Don't forget to keep track of the time so you can get your next drop." We nodded and thanked her for reminding us. I felt fuzzy, very irritable and extremely tired. All of a sudden it struck me. This was the same reaction I used to get at the theatre. I couldn't remember a play that I had ever lasted through. I was never able to stay awake from beginning to end. "Michael, I feel totally wiped out - the way I get at the theatre, in church or at the mall."

Ignoring my comments, Michael just stared at the children, bewildered by their erratic behavior. "Just look at them," he mumbled under his breath, "I wonder what they were tested for." They were so uncooperative he couldn't even take their pulses. He literally had to pick Max up and carry him into the testing room. Lori coaxed Nathaniel back, then asked him to write his name. She asked Emma to draw a picture. Then we each got another drop. It took almost an hour for everyone to get back to normal. It amazed me that once we got the right dilution, we returned to reasonable behavior almost immediately. It took only three drops for Max; for the other two, about five; and seven to bring me back to normal. Michael couldn't believe what he had witnessed. This is what their printing and drawing looked like:

| Before testing | During testing | After testing |
|---|---|---|

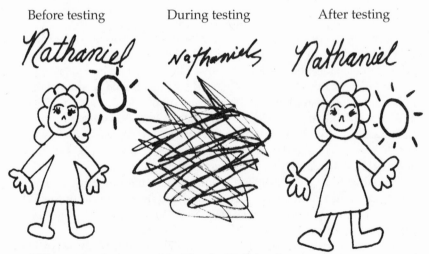

"What were they tested for?" asked Michael.
"Perfume."
" Jilly, you were right! Maybe it *is* Mrs. Allen's perfume."
"*Maybe?*"
"I mean . . . It must be! I just can't believe all this! This is amazing!"
"Ready for test number two?" asked Lori and Jaime, simultaneously.

"Let's go for it kids!" Michael herded them in to their chairs. I sat by Jaime's desk, holding Max on my knee while Lori gave the other two their drops.

We returned to the waiting area. The place was beginning to fill up with patients, from the very young to the elderly, all waiting their turn to be tested. The children began playing with some of the other kids while I buried myself in a magazine. Within minutes, I couldn't focus on a thing I was reading. I could hear Nathaniel and Emma picking at each other, their voices becoming louder, snarkier as each minute passed. It was embarrassing. I sensed everyone in the room staring at us. Then Max, still playing with blocks, stood up and kicked the entire structure down. They flew in all directions. The two older ones laughed at him. Totally distressed, Michael and I glanced sheepishy around the room, but quickly realized that no one seemed shocked or perturbed.

Dear old Mrs. Hilchie leaned over and said quietly, "Don't worry, this is what you're here for. There isn't anyone in this room who hasn't been through what you're now experiencing, except of course, newcomers like yourselves . . ."

At that moment, a boy about Emma's age came charging down the hall. "Matthew! Matthew! Come back in here!" called a voice from another room. He kept on running, clumsily bumping into anything in his way. My kids stopped dead in their tracks. They watched in amazement. A large woman, obviously another tester, emerged from a room down the hall, followed by a man and a woman. I assumed they were his parents. They tried to entice him to return. What ensued was right out of the Doris Rapp tapes.

The child became violent. He tore up anything he could get his hands on. His father had to restrain him while the tester pried his mouth open to give him another drop. It took three different drops, spaced five minutes apart to get the child back to normal. Once the correct dilution was administered, he became quite rational, cooperative, and pleasant - almost as if nothing had happened. The mother held her hands over her face, sobbing, "And I always thought he was a bad kid. They told me he'd end up in jail - that he was incorrigible, that there was no hope! My God! And to think he's sensitive to *oranges*! I'd give them to him every day, thinking they were good for him." My eyes began to tear. I felt her pain as a mother, wanting only the best for her child, but not having a clue about what was really going on all those years.

A staff member who had helped chase down the child, put an arm around her and said, "But Joan, just think, *now you know*! It's no one's fault. You did the best you could, and now you know for sure that his behavior had nothing whatsoever to do with the way you raised him." They all walked back down the hall, the boy now in control of himself.

Meanwhile, our time was up and we resumed our testing. Once again, it took several rounds to get us all back to normal. Lori told us that the last chemical we had received had been formaldehyde.

As she gave us our drops for the next test, Jaime reminded us, "Formaldehyde is found virtually everywhere - building materials, new carpeting, personal care and cleaning products, fabric treatments, and even school and office products like markers, paints and inks. It's a tough one to avoid."

As the day progressed, we both began to appreciate the value of this type of testing, painstaking as it was. It really enabled us to understand how each chemical affected our bodies - and our minds. Michael became fascinated with the process.

"How does this work?" he asked Lori during one of his many trips into the testing room with the kids.

"At the end of your testing period, you'll see Dr. Rowland. He'll explain it to you then. In the meantime, I can give you this information which gives a detailed outline of this procedure, better known as antigen therapy or, Provocation-Neutralization." She reached into her drawer and handed it to Michael.

Round three.

This time, Emma, Max and I seemed fairly level but Nathaniel began to fall asleep, complaining of a headache and nausea. When asked if he'd ever felt like that before, he replied immediately, "Yeah, in the car when we go on long trips."

Interestingly, the chemical we were tested for was auto exhaust!

While we waited for Nathaniel to return to normal, I struck up a conversation with some of the people in the waiting area.

"Is there testing going on in those other rooms?" I asked the gentleman who sat next to me.

"From my understanding, there are about six testers working at any given time. Are all of you being tested?"

"Everyone, except my husband." I nodded toward the door where Michael was escorting Nathaniel to see Lori.

"It must be quite stressful, having to sit through four days of this. I only have myself to worry about. I can't imagine being in charge of three other sensitive people. But you know, in the end, it's all worth it. My whole life has changed since I started coming here. Now I know what triggers what. Before that, I didn't have a clue."

Michael returned with Nathaniel. He seemed interested in our conversation. "What made you sick in the first place?" he asked, periodically glancing at the stopwatch.

"I was told for years that I had Chronic Fatigue Syndrome and that there was nothing I could do but live with it and wait it out. So, I did. I waited . . . and waited . . . and waited. Sixteen months later, nothing had changed. Then a friend told me about Dr. Rowland. When I mentioned him to my family doctor, he nearly laughed me out of his office! However, since coming here, I'm a new man."

"Are your symptoms environmentally triggered as well?" I asked.

"They definitely are. I had a long list of undiagnosed food and chemical sensitivities. The building I worked in also played a large part in my illness. It was one of those high-rise office towers with sealed windows and mechanical ventilation that was improperly operated. I was never the same after working there."

"Michael," I said, "check your watch. I think you have to go in."

"Right. Nathaniel, let's go." They headed back to the testing room.

Nathaniel was still a little confused and his speech was still slightly slurred. After seven more minutes, and another drop, he was back to normal. It was now lunchtime.

I had packed a large picnic cooler which we carried to the lunch room one floor up. There was a real feeling of camaraderie among the people there. We all chatted as if we had known one another for years. The woman beside us - tall, thin and attractive, with grey hair pulled into an elegant knot - introduced herself as Alice and told us her story.

"I'd had bowel problems since my early twenties. All I was offered were drugs and surgery. Dr. Rowland had me eliminate a few foods, take some supplements, and I haven't had a problem since. I just come here occasionally for checkups and some acupuncture for maintenance."

"And I was diagnosed with M.S.," said the man next to Alice. "I was told to take steroids whenever I had a flare-up. When I asked about diet and vitamins, the people at the Foundation took great exception. They didn't like me taking control of my own situation. They chastised me, somewhat like a parent talking to a child who doesn't know any better. Their attitude was very demeaning. They really need to become more educated, more knowledgeable about alternatives in dealing with this disease. Even my family doctor, whom I've known for years, thinks I'm crazy for coming here. He chalks up my progress to 'spontaneous remission' with no connection to my own efforts at getting better."

"You're sensitive to things too?" asked Michael.

"You betcha! In fact, it wasn't until I had my mercury amalgam fillings removed that my symptoms really improved. Up until that point, I rotated my diet like crazy, took vitamins, tried biofeedback and acupuncture. They all helped, but the removal of all that metal in my mouth brought about the greatest improvement. Homeopathy helped to drain the mercury toxins from my body. Had it not worked, my next course of action would have been chelation therapy. And, of course, the elimination of sugar, dairy products and yeasty foods from my diet also helped me regain my health."

"My God!" exclaimed Michael. "Even fillings can be a hazard?" He was absorbing story after story.

Everyone smiled knowingly. It was obvious they'd all been there in one way or another.

"Do you know," the man continued loudly, "there are over one hundred published scientific papers that directly implicate mercury toxicity with chronic illness!" He was incensed.

"And the Dental Association still endorses its use!" snorted the woman next to him. I assumed she was his wife. "Germany has prohibited the sale and manufacture of mercury amalgams since 1992, and Sweden has determined that such amalgams are toxic - advising against their use in pregnant women. In fact, as soon as a suitable replacement is found, they will be banned outright."

"That's right," continued the man. "And the Swedish government pays fifty percent of the cost for removal - a far cry from our approach here!"

"It's really outrageous to allow the use of a product that's clearly toxic to the human body!" Michael was appalled.

"How much suffering is connected with this routine practice is what I'd like to know!" exclaimed the woman.

"I can't believe that a substance designated by the EPA as a waste disposal hazard, one which I'm not permitted to throw in the trash, is okay to put in a person's mouth! And to make matters worse, when you want to have them removed and replaced with some other substance, you're treated as if you've lost your mind! Dentists who are more sympathetic are nervous about removing them because the dental associations have published literature which clearly states that the practice of removing amalgams for mercury toxicity is unethical. It's a no-win situation. It's just one more example of resistance to change being rooted in an organization and not necessarily in its members."

One thing I had noticed over the past months was that the people I met who had environmental sensitivities were usually well researched - up on the latest information. It was like being in an institution of learning.

A young woman introduced herself as Miriam. She was there with her daughter, Elise, who looked to be about thirteen. "I went to nearly every yoga ashram in the country to try to help myself, thinking that most of my problems were really 'in my mind', as so many of my friends and physicians had suggested. I could have meditated till the cows came home, and I wouldn't have been much further ahead. Not to say that meditation doesn't help - it does. But it was my *body* that was very sick."

"And what helped you?" I was most curious.

"For me, candida, parasites and food sensitivities were a major part of the problem. My new lifestyle took some adjustment, but I'm much stronger for it and would never even consider going back to my old ways. The meditation I learned along the way is the icing on the cake! I feel truly balanced for the first time in years."

I knew exactly where she was coming from. Only a few months ago, I would never have imagined that these things existed, let alone that I had them!

"Do you know, just about every doctor I ever went to asked me if I had a husband. When I'd answer 'No, I don't', they'd suggest I should find one - as if that were the root cause of my problems!"

A burst of laughter came from one corner of the room. A young woman in her early twenties, with a child on either side, exclaimed, "You know what I say when I'm given that line? I say, "No, I don't have a husband, I don't want a husband, and I'm *not* unhappy. *I'm* sick. So are you going to help or not? As it turned out, Dr. Rowland was the only one who could really help me since he was the only one who understood my problem."

I could see by Michael's expression that he was beginning to understand what I'd gone through for the past few years. Sometimes it takes other people voicing similar concerns to bring the point home.

Looking at Miriam's young daughter, Michael asked, "And does Elise have problems too?"

She nodded. " Like mother, like daughter. Only she's so lucky to be treated at such a young age. She won't have to go through the hell I went through most of my life simply because I was reacting to things I was exposed to on a daily basis. The most frustrating thing is that I suspected for years that foods were a large part of my problem, but every doctor I met pooh-poohed the notion, implying that I was just an overconcerned, distraught parent. They would always deny my experience, chalking up Elise's symptoms and my concerns to 'the neurotic mother syndrome'. When I asked for a referral to a specialist, one physician confronted me with: *There's only one cook in this kitchen*! I ask you, who knows their kids better than their own mothers!"

I nodded in agreement. She was right. Whenever I had tried to make some sense out of what was happening to me, I had often been met with comments such as 'You've been reading too much', and 'Maybe you need to get back to work'. It was little wonder that so much anger permeated the lives of those with this kind of illness. In turn, the anger was counterproductive to healing - just as Leah Irwin had suggested in our session.

My interest quickly turned to an elderly woman named Esther. She'd been crippled with arthritis for years until she began to follow Dr. Rowland's program. She was now symptom-free - as long as she adhered to the regime. I immediately thought of Mom and made a mental note to check with Emily to see if she had called for an appointment.

By the time we'd finished lunch, both Michael and I felt a kinship with these people, many of whom had stories similar to our own. They were so open, and willing to share their ideas, knowledge and experiences with us. It still amazed me that for so many years we had faithfully accepted what our doctors had told us about our health problems - no matter what. We had always accepted their advice as the gospel truth.

Our society had such a strong traditional belief in our physicians as the fountain of all knowledge - not only in medical matters, but even beyond. This value system was built on centuries of trust. It was a difficult concept to shake, but slowly it was beginning to sink in - I was the one who was primarily responsible for my own health. I needed to learn to question my doctors - to become more literate - to consider them as my medical advisors and not the final arbiters in matters affecting my health. I needed to accept more responsibility for important decisions that affected my life. Slowly, I rejoined the conversation.

Another woman about my age was recounting her experience. "Our family doctor told us that Henry had ear infections because his eustachian tubes were too small and that eventually they'd get larger and he'd outgrow the problem on his own. It was partly true, but by the time our second child was born, we learned there was so much we could do to prevent the problem in the first place - and most of it was related to diet! As a result, no antibiotics and no tubes."

Another parent, whose seven year old wet the bed every night, told us their doctor explained that the child had an 'immature' bladder that was a 'bit too small'. After putting her through several very uncomfortable procedures where they stretched her urethra, they were assured that she would eventually 'outgrow the problem'. I remembered reading in *An Alternative Approach to Allergies*, that although the bedwetting might stop, it would only be replaced by a new problem, because the original cause had never been addressed. Only the target organs changed. Of course, no one ever relates one problem to another. Just think of the years of humiliation that the child had endured due to a problem that could have been avoided from the start!

The woman continued. "She couldn't go to sleepovers for years. Then we heard about this clinic. Within *one week* of stopping dairy products, the bedwetting stopped!"

Another mother told us about her hyperactive son who'd been advised by the school to take Ritalin. A neighbor told her about the clinic. It turned out that her son was highly sensitive to table salt! No wonder he was hyper - just about everything he ate had salt in or on it! Who would ever have thought!

Then there was little Jessica's father who reprimanded her every Sunday in church for complaining about the incense.

"She'd tell me how the smell made her sick. I'd get so angry! She spent almost every Sunday afternoon in her room, punished for what I thought was insolence. And it was never her fault - it really *was* making her sick."

"I'll tell you one thing," said Earl, a middle-aged man sitting next to Michael. "This Dr. Rowland and Eva know their business. My wife and daughter had so many health problems, they'd been written off by umpteen doctors. They were also very overweight. They tried all kinds of diets, but it wasn't until Dr. Rowland suggested they go off wheat and dairy products that not only did their weight literally *fall* off, but their other chronic, long-standing problems cleared up. No more counting calories and no more starvation diets. It was clearly the foods to which they were sensitive that had caused their problems."

"So what brings *you* here?" inquired Jessica's father.

"Really bad migraines. But they totally disappeared since I changed my diet. I've decided to undergo the testing just in case I have more sensitivities of which I'm unaware."

"What helped your headaches?" asked Michael.

"Stopping coffee was a big one. It had also caused stomach upsets which I thought were normal - you know, a part of the aging process.".

Michael nodded, identifying with him.

And then there was Scott's mother who had been everywhere searching for help for his hyperactivity. "I was told his problems weren't connected to his diet in any way. In fact, when I mentioned my visit to this clinic, my doctor's words of wisdom were, 'If you want to go and pee off the end of a wharf, and it makes you feel good, then do it' . . ."

"That's a line I've never heard before!"

"Me neither - until then. With the clinic's help, we now know that foods are Scott's main problem. As long as he stays on his diet, he's a wonderful kid. Take him off it for a few days and he becomes prison material."

"Hey, that sounds a lot like one of our cats before we changed his diet," interjected young Elise. "He used to be cross - totally antisocial. Luckily we had another one who was cute and cuddly. Last summer, we went away on a two-month vacation and left both of them with a neighbor who just happened to be a patient at this clinic . . . "

"In fact it's through this neighbor that we eventually ended up here," added Miriam. "Sorry for interrupting, Elise. Please continue your story."

"By the time we returned, he was a new cat. In fact, we barely recognized him! His coat was twice as thick as before, and he was as calm and friendly as could be."

"What brought about such a dramatic change?"

"His diet had been switched from one that was highly processed to one without chemicals - no additives or preservatives. Our neighbor had also added brewer's yeast to his diet - which, by the way, is also a great flea repellent. He's never had them since!"

"An added bonus!" laughed Miriam. "That cat is fed better than most children!"

I didn't doubt it.

By the end of the day, we were all exhausted. We left the clinic with a handful of little bottles filled with antigens. Each bottle contained several different substances. For instance, one of the bottles contained chemicals - phenol, formaldehyde, auto exhaust, tobacco, chlorine and perfume. Another bottle contained foods; a third contained airborne antigens. Instructions on how to administer them were also enclosed as reminders.

The kids were cranky, partly from the testing and partly from being cooped up all day in a confined area. I hoped to bring Beth with us the next day to help with the kids. It would free me to keep a better record of our reactions. She could also keep them occupied when we had our appointment with Dr. Rowland on the last day of testing.

The kids and I fell asleep soon after we climbed into the car. Michael, also exhausted from the day, stopped at a drive-through for a coffee. He was awake most of the night with his first attack of heartburn since starting the diet. By morning, he was a convert through and through!

"Man! What a powerful reminder!" These were the first words Michael uttered upon waking, as he rubbed his swollen eyes and sore head. "I feel like I have a hangover."

As much as I empathized, I knew this was a big step forward in Michael's learning. I rubbed his head for a few moments. "Nothing like first-hand experience, is there? It really *is* incredible that foods can cause all this."

"What really bugs me is that the average person doesn't have access to this information. It should be common knowledge!" Michael was beginning to sound more like me every day.

"You should talk to Dr. Rowland about that . . . but right now, we've got to get the kids up. Testing starts at 8:30 sharp. Plus, we still have to give them their drops to make sure they're okay."

"How can we tell?"

"Jaime said that if the kids don't become reactive after taking them, we can assume the antigens will work. Apparently it can take anywhere from one to four weeks to see if they're helping or not. At this point, we only need to ensure they're not causing reactivity."

"Causing reactivity?"

"Well, we need to know whether or not the proper end points were found when the kids were tested. We'll know that by their response to the drops."

We were fine - no reactions at all.

We picked up Beth and drove to Bridgeport. The next few days were like the first, except that Beth was there to help us. Her assistance was invaluable.

We were tested for everything imaginable: Other chemicals, foods, dust, dust mites, molds, pollens, weeds and more - even candida! Needless to say, I tested positive. Apparently, one could not only have an overgrowth of this yeast, but one could develop a sensitivity as well. The kids handled the intradermal testing beautifully. I was so proud of them! Chlorine was definitely my worst. Both Emma and Nathaniel were also sensitive to it. No more indoor pools for them! Swimming lessons would have to wait for summer.

The tests for milk products brought back some unpleasant memories of not so long ago. Emma's chest tightened, the circles under her eyes darkened, and her face twisted into a pained expression. Then she started whining. Nathaniel and I felt our sinuses filling up as we both became sleepy and grumpy. Max's skin itched and he pulled at his ears. Wheat, yeast, corn, egg, sugar - we were sensitive to almost everything we ate daily. Suddenly, the logic of a rotation diet struck me! It was beginning to make sense.

On the final day of testing, Emily greeted us with her usual exuberance. Ushering us into the testing room, she mentioned, "Dr. Rowland would like to see you now. He thinks it might be easier in the morning while you're still fresh . . . "

"Great! Beth can you handle the kids?"

She looked a little concerned. "They'll be fine," smiled Emily, reassuringly. "The testing room doesn't fill up for another half hour. With Beth's help, Lori and Jaime will be able to handle everything. In any case, if there's a problem, you'll be just down the hall."

"That's true. Okay kids. We'll be back in a little while. Beth, you know the procedure. Call if you need us."

Don't worry about a thing," called Jaime from her desk, as she prepared drops for the day.

As we entered his office, Dr. Rowland greeted us with a warm smile. "Jillian, you look better every time I see you!" He reached out to shake Michael's hand. "And you must be Michael. I'm pleased to meet you at last."

Michael beamed. "Likewise . . . although I feel I already know you - especially after that horrendous chlorine episode. Dr. Rowland, I can't begin to thank you. My family's transforming before my very eyes . . . all thanks to you and your work."

"Thank you. But once again, I must emphasize that the congratulations should go to our patients for their hard work - they make the real difference."

He turned to me. "I can see you're well past that unfortunate incident with chlorine . . ."

"Yes. What a nightmare!"

"Now at least you'll have chlorine antigens. They'll help minimize your reactions should you be exposed to it in the future. But avoidance is the real key."

"I understand that. But it's good to know that the antigens will help in situations beyond my control. I don't ever want to go through that again, nor would I want the kids to see me in such rough shape."

He smiled sympathetically. "I understand . . . Jillian, how are your headaches and bladder problems? Has your abdominal gas and bloating subsided?"

"Well, now that I'm on the antifungal, acidophilus and yeast-free diet, much of it has cleared up."

"That's wonderful! What about your hair? Does it still fall out? Still feeling cold?"

"The flax oil really seems to help both my hair and skin, and I'm not as cold as I was, but I wouldn't go so far as to say I'm warm all the time."

"I'd like you to take your temperature every morning for the next few days. You may have an underactive thyroid . . ."

"Oh, Dr. Klamer already had my blood tested many times and all the tests came back negative."

"I'm sure they did, but you know, Jillian, many of these problems are often not picked up in bloodwork . . ."

"Are you serious?" said Michael with disgust. "You mean she could have a thyroid problem and the tests might not have detected it?"

"That's right. Although a test may give a normal reading, we're finding that many people with such readings are actually hypothyroid. Most blood tests just aren't sophisticated enough. What is commonly classified as 'low normal', may be asymptomatic for some, but for others it may mean the difference between sickness and health. So . . . here's what I would recommend. Every morning, hold a thermometer under your arm without moving for fifteen minutes - any motion can affect the reading. A consistent temperature of 97.6 F or lower may indicate an underactive thyroid. This is also known as the Broda-Barnes test. Keep a log. If, in fact, it turns out that you do have a sluggish thyroid, we'll try you on iodine drops, kelp or desiccated thyroid for a couple of months. Of course, there's always acupuncture, herbs and homeopathy. If these approaches don't solve the problem, then we'll try something stronger."

"That makes sense to me," mumbled Michael under his breath. "Try it and see what happens. I like that approach." He was becoming more involved by the minute. I'd never seen him so proactive - about anything! It made me feel good. He was becoming a true partner in my recovery. I felt so supported.

"How are iodine and kelp related to thyroid?"

"Iodine is a key mineral needed for a healthy thyroid gland and for the prevention of goiter. Kelp is an excellent source of iodine as well as other minerals. There's also a strong correlation between iodine deficiency and fibrocystic breast disease. A Dr. William Ghent of the Hotel Dieu Hospital in Kingston, Ontario found that eighty percent of women with this condition can be helped by increasing their intake of iodine. Studies also indicate that fluoridated and chlorinated water can block iodine receptors in the thyroid gland, which, in turn, can result in hypothyroidism."

"I wonder if this is responsible for the marked increase in this condition in so many young women. With so many women on Synthroid, it almost seems as if there's an epidemic." I could count at least six I knew personally who had underactive thyroid glands.

"Could be. There are so many factors these days - it's difficult to pinpoint a single cause. Probably it's a combination of many different things. Overgrowth of candida, for example, can suppress glandular function, including the thyroid."

"None of us will drink city water from now on," affirmed Michael. "Not after what we've been through."

"That's a good move. Jillian, I see from your file that you had a session with Leah Irwin. How was it?"

"It was incredible! She's an amazing woman - so full of wisdom. I felt empowered after that session. In fact, Michael and I will be seeing her together for the next while."

"I'm glad you liked her. She's a real asset to the clinic."

"Dr. Rowland, over the past few weeks I've witnessed miracles in our home. I've watched my wife go from being a sick, irritable, chronically-fatigued woman to that beautiful, self-confident, positive person I fell in love with fifteen years ago. Then, I watched my three kids become healthier, physically as well as mentally, in just a few short weeks. I still don't understand why this information isn't common knowledge."

"Well, Jillian and I have spent quite a bit of time discussing this very issue. You see, every new idea needs time to take hold. Just think about Darwin's Theory of Evolution. There was incredible resistance to that concept. Then there was the British doctor, Joseph Lister, who was attacked when he proposed that sterilization practices be used for surgical procedures. Today, we'd be sued if we did otherwise!"

"And what about that Austrian physician . . . I forget his name . . . who was persecuted for urging his colleagues to wash their hands before delivering babies?"

"Yes, yes . . . Ignaz Semmelweis - to prevent maternal deaths. And then, don't forget Louis Pasteur . . . you see, it's an age-old pattern. John Locke, the English philosopher said it beautifully: *New opinions are always suspected, and usually opposed, without any other reason but because they are not already common.*"

"But who could possibly be opposed to this approach - one without side effects, and one that even *cures* long-standing conditions when all else fails?"

"Well, some of the most vocal critics in the medical community are allergists, although they're not the only ones. Then of course, there are the pharmaceutical companies, food marketing boards and the processed food industry. They stand to lose billions of dollars if everyone were to follow the basic principles of holistic health . . ."

"Among physicians, why allergists in particular?"

"I suspect it may be the realization that environmental medicine is really a more sophisticated, more refined version of their own work and they see it as a direct threat. It is rather ironic though, that it was only thirty years ago that *they* were under attack for their particular approach to medicine."

"Jillian has seen every allergist in town and out of . . . how many did you see, Jilly?" Michael turned toward me.

"Oh, at least two at home and one in Ellsworthy . . ."

"So out of three, I can recall only one who even *considered* food as a possible reason for her symptoms. *Not one* ever brought up the idea of chemical sensitivity. Isn't that right, Jilly?" asked Michael.

I nodded, recalling the time I had spent running around to those appointments.

"But don't despair," continued Dr. Rowland. "It isn't all doom and gloom. While it's true that many of my colleagues who practice under the umbrella of holistic medicine are frequently harassed for using progressive therapies - several being persecuted by their medical boards as we speak - they are, at the same time, forging ahead with great success, paving the way toward acceptance. Unfortunately, before acceptance, there often has to be a struggle."

"But why would they be harassed for helping people get better?" Michael was incredulous.

"Good question."

"What's the basis for the harassment?"

"Things you wouldn't believe! For example, one of my colleagues is being charged by his medical board for advising patients to purchase air filters for their homes so they can improve the quality of their lives . . . oh yes, and for suggesting they take vitamins, minerals and other supplements to boost their immune systems. Another is being harassed for practicing homeopathy and for giving sound dietary advice - simply, I believe, because it's too far removed from standard dietetic practices . . ."

"Probably advising people to cut out sugar!" exclaimed Michael.

Dr. Rowland smiled, "I wouldn't be a bit surprised. The average person has no idea of what goes on. There are even police raids on private clinics across this continent. Although these types of events are more common in the U.S., the latest that comes to mind happened this past June in the province of Quebec . . ."

"The *police* actually raided a medical clinic?"

"I kid you not! And along with them were five 'inspectors' from The Quebec College of Physicians and Surgeons. This particular medical doctor was given a deadline to cease all natural treatments and terminate her association with her naturopathic colleague. Failure to do so would result in the loss of her license to practice medicine."

"Had there been any patient complaints?"

"Not one - ever."

"But what gives them the right to do that!" Michael could barely contain himself.

"They wield all the power. Ironically, the abbreviated version for College of Physicians and Surgeons is COPS."

"I wonder if these boards were aware of that when they came up with the name?"

Dr. Rowland shrugged his shoulders. "Most stories such as these are hushed, and often the physicians involved in these attacks are unable to amass the financial resources to properly defend themselves. Still others are being harassed for practising environmental medicine; and some for offering chelation therapy to their patients." Dr. Rowland held up a newspaper article. "I found this in the Parksville Qualicum Beach News a few months ago:

---

*Dear Patients:*

    *I regret to say that I am closing my practice as of April 22 due to health reasons. I am tired. I am tired of being persecuted for saving lives.*

    *I am tired of paying my lawyer $50,000 a year for keeping me out of jail. I hope that you can find it in your hearts to forgive me for letting it all go.*

    *I gave everything I had. In fact I gave it long after I had it.*

    *But before I go, I want to tell you a couple of things. The first thing is how I grateful I am to all of you. The only thing that I was good at was from my first night in medical school I had a bunch of people tell me just to listen. I did, and you all made me look brilliant and for that I am eternally grateful. Secondly, I am happy for your faithfulness in this therapy which was new and radical, and none of us knew when we started how good it was going to be, but now we know for sure because we've been there 15,000 times so you can decide for yourself.*

    *So now to you I throw the torch. If there is ever going to be permanent chelation therapy in British Columbia, Canada, or if there is ever going to be other alternative medicine therapies like Life Crystals and Chondriana and many, many other things I wish I could have tried, you will have to take responsibility for that. You will have to call your politicians, call the College of Physicians and Surgeons, and tell them that you want to be treated like you know your own bodies. I did my best.*

    *I love you. Take care. God Bless.*

                              *George Barber, M.D.*

---

"It's so sad," I whispered, choking back tears. "Very . . . very sad."

"It's absurd!" fumed Michael a little louder than he realized. "How antiquated! Dr. Rowland, you mentioned progress . . . where?"

"Five states - Alaska, Washington, North Carolina, Oklahoma and New York - have passed freedom of practice statutes, which allow physicians the freedom to practice complementary forms of medicine without fear of retribution from their medical boards. The State of Oregon was the sixth as of May, 1995. The Oregon House of Representatives passed the Alternative Medicine Bill by a vote of 56 to 1 . . . "

"The people have spoken," murmured Michael.

". . . and one of the more progressive moves in the U.S. was the development of an Office of Alternative Medicine at the National Institutes of Health in 1992. I'm told the phones haven't stopped ringing since it opened.   Hundreds of consumer groups are springing up everywhere, offering information on alternative therapies.  Then, in Nova Scotia, Canada, the Medical Society voted to establish a Complementary Medicine section for physicians who practice alternative or complementary therapies.  This includes approaches such as environmental, nutritional, and herbal medicine and treatments like acupuncture and homeopathy.  These new laws are forging the way toward medical freedom, providing people with real choices in medical treatment."

"What did it take to get to that stage?"

"It took at least one very persistent physician with a high public profile, a Dr. William LaValley, who refused to buckle under in the face of adversity. And it usually takes a group of very dedicated citizens banding together to form lobby groups such as Citizens for Choice in Health Care.  Put the two together, and you have the perfect equation for successfully challenging the system, the status quo, thereby paving the way for progress."

"And I'm ready for that!  Look out everybody, here I come!"  I could feel the words reverberate deep inside.

"Good for you!  Go get 'em!  Margaret Mead, the famous anthropologist once said: *Never doubt that a small group of thoughtful, committed citizens can change the world - indeed, it's the only thing that ever has.* So Jillian, shine that light!"

"And you can bet she will!"  grinned Michael.  He knew that when I became passionate about an issue, I'd follow through no matter who or what got in my way.

Dr. Rowland continued, "Then, there's the establishment of the first government-funded environmental treatment clinic in the world.  This implies progress."

"Where?"

"Again, in Nova Scotia . . ."

"Hey!  What's with this place?  Seems like everything happens there. They must be doing something right!" declared Michael.

"Or . . . they must have the largest collection of environmentally ill people on the face of this earth!" I joked.

"Put quite simply," replied Dr. Rowland, "a catastrophe had to happen. A very large group of people became environmentally ill from working in a new hospital subsequently identified as a sick building.  Most of the people were medical support staff.  It certainly brought the issue of environmental health into public focus.  And the work of Dr. Gerald Ross and the local chapter of the Allergy and Environmental Health Association (AEHA) must be given considerable credit for laying the groundwork in Nova Scotia. Put that together with an open-minded Dean at the local Medical School, and you've got a powerful mix!"

"So, would you say things are looking up?"

"They are . . . but ironically, at the same time this government-funded clinic was being set up there, a colleague practicing environmental medicine in Toronto, Canada, was being harassed by the Ontario College of Physicians and Surgeons - and once again, this occurred despite the fact there were no patient complaints.  It just doesn't make sense to have identical practices accepted in one province or state and persecuted in another. In fact, a few months prior to the advent of these charges, an environmental health research clinic was set up at a hospital in the very same city in which this particular physician practices!"

"It's absurd!" exclaimed Michael.

"Ultimately, public education is crucial. Ideally, the most significant focus should be on prevention, not intervention, although we mustn't minimize the necessity of the latter. This is where people like Jane Harding are invaluable. In fact, Jillian, I'm quite serious when I say I can easily see you doing some type of public education in the not-so-distant future. Parents, in particular, need to hear this message. It will give them and their children - the next generation - some hope. They must become more aware, which in time, will help them become healthier. It is critical to get out there and talk about how the environment impacts upon human health, behavior and learning. Medical doctors such as William Crook, Doris Rapp, Sherry Rogers, Carolyn Dean, William Rea and Gerald Ross have led the way in informing the public. But, more often, hearing it from a layperson who's been there, sends a more powerful message. It gives it that person-next-door credibility. People really relate to first-hand experience."

"And think about it," said Michael, "in about five years time, all this will probably be old news."

"Let's hope you're right. Speaking of old news, I read an interesting quote in the Toronto *Globe and Mail*. Let's see if I can find it." He rummaged in his top drawer and extracted a tattered photocopy. "Ah, here it is: *Holding a 1959 issue of the New England Journal of Medicine in his hand, Drummond Rennie, the deputy editor said: This was the finest medical research of it's time and most of it has already been proved wrong. The best that can be said about today's Journal is that we're publishing today's lies. We hope that next year's are a little better.*"

"That's one of the funniest, yet most prophetic statements I've heard in a long time!" laughed Michael.

"I agree," chuckled Dr. Rowland. "Going back to the issue of public awareness - there's a growing public disenchantment with mainstream medicine. A 1993 study published in that same prestigious medical journal reported that one in three Americans used at least one unconventional or alternative therapy during a recent one year period. In Europe, complementary medicine is widely embraced. For instance, it is estimated that 49 percent of the French population and 46 percent of Germans currently use some form of complementary medicine for treating their illnesses. The numbers of people embracing homeopathy in France grew from 16 percent in 1982 to 36 percent in 1992. In Great Britain, the use of homeopathic remedies is growing by 20 percent each year and in Greece and Portugal, by 30 percent. According to the *British Medical Journal*, conventional medical doctors are beginning to diversify their practices to accommodate more complementary approaches."

"Maybe people in Europe are more accustomed to paying their own expenses for these therapies," added Michael. I knew he was thinking of the cost of my visits and supplements. He held out his hand. "Don't get me wrong. Every cent has been well worth it! But there are those less fortunate than us . . ."

"Hopefully, in Canada, the government will see the light - that these therapies will save them millions of dollars in the long run. In the meantime, people need to establish their priorities. As a new patient recently commented in response to her initial consult fee - 'I spend that to get my hair highlighted!'"

"Isn't that the truth!" I declared. If only she knew what I'd just learned about perms and hair colors. I couldn't help but think that maybe that was part of her problem!

"In the area of private coverage," Dr. Rowland explained, "progress is also being made. For example, in the United States, Alexander Schauss, Executive Director of the non-profit health care advocacy groups, *Citizens for Health* and *American Preventive Medical Association (APMA)*, as well as many grassroots organizations, have contacted major medical insurance companies urging them to cover preventive, nutritional and exercise programs. Their efforts are paying off. Mutual of Omaha has indicated they would reimburse clients for a program developed by Dr. Dean Ornish, which is based primarily on diet and exercise."

"Well, I sure have my work cut out for the next few years! I think it's time to lobby governments into action. No wonder the medicare system is in dire straits!"

"Wow! Sounds like you'll be dynamite! The bottom line is that we must stop looking for the magic bullet. That approach hasn't worked and never will. What *does* work, as you've discovered, is a comprehensive review of our own lifestyle, and specifically, the role we play in it - and then finding a practitioner who can help guide us as partners, as equals, to greater awareness. Taking responsibility, as you have Jillian, is the answer." He closed my file and leaned back in his chair. "Now, let's get back to you. Do you have any issues you'd like to discuss before we end the session?"

"No . . . I think I'm on the right track. Do I just keep on doing what I'm doing?"

"It looks like it's working well."

"I must say, I was rather worried about parasites, but is it safe to say it's not an issue for me?"

"I would say so. If you experience any difficulties in the future, we can then explore that possibility with some lab tests or a trial with an antiparasitic herb." Dr. Rowland looked at me intently. "There's not much more I can advise at this point. You'll leave here today with the rest of your antigens and start your rotation diet in a couple of weeks . . ."

"How do those antigens work?" asked Michael. "From the handout Lori gave me, I gather that antigens are weakened dilutions of whatever makes you sensitive. Is that correct?"

"Antigen therapy or Provocation-Neutralization is really not a very new concept - it's simply a refinement of the therapy that began with conventional allergy shots. The only difference is that antigens are like well-aimed bullets instead of the shotgun approach of many traditional allergy practices. We simply find an effective neutralizing dose of the allergenic substances which provides symptomatic relief for the patient. Symptoms can be controlled by either injections or sublingual drops."

"So no medication is involved?"

"None whatsoever. Effective treatment requires total participation and cooperation from the patient who must make lifestyle changes - particularly in the area of diet and day-to-day environment. The two main ingredients in this approach are education and taking responsibility for one's own health."

"So a person can live a pretty healthy life as long as he or she follows certain principles."

"Right. Jillian is a prime example. Armed with this information, perhaps you'll join her in her crusade."

I laughed at the thought of Michael out there in a public forum fighting for freedom of choice in health care!

Dr. Rowland then said, "Jillian, you've done remarkably well. I really can't offer you much more . . . other than support whenever you need it. And you know where to find us."

"What about the thyroid check?"

"Call if your temperature is consistently low. Otherwise, you're definitely headed in the right direction. The one thing I urge you to do is to keep on searching. Try some different therapies such as acupuncture and massage. You might also find yoga, t'ai chi or meditation helpful as well. Homeopathy is especially wonderful for fine-tuning the immune system and helping to further detoxify the body. They're well worth trying. Then your sensitivities could take a back seat. Everyone responds differently. So you may have to try several approaches in order to find the best one for you."

"Can you recommend anyone?"

He nodded. "I'll have Emily give you names of practitioners we recommend. When do you finish testing?"

"Today is our last day."

"Good." He stood up. "Jillian, it's been a pleasure." Offering his hand, he looked directly at me and said, "You now have enough information to make a difference in your life. Awareness is where it's at. Galileo once said, *You cannot teach a man anything. You can only help him to find it within himself.* And you, Jillian Stowe, have not only learned an incredible amount in a short period of time, but you've actually *done it*! I've never met anyone who moved from victim to victor so quickly. I congratulate you. Good luck with your journey. I *know* you'll be successful!"

Tears of gratitude began to form. "Dr. Rowland, thank you for everything you've taught me. It's been quite a journey. But most important, thank you for giving me back my dignity."

With a wide grin, he nodded and headed off to see his next patient.

I knew Dr. Rowland was right. The rest was up to me. He had given me a map, now it was up to me to take the lead. As Leah had said, we must learn to go inward. We really are wiser than we think, and must learn to trust the inner teacher that resides within each and every one of us.

I felt liberated. I was ready to spread my wings!

# Testing for Allergies and Sensitivities

## Electro-acupuncture Bio-feedback Testing (EAV)

There are many different varieties of electro-acupuncture bio-feedback testing units on the market. They range from the simpler models such as the Vega to very sophisticated computerized systems such as the Omega AcuBase, Listen, and Best which not only can be used for screening purposes, but can balance the body by accessing thousands of remedies and nutritional supplements programmed into a computer. These devices measure energy at various acupuncture points on the fingers and toes. Readings that fall on the low end of what is considered 'normal' indicate fatigue or degeneration in the particular organ being measured, while high readings suggest that an irritation or inflammation may be present. These programs can also be used to detect food, airborne and chemical sensitivities; vitamin, mineral and enzyme deficiencies; and can detect the presence of Candida and parasites on an energetic level. The reliability of this test depends upon the skill and experience of the tester, so reputation and past results are your best guide. A follow-up appointment with a practitioner is also recommended if the E.A.V. tester is a technician only and not a qualified health practitioner.

## Muscle Response Testing (MRT) . . . or Applied Kinesiology

MRT identifies blockages in the electro-magnetic field of the body in relation to allergens and/or nutritional imbalances. When a suspected allergen is introduced to the body (either held in the hand; placed near the Thymus; or via drops under the tongue), the stong indicator arm muscle will weaken. If the item being tested is not allergenic, the arm will remain strong. This procedure can detect both hidden as well as acute sensitivities and can help to clarify which substances need to be treated or avoided. As with EAV testing, the accuracy of this technique depends upon the experience and clarity of the tester.

❊   ❊   ❊   ❊   ❊

NOTE: The beauty of these approaches is that they are non-invasive, take very little time, and you get results right on the spot! The accuracy of both of these testing methods rely heavily on a) the skill of the tester; b) prior exposure of the client to allergens; and c) the environment in which the test is conducted.

**For additional information on some newer methods of treatment, please refer to page 141 of this book.**

*The impact of the global total disregard*
*for our environment*
*affects all of us.*
*The problems of*
*worldwide chemical pollution*
*can no longer be ignored*
*by the public,*
*physicians, educators, or legislators.*
*We must insist upon measures*
*to protect the health*
*and wellbeing of this and*
*future generations,*
*even if the price is*
*a temporary economic loss.*
*We can no longer remain oblivious*
*of the increasing pollution of*
*our air, water, soil, food, clothing,*
*and homes.*

**Doris Rapp, M.D.**
**Is This Your Child?**

# 18

# For Whom the Bell Tolls

*The World Health Organization (WHO) estimates that about 30 percent of the nation's schools have indoor air quality problems and are suffering from the sick school syndrome.*

*L*ake of the Woods School was only an hour's drive from home. Michael decided to accompany me. After that memorable day of testing, he was with me all the way. Anyone who didn't believe that foods, chemicals and airborne irritants could cause health, behavior and learning problems should be required to sit in a testing room for a few hours. They wouldn't need any further convincing.

I dug a piece of paper out of my pocket. On it were written the names of the people we were to meet. As we entered the front door, several signs leaped out at us. One read, *Scent-Free Zone*. It portrayed a skunk holding a red heart with the words, *No Scents Please, We're Sensitive*. On the other wall was a blue school crossing sign put out by the Lung Association that read, *Scent-Free School*. The foyer was a beautiful atrium flooded with natural daylight. Colorful ceramic tile covered the floors and walls. The air smelled fresher inside than out - a far cry from our neighborhood school.

"Hello. May I help you?" called a voice from the nearest office.

"Yes," replied Michael, as he poked his head in the doorway, "as a matter of fact, you can. We have an appointment with the principal and a Ms.Theriault."

She looked in her appointment book. "Oh yes. Please have a seat." She gestured to an inner office. "They'll be with you shortly."

We had barely sat down when a booming voice greeted us. "Hi! You must be Jillian and Michael Stowe. I'm Paul Misener, and this is Suzanne Theriault."

The man was tall and lean, with a big bushy beard, and he looked not a day over forty. Suzanne was older but very trim and youthful looking. She wore wild designer glasses and her blonde hair was cut short on the sides.

"Hi. Welcome to Lake of the Woods School," she said, giving each of us a firm handshake.

"We've heard so much about this school. We're already impressed - that wonderful atrium to welcome us and fresh air too - rare commodities these days!"

"Yes, it is wonderful," said Suzanne. "We couldn't imagine working anywhere else. It's so important to keep indoor air clean, especially in a learning environment where youngsters spend much of their day. Not so long ago, I attended a national symposium that focused on the effects of environmental hazards on children. One of the experts said something that's remained with me: *Children are, in a sense, moving targets. Exposures which may be unnoticed or be relatively harmless in an adult, can be potentially devastating to a child.*"

"Children who are forced to sit in polluted classrooms," added Paul, "endure a form of abuse that differs little from mental or physical abuse - especially with respect to its impact on learning. We call it environmental abuse. Not only are they bombarded with poor quality air outside, but often by indoor pollutants as well - things to which we never give a second thought."

"What kinds of things?" Michael asked with genuine interest.

"Cleaning agents and building materials, perfumes, chalk dust, molds, unsafe supplies for art and science classes - you name it, most schools have them," replied Suzanne. "Other than intent, is there a difference between the child who's suffering from verbal or physical abuse and the one who's slowly being poisoned by products never proven to be safe for humans? This is especially true when the fumes from these products are mixed together, creating a chemical cocktail."

"You know, I never thought about it in those terms before," commented Michael, "but you're right, there really is little difference."

"That's right, one can only claim ignorance as a defence for a short while - after that, the abuse is deliberate." I thought of the example Andrew had given at Jane's place - the toddler strapped into a seat in a car full of cigarette smoke.

"Adults are one thing," said Paul, "but children are innocent victims. We're responsible for them. They depend upon us to provide a safe environment in which to grow up. What many parents don't realize is that when that school bell rings in the morning, their children could be entering classrooms filled with a wide range of pollutants, producing symptoms that are rarely linked to the air they breathe."

"At my previous school, many of the staff and students complained about not feeling well. The standing joke among parents every September was: *Here ends two months of good health!* And sure enough, within a few short weeks the sniffles began, along with nagging coughs, stuffy noses, headaches and changes in behavior. One ENT specialist commented that within weeks of the start of school, he saw a rash of children with ear infections. He certainly attributed many of these problems to the poor quality of the indoor air. But most of us rarely make these connections. We accept it as normal. Now that I know better, I can vouch for the difference that clean air, clean water and clean food make - especially in young children."

"Suzanne's right," said Paul. "The difference between children in schools with poor indoor air quality and our kids here at Lake of the Woods is astounding. By the way, what would an administrator with severe sinus problems, a librarian with chronic headaches and a grade four student with erratic behavior have in common?"

We both nodded. Michael said, "I give up. I was never good at quizzes."

"They each spend approximately six hours every day in the same environment - a sick school environment."

We all laughed, at the same time, acknowledging the seriousness of the problem.

"In my last school, several teachers were actually receiving allergy shots for molds, dust and other airborne irritants, yet they were forced to teach in polluted classrooms. They'd feel great in the summer, but virtually the moment they stepped into their classrooms in September, their old symptoms would resurface - sinus problems, headaches, fatigue - and the list goes on. It just didn't make any sense. And for fear of retribution, they were afraid to insist that the carpets be removed and the air quality improved."

"Wouldn't they have conducted air quality tests?"

"Sure, lots. But despite all the sickness, the tests showed everything was within acceptable limits . . ."

"The big problem," added Suzanne, "is that the so-called standards or limits for such tests are usually based on healthy adult males, not on women and small developing children. In addition, there's seldom any research on combined or synergistic effects." This was reminiscent of the conversation in Jane's workshop.

"Are there no standards for school children?" asked Michael.

"Not really. We have several standards for adults in the workplace. For instance, NIOSH is the most comprehensive set of chemical standards we have, but it fails to address children. Ironically, it's the standard we continue to use for our science labs. ACGIH, the code used by most provincial and state regulatory agencies such as Labor and Health, also doesn't have standards for children."

"But I understand from a workshop I just attended, that strides are being made in this area."

"Yes, some governments are in the process of developing Indoor Air Quality (IAQ) standards for non-industrial settings. I believe OSHA - the Occupational Safety and Health Administration - announced a proposal that would regulate indoor air quality in non-industrial workplaces, and that would include schools."

"What's NIOSH and ACGIH?" asked Michael.

"NIOSH, an acronym for the National Institute for Occupational Safety and Health, is one of the agencies that sets standards for safe exposure levels for humans. ACGIH stands for the American Conference of Governmental and Industrial Hygienists, another agency that also sets standards. Again, neither addresses the needs of children. But even if we had standards for children, would they be precise enough for those who are environmentally sensitive? Beyond this is the problem that little is known about the synergistic effects I mentioned a moment ago. For example, the combined effects of cigarette smoke and radon is 15-20 times more hazardous than when calculated separately."

"As one parent so aptly put it," said Suzanne, "*my child's body is far more accurate than any machine.* She was, of course, referring to the equipment used for measuring indoor air quality and the typical standards of measurement we accept as gospel."

I immediately thought of Jane and her chlorine story. "Ah yes," I said, "somewhat similar to the detection of chlorine in filtered water that's guaranteed free of this chemical. Experts tell you there's none detectable, yet your body continues to react to it. Then, you later discover that the standard kit measures parts per million and your body reacts to parts per billion. You're simply out of luck."

"Right. Not to mention that once you're sensitized to a particular substance in your environment, even minute amounts can elicit significant reactions," said Paul.

"The simplest definition of a sick building I've come across," said Suzanne, "is in the United States Environmental Protection Agency's publication, *Environmental Hazards in Your School: A Resource Handbook*. It states: *A building is characterized as 'sick' when its occupants complain of health and comfort problems that can be related to working or being in the building.*"

Paul chuckled. "I wonder if that was written *after* the EPA workers got sick. In any case, it's also very similar to the conclusion reached on a NOVA program aired on PBS in late December . . ."

"There's nothing quite like first-hand experience," I murmured. "I didn't see that program. What was it about?"

"It was an hour-long documentary titled *Can Buildings Make You Sick?*"

"The stories are as fascinating as they are scary. One of them dealt with the Registry of Motor Vehicles in Boston, a brand new multi-million dollar building which may never be repairable - or habitable by humans. Even after the lawsuits have ended, they may have no choice but to tear it down. After viewing the show, we found the whole video so compelling that we decided to buy a copy for our library. You might like to borrow it."

"Thank you. We'd love to. It might be a good one to use with parents at our school - you know, to increase their awareness of what could happen when buildings are not properly maintained. It should set the stage for a lively discussion."

"That same program also documented the battle with air quality fought by Brigham and Women's, a teaching hospital at Harvard University. Unlike the Registry building which was contaminated with mold, this hospital's problem, like so many others, was primarily chemical. In this case the offending substances were particles from latex gloves and liquids used for sterilization. Inadequate ventilation was also a significant factor in both situations - a common problem in public buildings, including many schools."

"So what differences have you observed in the children at Lake of the Woods?" asked Michael.

"We took some of the more difficult children in the school system, particularly those with learning and behavior problems," replied Paul. "You would never believe these are the same kids! Their overall health improved to the point where many have attendance records that are near perfect. Their ability to concentrate and retain information improved dramatically, as did their overall behavior. When their diet and environment at both home and school were changed from one full of food colorings, additives and refined sugars, to one which emphasized whole grains, fruits and vegetables, we observed even more positive results. Then we took it one step further. We dropped our milk program and switched over to purified water. Our overall rate of asthma dropped dramatically - from an average of ten percent to an all-time low of one percent!"

"That's impressive!" Michael exclaimed. "But how did you manage to get parents to cooperate?"

"We met with the parents to co-ordinate our efforts. Then we performed an experiment for a four week period - primarily for the students - so they could see the connection between what they ate, drank and breathed and their level of well-being. After two weeks, we didn't need to convince anyone of anything - they were sold. From that point on, this became our new lifestyle, at school and at home. Of course, there were a few families who chose not to participate."

"The changes were that dramatic?" Michael was incredulous.

"Indeed, they were. What they noticed most was that the children rarely needed to be reprimanded. Everyone was more relaxed and there was more time for fun. To prove our point, and with the parents' permission, we performed an experiment. We gave glasses of dark pop to half the students. To the other half, we gave water. By mid-morning, all kinds of strange behaviors began to happen - many of the kids who had been fed pop became hyperactrive, others got extremely tired, some even became aggressive. We recorded everything on videotape. Later, they were so embarrassed seeing themselves acting silly and out of control, that even if we'd tried, we couldn't have convinced them to go back to their old lifestyles."

"What a wonderful way to bring the point home. As I said a minute ago, there's nothing like experience."

"A bonus for this increased awareness is that our students are almost as alert mid-afternoon as they are first thing in the morning - a far cry from the other schools at which I taught. It makes teaching so much easier - so enjoyable!"

"It makes it easier for the kids to learn," added Paul. "And . . . I'm proud to admit, we don't have the fights they have at other schools."

It reminded me of the young offenders who were taken off pop and sugars and the rat studies mentioned by Dr. Rowland.

"What on earth do you do at Halloween?" I was curious to hear his reply.

"Our parties are called 'Horribly Healthy Halloween'. Veggie and fruit trays decorated with dried fruit, nuts and seeds seem to keep them quite happy. We encourage parents to set up a store at home on Halloween night. The kids go trick-or-treating just like everyone else, but the parents buy back the treats. That way the children have an incentive not to eat the junk. We found that most of them would rather take the money and buy themselves something they really want. In situations where kids insist upon eating what they've collected, we ask parents to limit it to the one night. As for the families themselves, they give out reasonably healthy snacks and novelties."

"What a grand idea! Michael, we should do that next Halloween."

"You're on!"

"I hate to change the subject, but one of my main concerns involves the perfumes, gels and hairsprays the kids douse themselves with - right from the lower grades straight through high school. From what I've read, these can affect kids in a big way." I was reminded of that distressing day at the school with Ms. Allen.

"They definitely can . . . and do," replied Paul. "Which is why this school has a scent-free policy. Anything that has a fragrance is prohibited. According to the FDA, fragrances cause thirty percent of all allergic reactions. When exposed to perfumes, more than seventy percent of asthmatics develop respiratory symptoms."

"I would never have made that connection - not in a thousand years!" exclaimed Michael, obviously thinking of Emma.

"Many perfumes contain chemicals which are known to be neurotoxic," continued Suzanne. "Scented fabric softeners are also a real problem. Get thirty kids in one classroom wearing that stuff and everyone's bouncing off the walls! We've been experimenting with some recipes for homemade gels using things like gelatin powder and lemons. The kids love to experiment. It's great fun!"

"And for those less inclined, we provide lists of commercially-available unscented products. You'll notice posters in the halls made by the kids - about how scents are 'uncool'. We spend a good deal of time discussing environmental issues and how they directly affect us. The kids themselves actually came up with the idea of having sniffers at the door of each classroom . . ."

"Sniffers? You mean to smell everyone?"

"Yes," Paul replied. "Because our school has a reputation for environmental health, we receive a large number of children with identified sensitivities, some quite severe. They need a clean environment at all times. Once the rest of the children are shown how devastating certain odors can be, they're more than willing to cooperate."

"Studies show," said Suzanne, "that most people are affected by odors, though they may be unaware of it. Did you know that some health clubs and churches actually compete for memberships by advertising scent-free policies?"

What next?

Paul chortled, "Did you folks happen to read yesterday's paper? Big headlines read, *Passenger Asked to Leave Bus Due to Scent.*"

"Are you serious?"

"Absolutely. The driver had a severe reaction to the woman's designer perfume which caused his eyes to water uncontrollably. When a substitute driver couldn't be found, she was asked to transfer to another bus for safety reasons. It was embarrassing for her, but they had no other choice."

"Sooner than you think, the demand for clean air will be as strong as the no-smoking lobbies," commented Michael. "Jillian, tell Paul and Suzanne about Nathaniel's school trip."

"I volunteered to be one of the chaperones on an overnight trip a few weeks ago. Several kids were spraying their hair next to their asthmatic classmates who were frantically gasping for air, trying to obtain relief with their puffers. It was a sad sight, indeed! I wish I'd had a video camera with me."

"Speaking of scents, did you folks hear about the teacher in Russell County who was forced out of his own classroom by his eighth grade students?"

"Forced out of his classroom!" we echoed.

"Yes, although this isn't particularly about violent behavior, as far as I'm concerned, it's just as bad. They all knew this particular teacher was extremely sensitive to perfumes and colognes. The students conspired to wear the most pungent of these to school on the same day. The teacher became violently ill and collapsed. Is this any less loathsome than overt physical abuse? It was deliberate, despicable!"

"It's downright cruel!" I was shocked that a group of kids would do such a thing.

Michael shook his head in disbelief. "What next? Just five years ago, would we ever have thought such a thing could even exist? Environmental abuse . . . God!"

"I know it may sound repetitive and perhaps even extreme," said Paul, "but I think it *is* a form of abuse when we put thirty youngsters in a classroom that's been cleaned with chemicals of dubious toxicity, or that has ceilings full of mold, or where renovations are done while the children are present."

"Not to mention putting them in brand new portables, knowing how toxic they can be . . ." I added, thinking of our discussion at Jane's about new mobile homes.

"Why would they be more toxic than a regular classroom?" asked Michael, looking somewhat puzzled.

"Because they're built essentially from synthetic materials which outgas for years, just like some mobiles," replied Paul. "An exception in Canada are the portable classrooms specially constructed by the Halton Board of Education, in an area west of Toronto. They built them completely with materials that were the lowest toxicity available. Very sensitive children can be placed in these multi-graded classrooms to do their work without fear of reactivity. These classes are often staffed by teachers who themselves have chemical sensitivities."

"Sometimes older portables can be a welcome change, especially if one has spent years in a toxic school. Ever since I can remember, a good friend of mine, a grade five teacher, had suffered from headaches and fatigue. They moved her into an older portable for the past two years and she's never felt better. She says her students also fare better. There's more ventilation and every time they have to use the washroom, which is in the main building, they have to go outdoors. This way they also get even more than their usual share of fresh air, and a good stretch to boot."

"So it was probably a situation where the main building was more polluted than the portable," replied Paul. "One caution is that some of the more poorly constructed older portables can harbor molds. They need to be regularly checked for leaks." Glancing at his watch, he suggested, "Let's take a stroll down to one of our classrooms. Recess is only minutes away."

"But there are kids outside already," observed Michael looking out a window.

"Oh, those are just a couple of classes getting their daily exercise, or DPA. We try to spend at least one hour a day out-of-doors, even in winter. We skate, snowshoe, cross-country ski - anything to get fresh air."

"Sounds good to me! The more fresh air, the better!" Glancing at the wall on my right, I broke into laughter. "Michael, take a look at this." I pointed to a poster entitled *Student of the Nineties* (fig. 19). It really was hysterically funny! "Who drew this?" I asked.

Bruce MacKinnon, the cartoonist for the Halifax Chronicle-Herald. A friend sent it to me a few months ago. It may seem pretty funny, but not very far from the truth, at least for some schools and some students. Let's take a peek into Ms. McNulty's class."

We walked in quietly, sat down, and observed. Instead of the regular black or green chalkboards, there were whiteboards on the walls. I noticed that the children were healthy-looking, robust, with bright faces. Not one had a runny nose! They were alert, focused and very involved with their work. Sunlight streamed in through the windows and skylights - the only artificial light was from a lamp on the teacher's desk. Suzanne leaned over and whispered, "I know a few minutes is hardly enough time to judge a group of kids, but they're basically always like this. I can't begin to tell you what a treat it is to teach children who are calm and balanced. You don't have to waste valuable time on discipline."

"I understand," I whispered. "I've spoken to numerous senior teachers in our own system and they agree that behavior problems have certainly increased over the years, especially since the mid-eighties."

"And so has the use of drugs like Ritalin and Cylert," said Paul out of the corner of his mouth. "In fact, their use has tripled over the last four years." He nodded toward the door. "Let's move along and see if we can find Jerry. He does most of the maintenance."

On our way, Michael asked Paul and Suzanne if there were any other things they had noticed before making the move to Lake of the Woods.

"I could cite hundreds of examples," Paul replied. "One child couldn't do her schoolwork on the days the floors were polished. Several others failed their tests and exams because their teacher insisted the entire class use correction fluid. Can you imagine thirty kids in a classroom all using this stuff at one time? I know my brain would quickly become mush! Another misbehaved only in music class. It turned out that his music teacher slathered himself in aftershave, and the child was very sensitive to fragrances . . ."

"Painting and other renovations caused many health and behavior problems," added Suzanne, "ranging from minor discomfort, such as headaches and the inability to concentrate, to severe and continuing illness, depending on the sensitivity of the child."

# Student of the 90's

## (fig. 19)

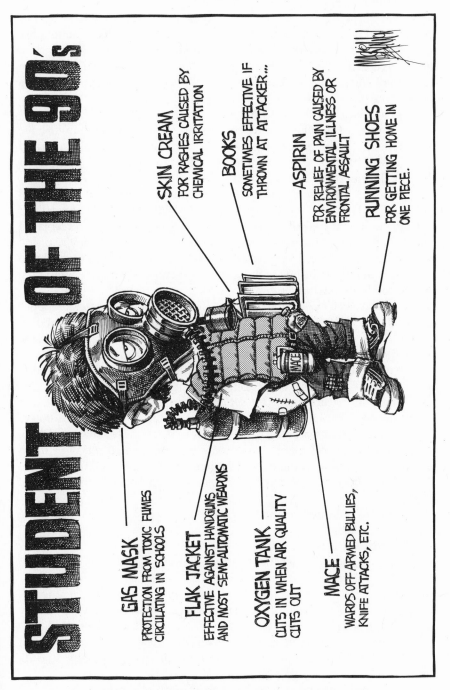

Courtesy of the Halifax-Herald and Mail-Star

"In my old school, gluing blackboards, tarring roofs, and refinishing gym floors were all done while the children were in class," added Paul. "Thank goodness that's a thing of the past."

Suzanne interjected. "Some of our kids previously attended a poorly ventilated, carpeted school. They were constantly plagued with headaches and fatigue. When the parents investigated, they discovered that not only were mushrooms growing in the carpets, but very high levels of carbon dioxide were found in the school. When they removed the children from that school and enrolled them here, their headaches and fatigue became a thing of the past."

"What about the kids who stayed?"

"Eventually the schoolboard got around to doing what should have been done in the first place. They removed the carpet, fixed the roof and put in new windows. No more leakage, no more mold. And fresh air for all. It really can be that basic."

"And then there were the kids who became sick from a newly carpeted classroom in Fitzville - remember, Suzanne? Within a couple of weeks of installing new wall-to-wall carpeting, it all had to be ripped out and replaced with tile. Several of those children are now in our school. They're doing much better, but are still very sensitive to chemicals found in carpets and glues. Carpeting can be one of the worst problems and must be avoided in schools at all cost - whether new or old."

"It sure was an eye-opener for me to learn about the hazards of house dust and dust mites at that seminar I attended. Just the thought that dust can harbor pesticide residues and linger in carpets was enough to turn me off for life." I could feel myself wince as I spoke.

We walked past a small room with a full-length glass door. I looked in and saw lots of plants, several cages and a large aquarium.

"That's our nature room. It's set apart from the rest of the school, and as you can see," Paul motioned to a large exhaust fan, "it's well ventilated. Furry and feathery creatures can cause severe reactions for some children, while aquariums and plants may create problems for those with mold sensitivities. This way, plants and animals are kept in isolation, yet the glass allows the more sensitive kids access to them, with minimal adverse effects."

"I noticed a whiteboard in the classroom we just left. Are you using non-toxic markers?"

"There really is no such thing as non-toxic. Because each of us has our own particular sensitivities, the product that may be fine for one person may not be tolerated by the next. So in effect, even what's labelled 'non-toxic' may be harmful for some. The more appropriate term is 'less toxic'. But, to answer your question, our markers are reputed to be low in toxicity and they are odor-free. And that's true for all of our teaching materials."

"I also noticed the lamp was the only lighting used. I realize it's bright today, but what kind of lighting do you normally use, especially on dull, winter days?"

"All of our lighting is broad-spectrum with electronic ballasts . . ." replied Paul.

Suzanne interrupted. "I used to get severe headaches from the fluorescent lighting in my classroom at the old school. I'd often turn them off and use natural daylight whenever possible. Then I noticed that on those particular days, my whole class was less irritable, seldom tired, and their overall behavior and concentration improved significantly."

"About that time, we began to research the effects of different kinds of lighting on children's behavior," added Paul.

"We delved into study after study," continued Suzanne, "and discovered that prolonged exposure to certain kinds of artificial light is known to cause fatigue, irritability, hyperactivity and other behavioral changes in children."

"And according to some of those studies," said Paul, "not only is the spectral range incorrect in most fluorescents, but the fixtures themselves produce an audible hum that has been connected to increased stress . . ."

". . . Not to mention that the flicker they produce can cause problems, ranging from visual irritation to seizures in more extreme cases. This is why we chose the electronic ballast. Not only does it eliminate the hum, but it reduces electromagnetic radiation and saves energy to boot."

"Is *anything* safe anymore?" lamented Michael.

"It really is important to be an informed consumer these days."

"Would it be correct to say that human beings have a wide range of vulnerability that's not, as yet, well understood, especially when it comes to children."

"That's well put," replied Paul. "Norma Miller, editor of *The Healthy School Handbook* - a new state-of-the-art book about environmental hazards in today's schools - sums it up best:

> Would you give a 50-pound child the same dose of medicine you'd give a 200-pound adult? Probably not. Yet many children are exposed at school to toxic substances that may not harm an adult, but which can be harmful to a developing child.

"And as we said earlier," commented Suzanne, "most studies are done with the adult male in mind, certainly not children. So they continue to be adversely affected, only no one connects their ailments to the root causes."

Paul looked over at Michael. "Do you realize how many children with A.D.D. suffer from chemical or food sensitivities?"

"A.D.D.?" Michael's eyes opened wider. It was obvious he was thinking of Nathaniel.

"Yes, Attention Deficit Disorder, another relatively new term for 'we're not quite sure what's wrong with you'. Mental confusion, inability to concentrate, behavior problems, inattentiveness - you name it, it's all lumped under this category. Would it not be far better to first rule out environmental or nutritional factors *before* these children are labelled and unnecessarily medicated? While not all A.D.D. is environmentally- induced, much of it can be - especially where a child has a history of colic, ear infection, eczema, asthma or other physical symptoms. And parents are told repeatedly by 'experts' that foods and chemicals have nothing whatsoever to do with their child's behavior. In our view, far too much is attributed to psycho-social causes and not nearly enough to environmental ones."

Suzanne piped up, "Just like canaries in the coal mine, small children are especially vulnerable to the effects of chemical exposure. They're at greater risk to illness from environmental pollutants than adults. Not only is their breathing more rapid than ours, but they are also less able to detoxify substances."

"And because childhood is a time of rapid cell division and growth, there's a greater probability of genetic damage," suggested Paul. "Not only are we slowly poisoning our children, but in all likelihood, we're damaging future generations as well."

"And add these exposures to the significantly high levels of pesticides in their foods . . ."

"How's that any different from what adults ingest?" I asked.

"Take for example, fruit. Children consume about six times as much fruit per body weight as we do," replied Suzanne. "They're the largest consumers of apple juice and sauce . . ." She noticed Michael's puzzled expression and continued. "Body weight, you know, is a very important factor. It affects the concentration of pollutants in the body."

"Then there's all the processed and fast foods they eat, full of additives, preservatives, sugars and fats . . ." I started to sound like Eva.

"Is it any wonder that so many children can't function properly?" quipped Paul. "And it's only getting worse. As Jillian pointed out, ask any of our staff whether teaching has become more difficult over the years. They'd readily agree that far too much time is spent disciplining kids, not teaching them."

"I know I couldn't even imagine trying to teach thirty kids a day, let alone ones with behavior problems!" I exclaimed, shuddering at the thought. "I really commend you for your efforts. Teaching these days must be very demanding."

"Thank you Jillian," smiled Suzanne. "Some days we need to hear that!" She turned away for a moment. "Ah, Jerry. Glad we found you. I'd like to introduce you to Jillian and Michael Stowe."

We shook hands with a burly older man with a shock of white hair. Nodding, he greeted us, "So, what do you think of the school so far?"

"We're impressed. We can't get over the freshness of the air in here. You must be doing something right!" Michael kidded.

He laughed. "Well, we do the best we can. You've probably noticed that there isn't a shred of carpeting to be found in this school - even the library has tile floors. Carpets are great traps for dust, mold, and even pesticides - not to mention bacteria when you have thirty kids tramping over them! I call them chemical sponges. Then, of course, you have to clean them, and if new, they can be toxic. You just can't win!"

I was impressed! It was obvious he knew his business.

"That's something I just learned at a workshop a few weeks ago. It's amazing what we don't know that can harm us."

I nodded, thinking of all we were learning. "And I noticed that the furnishings in the classrooms are older, wooden desks and chairs . . ."

"Good observation. There's a method to our madness at this school," smiled Jerry. "Newer furniture is built from pressboard and then laminated. It contains loads of urea-formaldehyde glues that can be a big problem."

"The most common chemicals in building materials, furniture and cleaning compounds are formaldehyde, toluene, phenols and ethanol. You'd be hard-pressed to find any significant levels of them in our school," beamed Paul with pride. "Sometimes the up-front costs of some of the materials we use may be higher, but because they're more durable and far safer in the long run, they become extremely cost-effective - especially taking into account fewer sick days among staff and lower substitute costs. We also use second-hand or surplus furniture."

"The timing of renovations is also very important," offered Jerry. "We're careful never to renovate during the school year unless it's an emergency situation. If we have no other choice, we use the least toxic materials available, and we never use oil paints or varnishes. Instead, we've gone to odorless, VOC-free latex and acrylics. On our floors we use water-based finishes that are about as durable as anything else on the market."

"That's great!" I exclaimed. "I'll never forget the day my daughter came home from school with a terrible headache and nausea. I thought she was getting a flu. Then I went to the school for a parent-teacher interview and was barely able to sit through it. They had just glued up blackboards while school was in session."

"Well, you'd never see that here," smiled Jerry. "And of course all of our cleaning products are not only odorless, but are as simple and basic as possible."

"What do you mean?" asked Michael.

"For instance," said Jerry, "to absorb odors in washrooms, we use open boxes of baking soda and bags of zeolite, a naturally-occurring mineral. Both absorb pollutants from the air. To prevent minor pranks, we put them in locked, vented boxes which are attached to the walls."

"A far cry from those intolerable air fresheners used in public washrooms, including those in many schools. I can barely stand to be in them!" I exclaimed.

"We use vinegar and water on our windows," continued Jerry proudly, "and products with the lowest possible toxicity in the washrooms. But almost as important as the products we use, is the *timing* of when we clean."

"Timing?"

"Yes. Practically all cleaning takes place after or long before classes are in session. As you know, some children can be sensitive to even the most innocuous products. Even dust can be a problem. After each cleaning, all windows are opened to air out the rooms."

"One of the simplest yet most important rules we have," added Paul, "is that of changing shoes from outdoor to indoor ones. This ensures that nothing is tracked into the classroom from outside."

"We also encourage teachers to open windows on a regular basis," said Suzanne. "They usually air out classrooms during recess and lunch. Each child keeps an extra sweater at school. This practice alone makes an enormous difference in the children's ability to think clearly."

"Mind you," added Paul, "we don't have the problem of neighboring wood smoke and auto exhaust that you have in the city."

"Agreed . . . I'm also very strict about idling buses," said Jerry. "In fact, we just instituted a no-idling policy. Now parents are trying to get it passed as a by-law in the local municipality."

"We haven't gone quite that far at work yet," said Michael, "but we do require cars to park in such a way that their exhaust faces away from the building. Prior to that, I could smell fumes in my office all day - even through the ventilation system! I must look into a no-idling policy."

"It's far too common to find the air intake vent right next to the air outlet vent - hard to believe but, nevertheless, a reality."

"That's ridiculous! Who are these architects, anyway?"

"Hopefully unemployed ones," replied Jerry. "And wherever possible, I try to schedule lawn mowing and snow removal before or after school hours. This way, we avoid problems that can arise from freshly cut grass, noise and exhaust fumes. A lot of our safety measures are simply a matter of careful scheduling - an easy practice for anyone to adopt."

Suddenly, a pleasant melody began to play over the intercom. Paul noticed our puzzled expression. "Oh, that's what we use instead of a loud, obtrusive bell or buzzer. It's our contribution to the reduction of noise pollution - much better for the nervous system!" We smiled, thinking back to our own days in school.

"Let's wander outside and see what the kids are up to," Suzanne suggested. "Jerry, maybe we could head over to the gardens and show the Stowes what we're doing in our ecology program."

"Good idea." As we walked down the hall, we passed an office. I noticed an enclosed room marked 'Photocopy Room'. "Usually, copiers are in the offices where people work," I said, pointing to the sign. "But you've separated your workspace from the equipment. Is that to reduce exposure?"

"Yes. And we also have a powerful venting system to the outside," replied Suzanne. "It is recommended that copiers be removed from areas where people work, and that they be properly vented. Otherwise, people are exposed to high levels of toner fumes as well as to ozone. And it goes without question that laminators be treated in a similar fashion. "

"What kind of health problems can ozone cause?" asked Michael.

"Impaired lung function and decreased resistance to infection. Those with asthma or other chronic lung diseases would be particularly susceptible."

"What about computers in schools? Do you use protective screens?"

"We certainly do," replied Paul. "Since most of our color monitors were designed and manufactured in the mid-to-late eighties - before current electromagnetic radiation (EMR) standards were set - they all have screen filters. We found that the filters best suited to our needs were manufactured by No-Rad. We also position students at least 50-60 centimeters - about arm's length - from the front of the computer screen. And we never permit students to sit directly behind or beside the monitors since the electromagnetic field (EMF) emissions are highest at this point. When replacing our equipment, we purchase only monitors with very low EMF levels - only those that meet the Swedish II standard."

"What's the Swedish II standard?"

"Well, the technical term is actually MPR-II and it's the internationally recognized standard for EMR emissions from computer monitors. In Sweden, the allowable standard is 2.5 mG (milligauss) at about one foot from the screen. But the United States EPA is also conducting the first comprehensive review of the literature on EMF health effects. The draft document suggests that the limit will be set at 2 mG, at least that's their goal. They're also looking at similar threshold limits for homes and public buildings near high voltage lines."

"If you're interested," suggested Suzanne, "both the New York City Public Schools and the Regina Catholic School Board in Canada have written comprehensive reports on the subject. Personally, I find the latter report very easy to read and understand."

"Another problem we've encountered," added Jerry, "are the fumes that outgas from the heated plastic of new computer monitors. For this reason, we purchase used models. As a result, our technology tends to be slightly behind others." He looked over at Paul sideways, and winked, "The boss says we're more interested in staying healthy than in keeping up-to-date with the latest and the greatest."

"It's impressive how thorough you are here. Lake of the Woods must be setting a precedent for other schools across the country."

"As a matter of fact, we are. Part of our mandate is to help any school or board that's willing to make changes. And we're very fortunate that we have our own board-managed maintenance and cleaning program. It's been our experience that contract cleaners - services hired from outside - will give you shiny floors but more often than not, they don't put a premium on the environmental health of the building and its occupants."

"Why is that?"

"I think it's because they're not really an integral part of the school. There's less involvement on a day-to-day basis. Another drawback is that there's little control over what and how things are cleaned."

Outside, we noticed children walking around with garden tools in hand. Some were squatting down, digging weeds from the lawn. Others were carrying buckets. I asked a particularly intense-looking little boy what they were doing.

"We're going to empty our compost buckets over by the garden. We do this twice a day."

"Here's where kids learn all about how food grows," explained Jerry, leading us to the gardens. One of the children, a little girl about Emma's age, skipped alongside of us. "We're almost ready for planting season, right Jennie?"

She nodded, as she dumped the contents of her bucket into the compost bin. "Right, Mr. Davis, and I can't wait! I'm in charge of the tomatoes."

I noticed a button she had pinned to her shirt. It was almost identical to the poster we had seen at the entrance to the school. "What's that button you're wearing?" I asked.

She held it out to me. It was a little wooden skunk holding a heart. "That's my *No Scents Please, I'm Sensitive* button. I picked a pink one, my favorite color. But you can get them in all colors."

"Isn't that sweet. Who makes them?"

"It's another fund-raising project for the school," replied Suzanne. "One of the parents tole-paints them." Looking at Jennie, she thanked her, and sent her on her way.

"Selling buttons to raise money sure beats selling candy bars!" I thought of all the organizations selling chocolate, including those raising money for the local Children's Hospital. What irony!

"Yes, we raise money with a variety of programs, based on ecology."

"And who tends these gardens in the summer?" asked Michael.

"Oh, we have it coordinated with parents and children from the neighborhood. Everyone is scheduled around summer vacations. It all seems to work out - especially when it comes to harvest!"

"And the children get a sense of growth cycles. They also learn to appreciate that food comes from the earth and not just from grocery store shelves," added Suzanne. "I'd recommend that any school adopt this program."

We watched the children for a few minutes. A couple of them wore masks while digging. Michael, puzzled and somewhat alarmed at the sight, asked why they needed them.

"Those kids are mold-sensitive. They wear the masks for protection while they're digging in the soil. A few are so sensitive they can't participate in the program at all. We find other interesting things for them to do so they don't feel left out."

"You know, in Japan, it's quite common for people to wear masks in public. You see it quite a bit on public transit systems. If someone suffers from flu or a cold, they'll don a mask to protect those who aren't sick. I find it's a very considerate practice. I believe you'll see increasing numbers of people in North America wearing masks - as protection against environmental contaminants."

"I find it very alarming that we've actually come to this," sighed Michael.

"Alarming perhaps, but nevertheless, very real."

"And what's this?" Michael asked, stooping to pick up a pink wooden tulip that read: *Support a Chemical Free Lawn.*

"I know!" I blurted. I felt like a kid in school who had the right answer. "I learned about it in Jane's workshop a few weeks ago. It's a program designed to promote pesticide-free lawns and gardens. It teaches people about the dangers of using chemicals on their property - you know, on lawns, trees and shrubs. If you're interested, I can tell you all about it on the way home in the car. We might want to start one in our own neighborhood."

"Jordan!" Paul called out to a young boy walking by. "Has your class completed the pink tulip project?"

"We just finished," replied the red-haired, freckled youngster. "We made over three hundred and sold them all. Nearly everyone in the neighborhood has one on their lawn." He beamed with pride.

Paul explained that it was a great learning experience for the kids and a program that helped unite the community, as well as a good fund-raiser for the school. I noticed that Jordan was also wearing a button. It read: *Fragrance Free, That's For Me!*

"Does the school make those buttons too?" I asked.

"Nope. I got this at the Children's Hospital. I used to be on a puffer every day - a mask every other day. Now, I never have asthma."

"Ever since you came to this school?" asked Michael.

"Yeah, and ever since I changed my diet. Dairy products were really bad for me."

Paul thanked the young boy. We began walking back toward the school.

"I'd like to add," said Jerry, "that chemicals including insecticides, herbicides, fungicides and chemical bactericides are never used in or around this school. Our entire focus is on prevention. Only in a crisis situation would we ever entertain using a pesticide and then, only with utmost caution."

"A big switch from schools like the one my daughter used to attend. They saturated the entire school ground with a herbicide one week before school was to be dismissed for the summer holidays. And do you know why they sprayed?"

Michael and I both blinked. "No, why?"

"Because of a few broad-leaf weeds! Apparently, the neighbors didn't want the seeds blowing onto their picture-perfect lawns. As a result, the asthma rate for that same week escalated by over fifty percent and behavioral changes were noted not only at school, but all around the neighborhood - in adults as well as in children."

"And remember, Suzanne? I couldn't think straight for at least two weeks after the spraying." Seeing Michael's puzzled expression, Paul explained. "I taught in the same school Suzanne's daughter attended. That stuff is dangerous! Not only was my mind affected, but my lungs took several weeks to get back to normal. So many people experience these symptoms, only they never make the connections."

I thought of Sam and her kids. "I recently met a young mother at a workshop who, along with her two children, became environmentally ill from a single spraying. She explained how the so-called inert ingredients can be even more dangerous than the active components."

"That's why our school decided not only to adopt a *no pesticide* policy, but to educate the neighboring community on their hazards as well."

"So what do you do about stinky sneakers?" I'd often heard this argument to justify the use of deodorizers.

"We have the children on a schedule. Each class takes their gym clothes and sneakers home at designated times to have them laundered."

"Makes good old-fashioned sense!" I commented.

As we rounded the corner, Michael pointed to a fair-sized outbuilding. "What's that used for?"

"Oh, that's our industrial technology shop," replied Jerry. "It's separate from the rest of the school. Although we only use materials of low toxicity, some airborne particles are unavoidable. The children wear protective masks and the building is well vented with a powerful exhaust system." He talked to us about how important it was to regularly maintain ventilation and heating systems. Then he went on to explain how vital it was to ensure that the water be safe as well - right from its source to the plumbing. He was so well-informed. "Jerry, where did you learn all this? Most people don't know a fraction of what you know."

"Couldn't have given me a better compliment!" He smiled. "I make a point of attending every conference I can on environmental health. I now spend a great deal of time helping other educational facilities make changes in the direction we've taken here at Lake of the Woods. But getting back to ventilation . . . a good system must be able to screen out the bulk of contaminated air brought into the building . . ."

"You mean pollutants like mold, smoke and pollen?" Michael was really getting into it!

"Well, mold and pollen are relatively easy to control, but smoke is another matter. Usually we shut off the external intake and re-circulate indoor air during these times. Although it's not perfect, it reduces the problem. The system must also be able to maintain proper temperature and humidity conditions. More important, it must be regularly checked for any microbial contamination - especially in coastal areas where the air is damp much of the year."

We were just about to enter the cafeteria when I noticed a collage on the far wall. It contained headlines from a variety of newspapers: *Perfumes Force Teacher From Classroom, Fungal Spores Scrubbed From Elementary School, Unknown Sickness Closes School, School Stays Shut Awaiting Air Check,* and *Many Schools Living on Borrowed Time.*

"Look at this." I gestured to Michael. "We really don't know where we're sending our kids every day, do we? We think they're in the best of hands. In terms of their education that may be true, but what about their health? I find this distressing, don't you?"

"I can't believe how I've been so much in the dark about all this. I keep thinking about Nathaniel's A.D.D. diagnosis and how much he's improved from the change in his diet alone. Now I can see, especially after that week of testing, that cleaning up the air in his classroom may be another part of the equation.

"I've witnessed so many children," began Suzanne, "who feel miserable from September to June, bless their little hearts. The connection is rarely made between how they feel and the environment in which they spend so much of their time."

"So how can we, as parents, help to bring about changes in our own schools?" I was certainly ready to become an active participant. "I know we have a group called the Joint Occupational Health and Safety Committee, but their main focus seems to be more directed at implementing safety measures such as the storage of lab chemicals, and examining fire doors, evacuation routes and first-aid kits."

"We also have an environment committee that deals with recycling and other related issues," added Michael.

"That's where you need to take the quantum leap from the environment 'out there'," said Paul, pointing to the outdoors, "to the one 'in here' - our indoor environment."

"And then, of course, equally important, is the environment 'in here'," said Suzanne, pointing to her body. "Speaking of which, welcome to our cafeteria."

I looked at the menu posted just inside the door on an easel - homemade vegetable soup, wholewheat sandwiches, salads, a stir-fry dish and fresh fruit. I thought of my own children's cafeteria and canteen, full of junk - right from the hot dogs, canned soups and high-fat tacos to the fruit punches full of dyes and sugars. Added to that were the disgustingly sweet desserts, including 'ice cream' sandwiches that Eva had cited as one of the worst examples of chemical factory foods. At that moment, making changes in our school seemed like a monumental task. Where would we begin?

"Michael," I whispered, "We've got to do something. I feel like we're living on another planet and that right now we're in some kind of time warp - a flicker of sanity in a very screwed-up universe."

"I think I know what you're saying, Jilly," he whispered back. Turning to Paul and Suzanne, he commented, "*This* is the way children ought to be living - at home, school and at play - the way our parents and grandparents grew up."

"You can bet," said Paul, "that in their time, behavior wasn't nearly the issue it is today. And no, it's not just that societal norms have shifted or that there are more pressures today than ever before. What we've proven here is that when children have access to clean food, clean water and clean air, they're much more receptive to learning. They're more balanced, they're happier, and of course, so are their teachers!"

"Couldn't have been better said!" exclaimed Suzanne. "Long ago we simply stopped debating whether present levels of contamination were acceptable or not. Instead, we asked ourselves how we could eradicate the problem once and for all. The results speak for themselves."

"That's right," added Paul. "We, as educators, have a much greater responsibility towards our children than simply teaching them math, science and spelling. It's equally important to teach them lifestyle skills and the concept of self-responsibility. These are the values that will shape future generations."

"With parental cooperation, of course," said Suzanne. "These values must extend both ways. For a program like this to be successful, there must be continual interaction among parents, children and educators. It *is* possible."

"I can vouch for that!" exclaimed Paul. "One recent example where parents and teachers cooperated was on the subject of head lice - always an emotional issue when it occurs . . . "

"Ah, yes, that's a great example!" said Suzanne.

"A new child arrived at the school. When the public health nurse examined her, she found a couple of nits - lice eggs. Notices were sent home promptly, but by then a few parents had already gotten wind of the situation. They began to panic. The general protocol was to use one of the shampoos developed for lice - even as a preventative measure."

I remembered the day, a couple of years ago, when Nathaniel came home with his notice. "That's pretty standard advice."

"Listen to this . . . We decided to have a meeting with parents so we could deal with the problem more calmly. Ironically and fortunately, between the time we made the decision and the actual meeting, CBS aired a program on lice and shampoos containing lindane, the active ingredient which kills lice. What we saw was pretty scary. We obtained permission to copy the news report and showed it at the meeting. The video gave parents sober second thoughts about using these shampoos indiscriminately."

"What did they see?" queried Michael. "Don't keep us in suspense."

"Well," continued Suzanne, "the program showed several children who were seriously affected by this chemical - which is actually an agricultural pesticide banned in eighteen countries, but commonly used here in North America. The symptoms ranged from rashes to seizures, to one child going into a thirty-six hour coma. The National Pediculosis Association has received thousands of letters citing illnesses attributed to using shampoos containing lindane. Dr. Sam Epstein of the Cancer Coalition argued that even a one-time exposure of short duration can be toxic."

"That's awful!"

"Wait, there's more," said Suzanne. "Dr. Epstein went on to say that the incidence of brain cancer is 4.5 times higher among those who had used lindane-containing shampoos. Although the US FDA defends its use, the agency has recently asked the three American producers of the chemical to do millions of dollars of research on the safety of their products."

"Yeah, right," interjected Michael. "Can you trust them to give us the truth, if it harms their profit margin? I doubt it. The FDA should conduct its own studies."

"I agree with Michael," said Paul. "But at least the manufacturers are now required to put strict warning labels on these products. Unfortunately, people are usually so caught up in the problem that they don't take the time to read labels. They assume that if it's on the market, it's okay to use."

I thought back to Martha's story about the cat and the flea collar. "So what happened in the end?" I asked.

"We had the public health nurse show parents how to examine their children for lice. For those who were still worried or discovered there was a problem, we recommended they use any regular shampoo containing sodium lauryl sulphate, and a thorough combing. It worked beautifully for the few who had the problem. Another option is to rub oil of rosemary on the scalp."

Suzanne interjected. "So the crisis ended and we now have a more literate group of parents in our community. It made the point about the danger of pesticides and other hazardous chemicals quite dramatically. Our PTA is now fully on board about most decisions. Really, I can't emphasize it enough - education is the key."

"Getting back to the story for a moment," said Paul, "one of the manufacturer's agents who was defending their product said they strongly recommended that users wear rubber gloves to apply the shampoo. Keep in mind, it was being applied to the children's heads! He couldn't even see the conflict - protecting the parent while exposing the child!"

Michael shook his head. He was obviously quite upset. "You mentioned cooperation. Where do we begin?"

My mouth hung open. I'd never heard him so eager to accept responsibility - to take charge. I was so proud of him! It was the second time in a week I'd had that feeling - it felt wonderful.

"Before this school became a reality," said Paul, "a group of interested parents and teachers got together to form an environmental health committee, as an adjunct to the existing JOHS Committee. Our mandate was to put together a report with recommendations for a truly healthy school environment. We came up with sixty-four of them, all outlined in this report." Paul handed Michael a thick, coil-bound book. "You're welcome to take this with you."

"I have to teach a class in a few minutes," said Suzanne. "It's been a pleasure meeting you and good luck in your endeavours." We thanked her for all her help. She said she'd be interested in helping us get the ball rolling at our own school.

"Well, I've got to get back on the job, too," said Jerry. "Those little munchkins will be back in before you know it."

"Thanks for all your help." Michael acknowledged Jerry's contribution. "You're a wealth of information. Keep up the good work!"

He grinned. "Thanks. If you need any more help, I'm only a phone call away."

Michael turned back to Paul. "For starters, I'm most interested in things we can do that would be of little or no cost to implement, such as instituting *no scents* policies and altering maintenance schedules. I would think schools and school boards would be more receptive to these types of suggestions. We could work on those right away. I just want to get a sense of what would be involved."

"It's all right here in this report," replied Paul. "Most of the points are ones which Jerry covered with us this afternoon - opening windows, and as you mentioned, rescheduling renovations. Some schools have installed state-of-the-art air purifiers in classrooms for children with known sensitivities. Others have gone as far as upgrading their air-exchange units. And let me tell you, everyone has felt the benefits of these improvements."

Suzanne jumped in. "However, I think it's vitally important to mention that in our experience, with our own colleagues, we've learned that the autocratic method is totally ineffective . . ."

"What do you mean?"

"Well, we've discovered that a far gentler and more intelligent way of making change is by educating people. Once they understand the issues, they're more apt to want to make changes. With understanding comes commitment. We've found that in-services are crucial."

"You mean through regular PTA meetings?"

"That's one good route. Also, bringing in specialists in the area of environmental health - like Dr. Rowland and Eva Sandor for example - would go a long way in creating awareness of how the environment affects health, learning and behavior."

"Eva would be great!" I exclaimed. "No one's better at explaining why proper nutrition is so important, especially for children."

"Once you have a working group on indoor pollution, you can create an on-going training program for staff, parents, and then students, on the latest issues in environmental health. You could use Lake of the Woods as a model. Often, regular in-services to maintenance crews on the latest, safest and best information possible related to indoor air quality would be another positive step."

"Should we work with our own school first, and then take it to the board if need be, or work the other way around?" asked Michael.

"If the principal of your school is interested and willing, work on that level first. If there's total disinterest, then obviously you have no other recourse but to take it to the board level. One very comprehensive book is the one we mentioned earlier, put out by the National Education Association. It's an invaluable resource. It covers many of the items we talked about today. It even contains a large chart in cartoon form depicting the potential environmental hazards in school buildings. Every school should have one - displayed on a prominent wall."

"That would move everyone to action!" I laughed at the prospect. "What's the name of the book?"

"*The Healthy School Handbook.* I'll give you the contact number before you leave. Another very powerful tool is Dr. Doris Rapp's tape, *Why An Environmentally Clean Classroom?* Focus your presentation on the part where it demonstrates children reacting to chemicals - school air in particular - and you'll have their undivided attention."

"We not only viewed that tape, but had first-hand experience with our own kids at Dr. Rowland's clinic. It's all quite new to me, but I'll tell you, I couldn't believe what I witnessed. If someone had merely described it, I'd never have believed it."

"So you can well appreciate," said Paul, "how difficult it is for the average person to understand what we're trying to do. Until you experience it yourself, it's nearly impossible to comprehend the enormity of the situation. However, that videotape will go a long way toward helping people understand these issues."

"When I think of how sick Jillian's been and how I doubted her simply because no one was able to connect her symptoms to her underlying problem . . ."

"And Jillian's an adult. Imagine a child who's less able to make these connections. All he can tell you is that he doesn't feel well. If poor behavior happens to be his particular reaction, his parents and teachers are kept busy trying to discipline him, or seeking psycho-social causes for his misbehavior. They never think to look at physical factors - diet and the immediate environment."

"Believe me, we've been there," said Michael. "And if it wasn't for this wonderful woman here," he squeezed my shoulders, "I shudder to think where we'd be today!"

His words touched me - deeply. Smiling, I turned to Paul. "Thanks for everything. Now that we're armed with all this information, believe me, we're ready to use it!"

"And knowing my wife, you can count on it!" said Michael with a hearty laugh.

Paul extended his hand. "It's been a real pleasure, folks. If there's anything we can do to help you make your children's school a safer place, remember, as Jerry said, we're only a phone call away."

As we drove off, I felt that Michael and I were now a team. I snuggled up to him, feeling supported and loved. "Jilly, we really have to get the show on the road. I'm now thoroughly convinced that Nathaniel and Emma are negatively affected by their school. I still remember the three-day headache I had after that meeting with Mrs. Allen! And you're right, it *is* always stuffy in that school."

"I know I can't go to any functions there - the odors are so bad. They set me back for days . . . But at least we now know what to do."

"And by God, we're going to do it!" He smiled and patted my hand reassuringly. I hadn't felt this happy in years.

"Michael, let's stop at the health food store for a minute. I have to pick up a few things."

He followed me around the store looking somewhat lost, but ever so curious. He touched everything, turning things over, reading labels. I picked up what I needed and headed for the check-out counter. As I waited in line to pay for my items, I noticed a book on their best-seller rack. It was entitled *Allergies: Disease in Disguise* by a Dr. Carolee Bateson-Koch. On the front cover were listed many of my symptoms of not so long ago. Just under the title, it said *How to heal your allergic condition permanently and naturally.* I quickly handed my things to Michael and began leafing madly through the pages. She talked about how enzyme therapy is a critical part of recovery from food allergies and that candida and parasites are two of the major underlying factors in the development of allergies. She sounded a lot like Dr. Rowland. I glanced at the back cover:

> *Allergies: Disease in Disguise* is the first book ever to explain how to achieve complete and permanent recovery . . . Following her program, you won't have to give up your pet, get allergy shots, rotate foods, keep diet diaries or cook allergy-free recipes for the rest of your life. You will not only recover and enjoy an allergy-free life, you will gain invaluable understanding of health and well-being.

Sold! I ran back to Michael who was just about to write out a check. "Here, buy this too! I think it's just what we need."

Michael looked at the salesgirl. "Can you add this on?"

"No problem." She looked at the book. "Good choice! Other than *Tired and Toxic* and *The Yeast Connection*, there's never been a book that's helped as many people as this one. They follow the instructions in here and return feeling better than they have in years." She grinned, "I'm sure you'll like it."

As we left the store, I grabbed Michael's arm, excitedly telling him about the book. I'd been quite prepared to permanently adjust our lifestyle to accommodate elimination and rotation, focusing on whole and raw foods. Now, here was a book suggesting that it could take us even further.

Could there be a cure?

*Science teaches that we must see*
*in order to believe, but we must also*
*believe in order to see.*
*We must be receptive to possibilities*
*that science has not yet grasped,*
*or we will miss them.*
*It's absurd not to use treatments*
*that work,*
*just because we don't yet*
*understand them.*

*Open-mindedness is the hallmark*
*of all physicians who are truly interested*
*in helping their patients.*

**Bernie Siegel**
**Love, Medicine & Miracles**

# 19

# Final Consult

*I thank God for my handicaps, for, through them, I have found myself,*
*my work, and my God*
**Helen Keller**


*I*t was exactly eight months to the day that Dr. Klamer had told me
there was nothing more she could do for me, other than refer me to a
psychiatrist - the appointment I never kept. Adhering to my routine, I felt
better than I had in years. As long as the candida was under control, my
chemical intolerances improved. Taking antigens and supplements
regularly, avoiding foods to which I was sensitive, and rotating the rest,
gave me a quality of life I had never dreamed possible. Meditation was a
bonus. It not only accelerated my recovery, but it gave me the strength to
cope with many of life's daily stresses. Not only did my physical symptoms
clear up, but gone too were the mood swings, panic attacks, irritability and
depression. I looked great - I felt great. In fact, we all felt great - even
Michael!

Dr. Rowland had suggested I go back to Dr. Klamer to update her on
my progress. I was so excited just thinking about how she'd be able to help
other patients who were experiencing similar problems. I knew there were
many who were suffering - especially children. I'd bought copies of *The
Yeast Connection and The Woman* and *An Alternative Approach to Allergies*.
They had become my source of inspiration - my support. I slipped them
into my purse as I left for my appointment.

"Well hello, stranger! You look great!" exclaimed Dr. Klamer, the
moment I stepped into her office.

"I *am* great! In fact, we all feel great! Max hasn't had an ear infection in
months and Emma has all but discarded her puffer - ever since we changed
our diets and started on an anti-yeast program." I pulled the two books
from my bag and handed them to Dr. Klamer. "These books are life-savers!"

"I'm not at all familiar with this one," she replied, pointing to *An
Alternative Approach to Allergies.*"I know about *The Yeast Connection,* and as
far as I'm concerned, there's absolutely no scientific basis for his approach."

"But what Dr. Crook says has helped thousands get better, when all else failed . . . "

"There's no proof of that. Jillian, in the seventies it was hypoglycemia, in the eighties it was yeast and Chronic Fatigue Syndrome, and now it's a toss-up between Fibromyalgia, Environmental Illness or Multiple Chemical sensitivity. Who knows what trend will come along next?"

My blood began to boil. "So to what do you attribute my recovery? Dr. Rowland has helped me more than anyone!"

"Dr. Gabriel Rowland . . . in Bridgeport?"

"Yes."

"He's considered to be a bit of a quack by most of my colleagues. It's a wonder he's still in practice. I hear he puts people on ridiculous diets . . . Jillian, the power of suggestion has a very strong placebo effect . . ."

*Power of suggestion . . . placebo effect* ! "Excuse me, but I've worked very hard at my recovery . . ." I looked directly at her. My frustration grew by the minute. "Dr. Klamer, can't you see I'm not the same person who was here only a few months ago? Don't you want to know what I did to help myself? Don't you want to share this information with your patients?"

"When I see double-blind studies, peer-reviewed in medical journals, I'd be happy to condone these techniques. Until such time, I can only look at all this popularized medicine as irresponsible. I consider myself to be a responsible physician and I'm certainly not prepared to experiment with my patients."

"But if the therapy works and causes no harm?"

"If it's not proven . . ."

"Proven by whom? Rats in a laboratory? What about the human experience! What about what *is* - what's happening right now? There are thousands out there who are still suffering as I did. Aren't you interested in helping them?"

"Of course I am . . ."

"Then why won't you at least phone Dr. Rowland and ask him about his protocols, or better yet, visit his clinic. You could at least try some of the basic steps outlined in these books."

"As far as I'm concerned, they're unproven and unscientific."

I could see the conversation had come full circle. There was no point in continuing. Glaring at her, I took my books back. "I'm going to have to find another family doctor who's more open - more willing to look at alternatives. I need someone to work with me on what I now know to be the truth. I'll send for my files."

"That's fine," Dr. Klamer said abruptly. She stood up in a gesture of dismissal.

I was in shock. I just stood there shaking my head. Here was an opportunity to learn, to grow, to expand her knowledge, and she wasn't the least bit interested! Her mind had shut down. There was nothing more to say. I left her office without looking back. As I walked down the hall, my only consolation was that at least this time I knew what to look for and what to ask when checking out potential family doctors. The clinic would be able to give me some leads.

That night I told Michael about my exchange with Dr. Klamer. He wasn't surprised.

"Don't you remember *my* reaction when you first told me about Dr. Rowland and Eva?"

"Yeah, but I hadn't started the program, so we didn't have any experience on which to base our judgment . . ."

"But really, it wasn't until we made the bet, and I went on the diet myself and *experienced* these changes first-hand that I believed it."

"But she's a doctor who deals with chronic yeast infections, asthma and ear problems day in and day out, offering little more than band-aid therapy. Then, to hear about something safe and effective that could actually resolve a problem and not try it - or even consider it? It's wrong!" I shouted. I could feel my outrage well up again.

"Jilly, just move on - forget about the Dr. Klamers of the world . . ."

"No . . . I can't . . . I won't! Michael, I'll promise you one thing - this experience will only spur me on to share this with everyone I meet! I feel I owe it to those who are still unaware - uninformed. And anyway, how could I ever go back to nursing knowing what I now know?"

"You might consider something similar to what Jane is doing . . ."

"Maybe . . . " I replied, the wheels turning. I slowed down long enough to think of how far Michael had come. "Michael, I do appreciate your support . . ."

He pulled me close and whispered, "Jilly, to see - *to know* - once again, that warm, caring, wonderful woman I fell in love with has been worth everything we've been through. And the difference in the kids . . . You're quite something, Jillian Stowe - you never gave up!"

It was so good to hear those words! I vowed right then and there to encourage others to keep on searching - to steer them in the right direction, to help them on their own journey toward wellness.

I finally understood . . .

Wellness is not a short trip - it's a lifelong journey.

I, the canary,

was finally

Free to Fly . . . . .

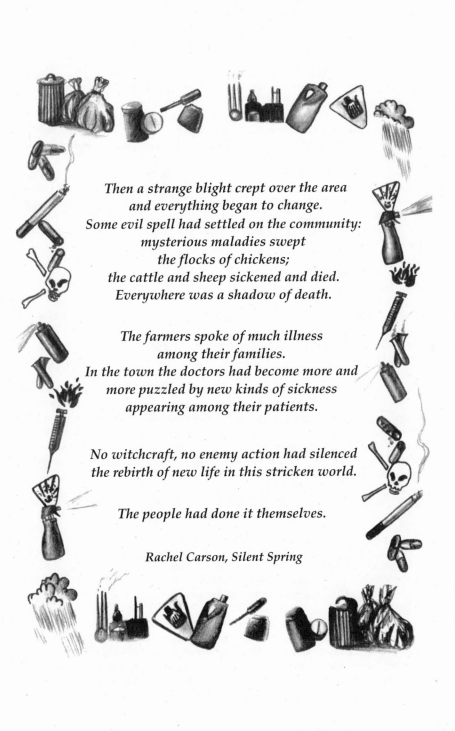

Then a strange blight crept over the area
and everything began to change.
Some evil spell had settled on the community:
mysterious maladies swept
the flocks of chickens;
the cattle and sheep sickened and died.
Everywhere was a shadow of death.

The farmers spoke of much illness
among their families.
In the town the doctors had become more and
more puzzled by new kinds of sickness
appearing among their patients.

No witchcraft, no enemy action had silenced
the rebirth of new life in this stricken world.

The people had done it themselves.

*Rachel Carson, Silent Spring*

# Last Words

For the past five years, I suffered from what was diagnosed as fibromyalgia. Symptoms included fatigue, headaches, sleep disruption, muscular stiffness and soreness, depression, sensitivity to cold, as well as some cognitive impairment such as forgetfulness, concentration problems and memory loss. Physiotherapy, acupuncture, exercise, psychological counselling and medication all helped somewhat, but were unable to relieve all my symptoms and prevented me from enjoying my job and family.

After one appointment with Judit, I couldn't believe the difference in my physical and emotional well-being. I eliminated wheat, sugar, yeast and dairy products from my diet, took some nutritional and homeopathic supplements and haven't looked back! I now have more energy and a better sense of well-being, and I lost more than twenty pounds! I continue to follow this program, and feel better than I had thought possible.

*Norah Muise, teacher*
*Dartmouth, N.S.*

When I was at my worst, I was so tired I couldn't get out of my own way. Every day, I had to force myself to go to work. During stressful times, I could barely walk. My asthma was so bad, I was on three different types of puffers. At times I had to use a mask every couple of hours. The fall was the worst time of year for me.

I heard about a lecture on allergies and candida. What jumped out at me were the words: What you like the most is what you're probably allergic to. It made sense. All my friends laughed at me when I began my elimination/candida diet. I cut out all dairy products, sugar and yeast and took a few supplements. Within six weeks I was off all medication! I have all kinds of energy, ready to take on projects at 11:00 p.m.! This year the fall was not a problem at all. I highly recommend this approach to health.

*André MacDonald, public servant*
*Antigonish, N.S.*

From a toddler, our five year old son had been an aggressive and at times unmanageable child and did not play well with other children. I consulted doctors, child psychologists, day care and nursery school workers, had his vision and hearing tested, read books on disciplining but all to no avail. We were not making any headway.

Finally, we were referred to Judit who became our saviour. Just days after being on a diet restricting mostly dairy and sugar products, we noticed physical changes, and after only one month we saw remarkable changes in our child's behaviour. Family members and friends have also commented on the changes they see in him. Now each time he has a food that his body has trouble dealing with, we see the effect almost immediately - it also helps reinforce that we are, indeed, on the right track.

*Donna Fancey, office manager*
*Upper Northfield, N.S.*

Since I was thirteen years old, I suffered from severe migraine headaches. As I got older my health problems increased. In my menopausal years, I suffered from insomnia, hot flashes, fatigue and recurring sore throats. I felt terrible. To combat these symptoms, I took a variety of medications, including estrogen, sleeping pills, headache preventatives and pain killers.

I saw Judit on September 22, 1995. This day marked a new beginning for me. During the consultation, she suggested a complete change of diet. I had to eliminate sugar, dairy products, yeast and caffeine. She also recommended acidophilus, an antifungal, digestive enzymes and calcium/magnesium. At first, I was very skeptical. However, once I got through the initial 'withdrawal period' which lasted about 8 days, I actually began to feel better. It's been four months since I started this program. I no longer experience migraines, hot flashes, insomnia or fatigue. I have a tremendous amount of energy and walk 5 - 6 miles daily. Another major outcome of this program is that I have lost 35 pounds! I continue to follow the diet and take my enzymes and calcium/magnesium, along with garlic. I finally feel in control of my life, I feel absolutely wonderful!

*Mary Miles, homemaker, mother of three*
*Mulgrave, N.S.*


I am 62 years of age. For over ten years, I felt constantly fatigued and had no energy whatsoever. Doctors could not identify the cause of my condition and wrote it off as being "all in my mind". I became progressively weaker, ballooned from 136 to 208 lbs., and went through terrible mood swings, including periods of depression. In desperation, I turned to holistic nutrition.

Judit immediately identified food sensitivities and Candida as my problems and put me on a diet. Within mere weeks, I felt human again. Now, sixteen months later, I wake up feeling refreshed and am enrolled in a daily exercise program. I lost a total of 50 lbs. by just eliminating foods that I was sensitive to. I now feel better than ever!

*Kathleen Bezanson, homemaker*
*Dartmouth, N.S.*


Since starting work as a teacher, and even as a student, I can remember coming down with regular bouts of severe head colds which developed quickly into chest infections every year. I used to regularly lose a week of work each fall and again in mid-February. Since eliminating foods such as dairy, reducing grains, and removing scented products from my personal and home environments, I have not been afflicted by this type of illness in two years. In fact, the only serious bout of sinus and chest infection I have experienced in almost five years occurred three years ago when the school was painted inside, and the roof was re-tarred outside - while school was in session!

*Mike Coughlan, teacher*
*Halifax, N.S.*

Amanda was a colicky baby. At about two years of age, she developed regular episodes of chest and ear infections, eczema and general irritability. Her facial appearance was pale with dark circles under her eyes. For an entire year, she was on antibiotics and finally diagnosed and hospitalized with asthma. Her drug regime included inhaled medication (puffers) and steroids. Her pediatrician didn't feel allergies were implicated. My G.P. maintained that Amanda was sick so much because she attended day care.

Because of my own struggle with Environmental Illness, I began researching and experimenting with our home environment and diet. We stopped eating dairy products, yeast and sugar and supplemented our diet with the vitamins and minerals she needed. Within three months, Amanda was drug free! Today, she's a healthy five year old who rarely becomes ill. Awareness of these issues has given us control over our health - our lives.

*Ann Thompson, nurse*
*Dartmouth, N.S.*

Goodbye yeast, dairy and sugar.
Goodbye fat, tired, achy body.
Goodbye dull, pale, acne-infested face.
I love my new physically, emotionally and mentally healthy, energetic body. And the transformation took only three months! Thanks Judit!

*Susan Pottie, salesperson*
*Sackville, N.S.*

For over thirty years, I suffered from depression. Since the age of twenty-four I was on medication. If I were to describe myself in two words or less, it would be 'tired and sad'. The doctor said I was born tired. Weight gain, fluid retention, headaches, gastritis and sinus infections also plagued me. In the mornings, I felt stiff and lame, having a difficult time getting my body mobilized.

Upon a friend's suggestion, following a seminar by Dr. William Crook, I went to see Judit. I eliminated dairy products first. After the third day, my sinuses were clear and within a couple of weeks, I was no longer stiff when I got up in the morning. I decided to test myself and ate pizza with lots of cheese, followed by ice cream. I awoke very tense, anxious, and became quite weepy. By afternoon I was depressed and crying - totally miserable. I haven't had dairy products since, nor have I had any sign of depression. Then I eliminated yeast and sugar. I'm not tired anymore, look forward to the day, and instead of becoming overwhelmed, can meet the challenges. In fact, I feel revitalized!

*C. Evangeline Leslie, self-employed*
*Dartmouth, N.S.*

At the beginning of treatment, I felt sluggish, tired and weak. I was irritable and had difficulty concentrating. After removing sugar, wheat, yeast and dairy products from my diet, I felt stronger with a lot more energy and vitality. I continue to experiment with foods, but feel best when I keep as close as possible to the prescribed diet.

*John Cotton, public servant*
*Judique, Cape Breton*

When I was eight months pregnant with Andrew, I was treated with antibiotics for a urinary tract infection, which ended up in a yeast infection. Andrew was only two weeks old when large pus-filled blisters invaded his diaper area. The doctor prescribed an antifungal cream. At one month of age, Andrew had his first of many ear infections, all of which were treated with antibiotics. By the time he was four, I was desperate for help. He was very thin, pale with dark circles under his eyes. He had asthma, sores on his face, itchy, sore genitals, and was always constipated. He couldn't sit still, barely slept, had very poor attention span, couldn't obey anyone and couldn't get along with other children. All we were offered was Ritalin.

I picked up a book by Dr. William Crook called *Help for Your Hyperactive Child*. It was all about Andrew! All of his symptoms were described in this book. I finally knew what was wrong. With the help of a holistic doctor, we took away all processed and packaged foods, switched to organic, and followed a caveman diet. He began taking acidophilus and an antifungal. Within *two weeks* Andrew was a totally different child! He is now ten, still avoids many foods and continues to take supplements. His health problems are still absent. He does very well in school, gets excellent marks, and is calm and kind - a far cry from before. He plays the violin - something I would never have believed possible five years ago!

*Twila Touesnard, homemaker*
*Halifax, N.S.*

I would return from school, watch television, maybe get up and have a few cookies. Then I'd have my supper, do my homework and lay down again. That pretty much was a day for me. I also had asthma, a continuous stuffed up nose and dark circles under my eyes. My Mom decided I should see Judit.

After seeing her and being on my 'special' diet for a month now, I'm feeling a lot better. This doesn't mean I stick to my diet 100 percent. It's hard for an eleven - almost twelve - year old girl, but I do my best. I still receive sympathetic looks from friends when I turn down cupcakes because of what's in them. All I care about is I was totally maxed out then and I have (almost) boundless energy now and can breathe freely! I used to dislike gym and am now actually enjoying it. But the best part is that if I follow my diet, I don't need to use my puffer!

*Nicole Francis-Brooks, grade six student*
*Dartmouth, N.S.*

Five years ago, at the age of 35, I was exhausted, had bowel problems, suffered from pains in my lower abdomen, multiple yeast infections, a lump in my throat, had no sex drive and was depressed a good part of the time. I gained 18 pounds and diets were of no help at all. I had ultrasounds of my kidney, bladder and ovaries, nuclear x-rays of my throat, an ongoing prescription for Monistat for yeast infections. My depression was treated with drugs and my low energy was attributed to stress.

I then chose alternative therapies. I was told I had candida, possibly parasites and a thyroid problem. I altered my diet, eliminating foods to which I was sensitive, and took specific supplements. Within a month I felt well enough to rake leaves. By Christmas I returned to my normal 128 lbs. and felt terrific. My brain could handle things efficiently once again and my memory returned. Being forty is great! I feel like a teenager again.

*Susan Stewart, stockbroker's assistant*
*New Germany, N.S.*

Ever since I can remember, prior to meeting Judit, my usual routine was filled with various, almost continuous, illnesses. Infections, viruses and bronchial colds usually led to antibiotic treatment. Asthma developed around age six with ventolin treatments, steroids and recently, four different types of inhalers. Stomach aches, headaches, and a general feeling of tiredness were common.

After Judit recommended a diet eliminating some major food allergy components, I was slowly able to stop using the inhalers. In summary, my energy level has increased dramatically and I seldom attract all those illnesses I was so used to getting. Recently, the inhalers were disposed of altogether!

*Julia Goodall, high school student*
*Bedford, N.S.*

For over six years, I suffered from symptoms ranging from irritability, dry, itchy eyes, depression, extreme chronic fatigue and facial acne. I went to twelve different doctors and allergists, took their prescribed medications, but nothing really helped

I was taken off dairy products, corn and cucumbers. Within only a few days of stopping these foods, almost all of the symptoms disappeared! It's been almost four months and I've only suffered minor reactions on two or three different occasions.

*Zuhier Hammude, entrepreneur*
*Halifax, N.S.*

Most of my life I had bowel and sinus problems, pains in my stomach and trouble sleeping. By the time I was sixteen, I suffered from hot flashes, heartburn, weakness, more insomnia and constant stomach pains. I had to miss three months of school. The doctors couldn't find anything and suggested I was having anxiety attacks and that I'd have to learn to live with the pain.

I was treated for candida and parasites and was told to remove sugar, dairy products and yeast from my diet. I took plant enzymes to help my digestion and was given supplements to support my thyroid gland and to help rebuild my immune system. Within four months I felt great! I am so thankful for my health. I can now be a 'normal' teenager.

*Shannon MacDonald, high school student*
*Port Hawkesbury, Cape Breton*

For the past three years, I felt exhausted. I functioned between 10 a.m. and 3 p.m. on a *good* day. I had a lot of gas and bloating, heartburn, nausea and headaches. My skin was very dry and my arms and legs felt weak, rubbery. Every night I coughed and my sinuses would fill up. If this wasn't enough, I was also overweight. I had every test going - blood tests, scopes, and had just about every part of my body x-rayed. Everything came back normal. According to medical diagnoses, I was as healthy as a horse.

Eight weeks ago, I was treated for candidiasis, Epstein-Barr virus and food sensitivities - dairy products, sugar, wheat, yeast, salt, chicken and peanuts. By the second week of my new regime, I felt considerably better. Now I feel energetic, positive, healthier than I've been in years - and lost 22 1/2 pounds to boot! It seemed effortless. My husband can't believe the difference. Neither can I!

*Nancy Wentzell, sales representative*
*Lake Echo, Nova Scotia*

I never thought I could be like other people - not even in my wildest dreams. I had less energy than most, dreading bedtime, because waking up and never feeling any better was such a disappointment. I also dreaded the summer pollen season, taking two and one-half times the recommended dosage of antihistamines just to make myself drowsy enough to have a restful night's sleep. Every summer I got sore throats and lung infections. No doctor ever helped me. One even wrote 'hypochondriac' in my file!

I was 34 when I found out what caused allergies and decided I had nothing to lose in trying out what I'd learned. I stopped eating wheat, sugar, dairy products and took a natural antifungal and an herbal antiparasitic. Within 3 days I began to feel rested by morning! Instead of taking two antihistamines at once, I would cut one in quarters and it would last me for days. Halfway through July, I threw them out. I had boundless energy and literally gardened until sundown every day. The pollen count was twice that of the previous year and I went around feeling sorry for all the poor people with hay fever. For the first time in years I wasn't one of them!

Imagine the implications for pharmaceutical and marketing companies if everyone found out that they could eliminate their hay fever pills and cure many other things at the same time!

*Sam Kaiser, gardener*
*Beckerton West, N.S.*

Before I embarked on this program, I had a host of complaints. I was constantly fatigued, suffered from heartburn, rhinitis, constipation, mood swings, weight gain and insomnia. My short-term memory was at an all-time low, creating periods of panic. I never realized the significance of the symptoms I was suffering, as they had become second nature to me. I didn't know how badly I was feeling until I was feeling better.

I was advised to eliminate sugar, yeast and dairy products from my diet and was put on an anti-fungal regimen to combat Candidiasis. I endured the initial withdrawal symptoms, and within one week I noticed a great lessening in many of my complaints. I felt like I had enough energy to fly to the moon! And . . . to my great surprise, an added bonus for me was the natural weight loss that I have incurred. I feel positively jubilant at my new-found sense of well being!

*Ethel Jack, librarian*
*Dartmouth, N.S.*

Jared spent his first three years being itchy, pale, lethargic, bloated, insecure and very aggressive. At age three, he developed seizures. His appetite was limited to ten foods. Strict adherence to an eight week Candida diet, and taking a variety of nutritional supplements has given Jared new found health. Bright-eyed, inquisitive, energetic, loving and content are words that come to mind now when I think of my little son. And no more seizures! Many thanks to Judit and holistic nutrition.

*Scott Little (Jared's dad), loss control manager*
*Bedford, N.S*

I had suffered for years with the slow deterioration of osteoarthritis, when the School Board moved my department to a school which had been used as a warehouse for cleaning chemicals. Once, I thought I had forgotten to deliver a report to the downtown office and took a city bus to get there. As the bus turned a corner I thought I was in a city I had lived in as a teenager. I had no idea of how I had gotten there, why I was on a bus, or how long I had been away. I endured several minutes of absolute panic as thoughts of amnesia, homelessness, and the impossibility of explaining what had happened raced through my head. Finally, I recognized the town clock and knew I was in Halifax, but I did not know why I was on a bus. I was totally shaken. The next day I found out that I had not forgotten the report, but had delivered it the day before. Soon after this, I entered the hospital for hip replacement surgery. During the extended recovery period, I began to realize how "brain fogged" I had been. Others in the building were getting sick and complaining of a variety of symptoms. Tests were conducted for molds but not for the toxicity of the cleaning compounds. They issued a report which stated that what they had tested for had been "within acceptable limits". However, since I have been out of the building, I am more alert, able to concentrate, and focussed. I no longer go to bed at 8:30, totally exhausted and wake up groggy. I no longer have constant pain in my hip and in my hands - Judit's recommended diet has helped. As I educate myself (helping with this book) I am finding how important diet and environment are to my health. I am worried about re-entering the building to work.

*Fred Daugherty, resource centre manager*
*Halifax, Nova Scotia*


Imagine yourself not being able to get out of bed without being short of breath. Imagine being so tired you're unable to function. If that's not enough, imagine everything you're eating and breathing making you sick. I felt as if I was going to die. Finally, I was diagnosed as having Environmental Illness or Chemical Sensitivities. My doctor didn't know what to do with me. I did some detective work on my own

Then I went to see Judit Rajhathy of New Directions In Health. It was one of the best decisions I've ever made. When she said I'd feel better in two weeks, I thought . . . right! But Judit *was* right. Within a few weeks, I felt physically and mentally stronger. Symptoms such as headaches, fatigue, depression, sinusitis, gas and bloating and my inability to make decisions vanished. Although I still have a way to go, I am definitely on the mend. Thanks Judit!

*Sandra Francis, federal government employee*
*Dartmouth, N.S.*

It is most rewarding to witness the health benefits that my clients experience when the impact of their total environmental picture, including *Candida albicans*, is considered in their nutritional assessment and treatment plans. It is the magic combination that opens the door to healing for many caught in a chronic, static state of ill health. As a profession, we need to be open to this new era in nutrition, listen attentively to our clients, trust these experts and be courageous to support them within safe limits.

*Anna Protheroe, dietician*
*Halifax, N.S.*

It was the spring of 1989 when we made the overnight journey from our existing North American diet to a more natural one. What prompted this drastic change? Our 'normal' family life was becoming crazy and out of control. Our five year old son Nathan was somewhat hyper; Cassandra, our three year old daughter, developed ear, bladder and yeast infections and had a Jekyll-Hyde personality; and my new baby, Thomas, had a host of problems - from diaper rash, diarrhea, to terrible eczema - all of which began with the introduction of dairy foods to his diet. We went from one doctor to another trying to find help.

One visit with Judit and overnight changes took place. Dairy, sugar, wheat, corn, processed foods, colorings, additives, etc. were gone! It's now 1996, seven years later, and the growth of this family has been fabulous and exciting. Nathan now knows that any form of sugar and wheat changes his personality. Cassandra hasn't had an infection requiring antibiotics since our diet change. Her main food culprits are wheat and dairy, causing her to change from a happy, lovable child to one who is moody, cranky and stubborn. Once taken off dairy products, Thomas' symptoms resolved within a week. We also found out that perfume, cigarette smoke and other chemicals were significant factors in his stuttering.

In addition my chronic vaginal infections and irritable bowel ended, and my husband, Chuck, stopped snoring shortly after stopping dairy. He even lost 26 pounds within two months of stopping yeast and wheat products. We are definitely advocates of this quality of lifestyle and recommend Judit's expertise to many families. There has yet to be a disappointed family! What a family eats can be the difference between harmony and dysfunction. You really *are* what you eat!

*Kim Given, teacher*
*Co-founder of Back to Basics Allergy Support Group*
*Halifax, N.S.*

My three years at junior high were very difficult. I had a handle on my food sensitivities, but poor air quality at school, including perfumes and colognes my classmates wore, gave me splitting headaches and I couldn't concentrate on anything. By grade nine, I developed breathing difficulties. There were times my face would turn bright red and my cheeks and ears would almost burn up. Finally, it got to the point where a home study program was the only option. After only a few days at home I began to notice a remarkable improvement in my health. Unfortunately, my principal and the School Board never really understood environmental sensitivities - nor do I think they even cared about my difficulties.

This year I started grade ten at a new school. Although I still have problems with scented products, at least the building itself is much cleaner than my junior high. Also, my teachers are more receptive and supportive concerning my sensitivities. I have been relentlessly encouraging other people not to use scented products. It is most unfortunate that more people do not realize that this type of daily pollution might also be affecting them and many others.

*Matthew A. MacDonald, high school student*
*Halifax, N.S.*

# Appendix 1
# Reading List

## Environmental Sensitivity (overview)

*An Alternative Approach to Allergies* - Theron G. Randolph, M.D. and Ralph Moss, Ph.D., Rev. ed. 1989. Perennial Library, Harper & Row, Publishers, Inc., 10 East 53rd Street, New York, NY. 10022. ISBN 0-06-091693-1

*Why Do I Feel So Awful?* - Dr. David R. Collison, MB BS FRACP, 1989. Angus & Robertson Publishers, London, UK. ISBN 0-207-15731-6

*The Allergy Connection* - Barbara Paterson, 1985. Thorsons Publishers, Inc., Park Street, Vermont, 05767. ISBN 0-7225-0984-7

*Brain Allergies: The Psychonutrient Connection* - William H. Philpott, M.D. and Dwight K. Kalita, Ph.D., 1980. Keats Publishing, Inc., 27 Pine Street, New Canaan, Connecticut, 06840. ISBN 0-87983-426-9

*Allergy and Intolerance: A complete guide to environmental medicine* - George Lewith, Julian Kenyon and David Dowson, 1992. Green Print, The Merlin Press, 10 Malden Road, London, UK. ISBN 1-85425-0671

*Coping With Your Allergies: Discover How Clinical Ecology Can Help You* - Natalie Golos and Frances Golos Golbitz, 1986. A Fireside Book, Simon & Schuster, Inc., New York. ISBN 0-671-60199-7

*Tired or Toxic: A Blueprint For Health* - Sherry A. Rogers, M.D., 1990. Prestige Publishers, Box 3161, 3502 Brewerton Road, Syracuse, N.Y. 13220. ISBN 0-9618821-2-3

## Food Allergy/Sensitivity

*Allergies: Disease in Disguise* - *How to heal your allergic condition permanently and naturally* - Carolee Bateson-Koch, DC, ND, 1994. Alive Books, 7436 Fraser Park Drive, Burnaby, B.C. Canada. ISBN 0-920470-42-4

*Dr. Braly's Food Allergy & Nutrition Revolution* - James Braly, M.D., 1992. Keats Publishing Inc., 27 Pine Street, P.O. Box 876, New Canaan, Connecticut. ISBN 0-87983-590-7

*Tracking Down Hidden Food Allergy* - William G. Crook, M.D., 1980. Professional Books, P.O. Box 3494, Jackson, Tennessee, USA. ISBN 0-933478-05-4

## Children, Sensitivities and Behavior

*The Impossible Child: In School, At Home* - Doris Rapp, M.D., and Dorothy Bamberg, R.N., Ed.D., 1986. Practical Allergy Research Foundation, P.O. Box 60, Buffalo, N.Y. ISBN 0-9616318-0

**Is This Your Child?** *Discovering and Treating Unrecognized Allergies* - Doris Rapp, M.D., 1991. William Morrow and Company, Inc., 1350 Avenue of the Americas, New York, N.Y. ISBN 0-688-08623-3

**Solving the Puzzle of Your Hard-to-Raise Child** - William G. Crook, M.D. and Laura J. Stevens, 1987. Random House, Inc., New York, N.Y. ISBN 0-394-56054-X

**Help for the Hyperactive Child** - William G. Crook, M.D., 1991. Professional Books, Inc., 681 Skyline Drive, Jackson, Tennessee. ISBN 0-933478-18-6

**Core Diet For Kids** - Stephen J. Gislason, M.D., 1989. PerSona Audiovisual Productions, 1601 Yew St., Suite 200, Vancouver, B.C. V6K 3E6. ISBN 0-9694140-1

**Videos by Dr. Doris Rapp:**

*The Impossible Child Videos*

Video 1 - How You Can Recognize Unsuspected Allergies
Video 2 -Make the Connection - What Causes Allergies and What You Can Do About It
Video 3 -Clues to Predict Possible Allergies

**Why An Environmentally Clean Classroom** - Available from: Practical Allergy Research Foundation, P.O. Box 60, Buffalo, N.Y. tel: 716-875-5578

# Alternatives to Ongoing Antibiotic Therapy

**Childhood Ear Infections:** *What every parent and physician should know about prevention, home care, and alternative treatment* - Michael A. Schmidt, 1990. North Atlantic Books, 2800 Woolsey Street, Berkeley, California. ISBN 1-55643-089-2

**Beyond Antibiotics:** *Healthier Options for Families* - Michael A. Schmidt, Lendon H. Smith, Keith W. Sehnert, 1993. North Atlantic Books, 2800 Woolsey Street, Berkeley, California. ISBN 1-55643-134-X

*Also, any books on homeopathy would be useful.*

# Optimum Health for Your Child

**SuperImmunity for Kids** - Leo Galland, M.D., 1988. Bantam Doubleday Dell Publishing Group, Inc., 666 Fifth Avenue, New York, N.Y. ISBN 0-385-29827-7

**Feed Your Kids Right, Foods for Healthy Kids, Improving Your Child's Behaviour Chemistry, and Dr. Lendon Smith's Diet Plan for Teenagers-** all books by Lendon Smith, M.D.

**Homeopathic Remedies for Children's Common Ailments** - Carolyn Dean, M.D., 1995. Keats Publishing, Inc., 27 Pine Street (Box 876), New Canaan, Connecticut 06840-0876. ISBN 0-87983-668-7

# Chronic Candidiasis and Parasites

**The Yeast Connection and the Woman** - William G. Crook, M.D., 1995. Professional Books, Inc., Box 3246, Jackson, Tennessee, 38303 ISBN 0-933478-22-4

**The Yeast Connection Handbook** - William G. Crook, M.D. ,1996 Professional Books,Inc.,Box 3246, Jackson, Tennessee, 38303 ISBN 0-933478-23-2

**The Yeast Syndrome:** *How to Help Your Doctor Identify And Treat The Real Cause Of Your Yeast-Related Illness* - John Parks Trowbridge, M.D. and Morton Walker, D.P.M., 1986. Bantam Books Inc., 666 Fifth Avenue, New York, NY. ISBN 0-553-26269-6

**Back to Health:** *A Comprehensive Medical and Nutritional Yeast Control Program* - Dennis W. Remington, M.D. and Barbara W. Higa, R.D., 1986. Vitality House International, Inc., 3707 North Canyon Road #8-C, Provo, Utah. ISBN 0-912547-030

**Candida** - Luc De Schepper, M.D., Ph.D., C.A., 1986. LDS Publications, 4318 Beaucroft Ct., West Lake Village, California. ISBN 0-9614734-1-X

**Guess What Came to Dinner:** *Parasites and Your Health* - Ann Louise Gittleman, 1993. Avery Publishing Group, Inc., Garden City Park, New York ISBN 0-89529-570-9

## Chronic Fatigue Syndrome

*Chronic Fatigue Syndrome and the Yeast Connection:* A *"Get-Well" Guide for People with This Often Misunderstood Illness - and Those Who Care for Them* - William G. Crook, M.D., 1992. Professional Books Inc., Box 3246, Jackson, Tenessee. ISBN 0-933478-20-8

*The Canary and Chronic Fatigue* - Majid Ali, 1994. Life Span Press, 95 East Main Street, Denville, New Jersey. ISBN 1-879131-04-8

## Holistic "Bibles" for Your Home

*Prescription for Nutritional Healing: A practical A-Z Reference To Drug-Free Remedies Using Vitamins, Minerals, Herbs & Food Supplements* - James F. Balch, M.D. and Phyllis A. Balch, C.N.C., 1990. Avery Publishing Group Inc., Garden City Park, New York. ISBN 0-89529-429-X

*Return to the Joy of Health* - Zoltan P. Rona, M.D., MSc., 1994. Alive Books, 7436 Fraser Park Drive, Burnaby, B.C. ,Canada V5J 5B9. ISBN 0-920470-62-9

*When You Can't Reach the Doctor* - Carolyn Dean, M.D., 1989. Perfect Pitch Editions, 598 St. Clair Ave. West, Toronto, Ontario, Canada. ISBN 0-9694528-0-2

*Dr. Carolyn Dean's Complementary Natural Prescriptions for Common Ailments* - Carolyn Dean, M.D., 1994. Keats Publishing, Inc., 27 Pine Street (Box 876), New Canaan, Connecticut 06840-0876. ISBN 0-87983-632-6

*Better Health Through Natural Healing: How to Get Well Without Drugs or Surgery* - Dr. Ross Trattler, 1985. McGraw-Hill Book Company. ISBN 0-07-065172-8

*Alternative Medicine: The Definitive Guide* - *compiled by The Burton Goldberg Group*, 1993. Future Medicine Publishing, Inc., Puyallup, Washington. ISBN 0-9636334-3-0

## Women's Health

*Take Charge of Your Body* (6th Edition) Carolyn DeMarco, M.D., 1989; 1996 R&R Bookbar, 14,800 Yonge St., #195 Aurora, Ontario L4G 1N3 ISBN 0-9694766-1-2 Tel: 1-800-387-4761 (Supplements Plus)

## Vitamins, Minerals, Essential Fatty Acids & Other Supplements

*The Real Vitamin & Mineral Book: Going Beyond The RDA For Optimum Health* - Shari Lieberman & Nancy Bruning, 1990. Avery Publishing Group Inc., Garden City Park, New York. ISBN 0-89529-449-4

*Vitamin Bible* - Earl Mindell, 1985. Warner Books, Inc. 666 Fifth Avenue, New York, NY. ISBN 0-446-32765-4

*Minerals and Your Health* - Len Mervyn, Ph.D., 1980. Keats Publishing, Inc., New Canaan, Connecticut. ISBN 0-87983-402-1

*The Omega 3 Phenomenon: The Nutrition Breakthrough of the '80's* - Donald O. Rudin, M.D. & Clara Felix with Constance Schrader, 1987. Collier Macmillan Canada, Inc. ISBN 0-89256-314-1

*Fats That Heal: Fats That Kill :* *The complete guide to fats, oils, cholesterol and human health* - Udo Erasmus, 1993. Alive Books, 7436 Fraser Park Drive, Burnaby, B.C. ,Canada. ISBN 0-920470-40-8

## Your Healthy Home, School and Workplace

*Your Home, Your Health, and Well-Being* - David Rousseau, W.J. Rea, M.D., Jean Enwright, 1988. Hartley & Marks, Ltd., 3663 West Broadway, Vancouver, B.C. ISBN 0-88179-017-6

*The Healthy House :* *How to Buy One, How to Build One, How to Cure a "Sick" One* - John Bower, 1989. Lyle Stuart Book, Carol Communications, 600 Madison Avenue, N.Y., N.Y. ISBN 0-8184-0494-9

*The Nontoxic Home & Office:*
*Protecting Yourself and Your Family from*
*Everyday Toxics and Health Hazards* -
Debra Lynn Dadd, 1992. Jeremy P. Tarcher,
Inc., 5858 Wilshire Blvd., suite 200, Los
Angeles, CA. ISBN 0-87477-676-7

*The Healthy School Handbook* - Norma
L. Miller, Ed.D, Editor, 1995. National
Education Association (NEA) of the United
States Professional Library, P.O. Box 509,
West Haven, CT. ISBN 0-8106-1863-X

*Report of the Committee on Environ-*
*mental Health* - Halifax District School
Board, July 1994. P.O. Box 370, Halifax,
N.S. B3J 2R1 (902) 421-6834

*The '90s Healthy Body Book* - Gary
Null, Ph.D., 1994. Health Communications,
Inc., 3201 S.W. 15th Street, Deerfield Beach,
Florida. ISBN 1-55874-303-0

*Your Health & Your Home: a resource*
*guide* - Nina Anderson & Albert Benoist,
1994. Keats Publishing, Inc., 27 Pine Street,
Box 876, New Canaan, Connecticut.
ISBN 0-87983-630-X

*The Green Home Handbook: A Guide*
*to Safe and Healthy Living in a Toxic*
*World* - Gillian Martlen and Shelley Silver,
1991. Fontana, Harper Collins Publishers,
Hammersmith, London, ISBN 0-00-638132-4

*Clean & Green: The Complete Guide to*
*Nontoxic and Environmentally Safe*
*Housekeeping* - Annie Berthold-Bond,
1990. Ceres Press, P.O. Box 87, Woodstock,
N.Y., USA ISBN 0-9606138-3-8

*The Zapping of America* - Paul Brodeur,
1977. W.W. Norton & Co., Inc., 500 Fifth
Avenue, New York. ISBN 0-9606138-3-8

*The Clean Air Guide - How to Identify*
*and Correct Indoor Air Problems In Your*
*Home; Building Materials for the*
*Environmentally Hypersensitive; How*
*to Improve the Quality of Air in Your*
*Home; and Investigating, Diagnosing*
*and Treating Your Damp Basement;*
and the video, *This Clean House* - all
available from Canada Mortgage and
Housing Corporation, 700 Montreal Road,
Ottawa, Ontario, Canada K1A 0P7
(613) 748-2367

# Our Contaminated Food Supply

*Diet for a Poisoned Planet* - David
Steinman, 1990. Harmony Books, Crown
Publishers, Inc., 201 East 50th Street, New
York, New York 10022. ISBN 0-517-57512-4

*May All Be Fed* - John Robbins, 1992.
William Morrow and Company, Inc., 1350
Avenue of the Americas, New York, New
York 10019. ISBN 0-688-11625-6

*Additive Alert!* - The Pollution Probe
Foundation, 1994. McClelland & Stewart
Inc., The Canadian Publishers, 481
University Avenue, Toronto, Ontario,
Canada M5G 2E9. ISBN 0-7710-7139-6

# Yeast-Free, Rotation and Allergy Diet Cookbooks

*Freedom From Allergy Cookbook* - Ron
Greenberg, M.D. and Angela Nori, 1990.
Blue Poppy Press, 212-2678 West Broadway,
Vancouver, B.C., Canada V6K 2G3.
ISBN 0-88925-905-4

*Full of Beans* - Violet Currie and Kay
Spicer, 1993. Mighton House, Box 339,
Campbellville, Ontario, Canada L0P 1B0.
ISBN 0-9695688-1-9

*The Self-Healing Cookbook* - Kristina
Turner, 1987. Earthtones Press, P.O. Box
2341-B, Grass Valley, California 95945.
ISBN 0-945668-10-4

*Mrs. Mouse's Cookbook* - Joy
Underwood, 1987. Allergy Educational
Services, 1202-1175 Broadview Ave.,
Toronto, Ontario, Canada M4K 2S9. ISBN

*The All Natural Allergy Cookbook* -
Jeanne Marie Martin, 1991. Harbour
Publishing, P.O. Box 219, Madeira Park,
B.C., Canada V0N 2H0.
ISBN 1-55017-044-9

*Rotational Bon Appetit!* - 1986
Environmental Health Center, 8345 Walnut
Hill Lane, suite 205, Dallas, Texas 75231 tel:
(214) 368-4132 fax: (214) 691-8432.

*Recipes for Health, Candida Albicans*
- 1995. Thorsons, HarperCollins, 77-85
Fulham Palace Rd., Hammersmith, London
W68JB, UK ISBN 0722529678

*The Candida Albicans Yeast-Free Cookbook* - Pat Connolly and Associates of The Price-Pottenger Nutrition Foundation, 1985.
Keats Publishing, Inc.,
27 Pine Street,  Box 876
New Canaan, Connecticut 06840.
ISBN 0-87983-409-9

*Naturally Sweet Desserts, The Sugar-Free Dessert Cookbook* - Marcea Weber, 1990.  Avery Publishing Group, Inc.
Garden City Park, New York.
ISBN 0-89529-443-5

*Just Desserts* - Steve Parsons, 1989.
Lancelot Press, Ltd.
Hantsport, Hants County
Nova Scotia, Canada.
ISBN 0-88999-424-2

*Cookies Naturally*,1989 and *Muffins from the Heart,* 1993.
Shirley M. Hartung.
Cookies Naturally
32 Layton Street,
Kitchener, Ontario, Canada.
ISBN 0-969411510

# The Politics of Holistic Medicine

*What Your Doctor Won't Tell You: The Complete Guide to the Latest in Alternative Medicine* - Jane Heimlich, 1990.  Harper Collins Publishers
10 East 53rd Street
New York, N.Y.
ISBN 0-06-096539-8

*Racketeering in Medicine: The Suppression of Alternatives*
James P. Carter, M.D., Dr. P.H., 1992.
Hampton Roads Publishing Company, Inc.
891 Norfolk Square, Norfolk, VA.
ISBN 1-878901-32X

*The Medical Mafia*
Guylaine Lanctôt,  M.D.
1995.  Here's The Key Inc.
P.O. Box 830 850
Miami, Florida.
(819) 835-9520
ISBN 0-9644126-0-8

# Living in the Moment - mind over matter

*Peace Is Every Step*- Thich Nhat Hanh, 1991. Bantam Books, 666 Fifth Avenue
New York, N.Y.
ISBN 0-553-07128-9

*The Language of Letting Go* - Melody Beattie, 1990.  Hazelden Foundation, Pleasant Valley Road, P.O. Box 176
Center City, MN 55102-0176.
ISBN 0-89486-637-0

*Love, Medicine & Miracles* - Bernie S. Siegel, M.D., 1986.  Harper & Row, Publishers, Inc., 10 East 53rd Street, New York,  N.Y. 10022.
ISBN 0-06-091406-8

*The Healing Journey* - O. Carl Simonton, M.D. and Reid Henson, 1992.
Bantam Books, 666 Fifth Avenue
New York,  N.Y. 10102.
ISBN 0-553-08282-5

# Information on NAET

*Winning the War Against Asthma and Allergies: a drug-free cure for asthma and allergy sufferers* -Ellen.W. Cutler,D.C.
1998. Delmar Publishers
3 Columbia Circle, Box 15015
Albany,  N.Y. 12212-5015
ISBN 0-8273-8622-2

*Say Goodbye to Illness* - Dr.Devi S. Nambudripad, D.C., L.Ac.., R.N., Ph.D.
1993.  Delta Publishing Company
7282 Melrose Street,  Suite F
Buena Park, CA 90621
ISBN 0-9637570-0-8

# Appendix II

# Resource List

## Locating a Practitioner

*American Academy of Environmental Medicine*, 4510 West 89th Street, suite 110, Prairie Village, Kansas 66207 tel: (913) 642-6062 - an international referral service for doctors practicing Environmental Medicine, $3 donation requested.

*Canadian Society for Environmental Medicine*, P.O. Box 62058 Convent Glen Postal Outlet, Orleans, Ontario K1C 7H8 fax: (613)-837-8896 - the Society's main purpose is to raise awareness of the link between environmental exposures and human health - will refer to local organizations who are familiar with these problems.  By fax only.

*American Holistic Medical Association*, 4101 Lake Boone Trail, suite 201, Raleigh, N.C. 27607 tel:  (919) 787-5146  fax: (919) 787-4916 - for an $8 charge, provides a directory that lists physicians practicing holistic medicine throughout the U.S.

*Canadian Holistic Medical Association*, 42 Redpath Avenue, Toronto, Ontario M4S 2J6 Will accept mail enquiries only.

*American Association of Naturopathic Physicians*, 2366 East Lake Avenue East, suite 322, Seattle, Washington 90102  tel: (206) 323-7610 - recorded message instructs you to send $5 in order to receive a referral and information directory listing naturopaths practicing in the U.S. and Canada. Or fax: (206) 323-7612 with your Visa or Mastercard number.

*Canadian Naturopathic Association*, 4174 Dundas St. West, suite 304, Etobicoke, Ontario, Canada M8X 1X3  (416) 233-1043 fax: (416) 233-2924 - provides names of practicing naturopaths in your area.

*EDTA Chelation Lobby Association of BC*, P.O. Box 67514, Station O, Vancouver, BC V5W 3T9 (604) 327-3889 - provides information and referrals.

## Information and Support

*Allergy and Environmental Health Association of Canada*, Mic Mac RPO, Box 24030, Dartmouth, Nova Scotia, B3A 4T4 tel: 1-800-695-9271- for $25 a year membership, list of local support groups, information and resources regarding the environmentally sensitive as well as health-conscious individuals, and *The National Update*, a quarterly magazine, full of up-to-date information on environmental health - from strategies in dealing with the problems of sensitivities to sources of safe products.

*Human Ecology Action League (HEAL), Inc.*, P.O. Box 49126, Atlanta, GA 30359-1126 tel: (404) 248-1898 fax: (404) 248-0162 - referrals to local HEAL chapters and other support groups for those whose health has been adversely affected by environmental exposures.  Resource lists, quarterly magazine, reading lists, etc.

*Consumer Health Organization of Canada*, 250 Sheppard Avenue East, suite 205, Willowdale, Ontario M2N 6M9 tel: (416) 222-6517  fax (416)-225-1243 - for $38 (Cdn) a year membership, offers a bi-monthly magazine, *Health Freedom News* (from above umbrella group), and a monthly newsletter. CHOC puts on a Total Health Conference once a year in Toronto, sells health books, and provides information on holistic health practitioners. Freedom of choice in healthcare is a mandate.

*International Health Foundation, Inc.,* Box 3494, Jackson, TN 38303 tel: (901) 427-8100 - Founder and President: William Crook, M.D. - will respond to people seeking help for health problems related to the yeast, *Candida Albicans.* It provides an international roster of physicians who have expressed an interest in candida-related disorders.

*Candida Research and Information Service,* 575 Avenue Road, Apt. 601, Toronto, Ontario M4V 2K2 tel: (416) 928-1844 fax: (905) 731-7605 Founder: Maggie Burston - CRIS is part of an international network that keeps up-to-date on all therapies and the latest research related to parasites and candidiasis in particular. CRIS has the largest medical library on candidiasis in Canada - physician referrals are available. Telephone consultations are $75.

*Back to Basics Allergy Support Group,* 59 Westridge Drive, Halifax, N.S. B3M 3K3 tel: (902) 445-4558 fax: (902) 443-2542 - was formed by a small group of people who were struggling to provide safe food and safe environments for themselves and their children. Provides support and a listening ear. Also have available 'tried and true' recipes, particularly for those with restricted diets (e.g. candida).

*The Health Resource, Inc.,* 564 Locust Street, Conway, Ar 72032 tel: (501) 329-5272; 1-800-949-0090 fax: (501) 329-9489 - is an international medical information service that provides individualized comprehensive reports on specific medical conditions. They contain the latest treatment options - both conventional and alternative - and information on current research, nutrition, self-help measures, specialists and resource organizations. Prices dependent upon whether condition is cancerous or non-cancerous.

*CFIDS (Chronic Fatigue Syndrome) Association of America, Inc.,* P.O. Box 220398, Charlotte, N.C. 28222-0398, tel: 1-800-442-3437 1-900-896-2343 fax: (704) 365-9755 - is the largest patient-based non-profit organization dedicated to conquering chronic fatigue and immune dysfunction syndrome (CFIDS) through its

public policy, education and research programs. Membership is $35 annually, which entitles members to a subscription to *The CFIDS Chronicle,* a 64-page quarterly publication, and other benefits. Free information packet available.

*The M.E. (Chronic Fatigue Syndrome and Myalgic Encephalomyelitis) Association of Canada,* 400-246 Queen St., Ottawa, Ontario K1P 5E4 tel: (613) 563-1565 fax: (613) 567-0614 - a clearing house of information, providing legal help, medical counselling and information packages free of charge. Membership is $40 a year and includes a 20-24 page monthly newsletter.

*Nightingale Research Foundation,* 383 Danforth Ave., Ottawa, Ontario Canada K2A 0E1 tel: (613) 728-9643 fax: (613) 729-0825 - provides network of support groups throughout North America and Europe. Compiles and publishes articles, pamphlets, and books.

*Practical Allergy Research Foundation,* P.O. Box 60, Buffalo, N.Y. 14223 tel: (716) 875-5578 fax: (716) 875-5399 - Founder and President: Doris Rapp, M.D., F.A.A.A., F.A.A.P. - under Dr. Rapp's direction, PARF has published pamphlets, books, and very reasonably priced educational audio and video tapes for the public and physicians (for some subjects, see book list). The focus of this information is environmentally-related health, learning, and emotional illnesses in children.

*Cancer Control Society,* 2043 N. Berendo St., Los Angeles, CA 90027 tel: (213) 663-7801 - information on alternative therapies and nutritional approaches to cancer and other diseases.

*Environmental Dental Association,* 9974 Scripps Ranch Blvd., Suite #36, San Diego, CA tel: (619) 586-1208 fax: (619) 693-0724 - research, education, referral and other resources for less-toxic dentistry.

## Pesticide Information

*National Coalition Against the Misuse of Pesticides (NCAMP),* 701 E Street, SE, suite 200, Washington, DC 20003 tel: (202) 543-5450 fax: (202) 543-4791- NCAMP is a non-profit membership organization dedicated to providing the public with information on pesticides and nonchemical methods of pest control. Membership entitles you to a year's subscription to a newsletter, *Pesticides and You.*

*The Pink Tulip Program,* c/o *Ecology Action,* 1555 Granville St., Halifax, Nova Scotia tel: (902) 429-2202/425-3737 - information on the 'get your lawn off drugs' project includes a brochure and a pink wooden tulip '- support a chemical-free lawn'.

*Northwest Coalition for Alternatives to Pesticides (NCAP),* P.O. Box 1393, Eugene, OR 97440 tel: (503) 344-5044 fax: (503) 344-6923 - a non-profit member-ship organization dedicated to providing the public with information on pesticides and nonchemical methods of pest control. Membership entitles you to a year's subscription to a quarterly magazine, the *Journal of Pesticides Reform.*

*American Pie (American Public Information on the Environment),* 31 North Main St., P.O. Box 460, Marlborough, CT 06447-0460 tel: (203) 295-6117 fax: (203) 295-6127 - a non-profit corporation dedicated to answering all your questions concerning the environment. They will redirect your questions to the appropriate groups.

## More Information and Political Action

*The National Health Federation,* P.O. Box 688, 212 West Foothill Blvd., Monrovia, California 91017 tel: (818) 357-2181 fax: (818) 303-0642 - regular membership is $36 (U.S.) a year and benefits include a bi-monthly magazine, Health Freedom News that has a 70,000 plus readership; *Shedding Light on Legislation,* a political action newsletter, dealing with legislation which impacts our health freedoms; Natural Health Shows discounts; an Alternative Medicine Library. Also available is an Alternative Health Care Provider Referral Service.

*My Health, My Rights,* 2309 Horton Street, Ottawa, Ont. K1G 3E7 tel: (819) 684-3060 fax: (819) 684-6351 In Toronto: 16 Marquis Avenue, Etobicoke, Ont. M8X 1V4 tel: (416) 233-1689 - is a society formed to inform Canadian consumers on their rights in health-related matters and to promote freedom of choice, unbiased and dissociated from any industry, political party or religious group. Membership is $25 a year ($35 for families) and includes a membership card, package and quarterly newsletter.

*Citizens for Choice in Health Care,* 128 Queen Street South, Box 42264, Mississauga, Ontario L5M 4Z0 tel: (905) 826-9384, fax: (905) 895-5621 and *Citizens for Choice in Health Care,* 14 O'Hara Drive, Halifax, N.S. B3M 2E6 tel: (902) 868-2108 - a grassroots advocacy group formed to take direct action to ensure freedom of choice in health care and access to safe and effective medical treatment for all people. CCHC neither endorses nor rejects any specific form of therapy.

## Products for the Environmentally Conscious

*The American Environmental Health Foundation,* 8345 Walnut Hill Lane, suite 225, Dallas, Texas 75231-4262 tel: 1-800-428-2343 - is a non-profit organization founded in 1975 by William J. Rea, M.D., at the Environmental Health Center in Dallas, Texas. It has funded over 13 major medical projects, and carries over 1100 environ-mentally safe products in its mail-order department, including air filters, bedding, personal care items, etc.

*Healthy Environmental Alternative Lifestyles (H.E.A.L),* 5568 Falkland Street, Halifax, N.S. Canada B3K 1A5 tel/fax: (902) 425-0133 E-mail address: aco53@ccn.cs.dal.ca H.E.A.L.- is a mail-order catalogue service serving the environmentally sensitive and health-conscious. Specializing in allergy masks, bedding, personal/home care prod-ucts, air/water filtration supplements, etc.

*Austin HealthMate Air Purifiers.* For direct delivery anywhere in the U.S., Canada, or abroad: H. Lofgren, Air and Water Purification Systems for the Environmentally Sensitive tel: (902) 477-4022 E-mail: Helen_Lofgren@mmcs.com,Internet

*P'lovers Environmental Store,* Park Lane, 5657 Spring Garden Road, Halifax, Nova Scotia, Canada B3J 3R4 tel: (902) 422-6060 fax: (902) 425-2990 Internet-http:// emporium.turnpike.net/A/AAlen/ plovers/ For free catalogue call 1-800-565-2998 - carries a wide range of alternative products for everything from non-toxic personal care and household cleaning needs to natural and organic unbleached clothing and bedding.

Skunk signs and tole-painted wooden skunk pins, "No Scents, I'm Sensitive",
Ildi Isenor, Box 102, Lantz, N.S., Canada
BON 1RO  (902) 883-9629

Your Local Healthfood Store or Alternative Pharmacy are the best places for information
about holistic practitioners, support groups, health publications as well as nutritional and
environmentally safe products in your area.

> If you know of a group with national or international
> reach that is not in this directory, please let us know.
> **The Staff**
> **New World Publishing,**
> **P.O. Box 36075,**
> **Halifax, Nova Scotia,**
> **Canada B3J 3S9**
> **tel: (902) 466-0000 or 466-5000**
> **fax: (902) 466-0005**
> **e-mail: info@newworldpublishing.com**

# Appendix III

# Laboratories and Testing Information

*Anamol Laboratories*, P.O. Box 96, Concord, Ont., Canada L4K 1B2 or 83 Citation Drive, unit 9, Concord, Ontario L4K 2S4  tel: (905) 660-1225 - Hair analysis for minerals, dietary survey and risk factor analyses.

*Accu-Chem Labs*, 990 North Bowser Road, suite 800, Richardson, Texas, USA 75081  tel: 800-451-0116/214-234-5412 - Performs a complete array of pesticide and industrial chemical analysis on blood, urine and body tissue.

*Doctor's Data Inc.*, P.O. Box 111, 30 W. 101 Roosevelt Rd., West Chicago, IL USA 60185  tel: 800-323-2784 - Performs amino acid testing; hair, urine, whole blood; and Red Blood Cell Mineral Analysis (RBC).

*Great Smokies Diagnostic Laboratory*, 18-A Regent Park Blvd., Asheville, NC USA 28806  tel: (704) 253-0621 - Comprehensive digestive stool analysis, comprehensive ova and parasite detection; immune competence; secretory IgA; functional liver detoxification profile, etc.

*Meridian Valley Clinical Laboratory*, 24030 132nd Ave. SE, Kent, WA USA 98042 tel: (206) 631-8922 or 1-800-234-6825 - Tests blood for food allergies, urine for hormones and osteoporosis, stool for digestion, dysbiosis, parasites and hair for toxic metals.

*Pacific Toxicology*, 1545 Pontius Avenue, Los Angeles, CA USA  tel. 310-479-4911 or 1-800-TOXIC - Performs a complete array of pesticide and industrial chemical analysis on blood, urine and body tissue.

*Serammune Physicians Laboratories*, 1890 Preston White Dr., Suite 201, Reston, VA USA 22091  tel: 1-800-553-5472 - ELISA/Act can determine the immune system's sensitivities to up to 300 different foods and chemicals.

# *About the Author*

Born in Hungary, Judit Rajhathy and her family emigrated to Canada during the 1956 revolution. Growing up in Ottawa, she completed her high school education at Campanile Notre Dame and graduated in 1975 from Carleton University with a Bachelor of Arts with distinction. After living for a short time in Toronto, she moved to Nova Scotia in 1978.

Judit is a registered nutritional consultant, licensed acupuncturist and NAET practitioner in private practice in Dartmouth, Nova Scotia, Canada. She specializes in food and environmental sensitivities, as well as in Candida protocols. A noted speaker and health educator, she regularly tours from coast-to-coast lecturing on environmental health within school systems, to corporate and service organizations, as well as to the public at large. She appears on television and radio; is a dynamic lecturer and health promoter; and writes for a variety of Canadian health and wellness publications. Judit has also produced and hosted two successful local television series on holistic health. She is particularly well known for her work in preventative/environmental health, her specific focus being to help others take responsibility for their own health through dietary and environmental management.

Judit became ill in 1985 and began searching for answers for her poor state of health and that of her children. It was this quest that sparked her interest in orthomolecular nutrition, environmental health, and personal growth. Since that time, Judit has read, studied and researched extensively in these fields. She also studied through the Canadian Nutrition Institute and in 1990, became certified as a practitioner through Nutritional Consultants Organization of Canada (NCOC). More recently Judit became certified as an acupuncturist and NAET practitioner.

Judit's commitment to help others help themselves is reflected in her many accomplishments, which included her two popular local television series - *It's Your Health* and *Health Talk*. She also founded *Dartmouth Citizens Against Incineration* and co-founded *Citizens for Choice in Health Care*, both highly successful undertakings. She is a former vice-president of the *Allergy and Environmental Health Association of Nova Scotia* and currently is the President of *New Directions In Health*, a company dedicated to bringing up-to-date health information to the public. She also regularly delivers workshops to schools and educational institutions entitled *The Effects of Diet and the Environment on Health, Learning and Behavior.*

Judit is a dynamic and entertaining speaker, intricately weaving factual information, research and anecdote into the fabric of her presentations. She keeps audiences riveted to their seats, often eliciting bursts of laughter as she intersperses humor with the harsh realities of life in the nineties - a reality she knows only too well, having travelled her own path from sickness toward wellness. The release of *Free to Fly: a journey toward wellness,* added the title 'author' to Judit's growing list of credits.

# Free to Fly
## *a journey toward wellness*
### *by Judit Rajhathy*

## Ordering Information

In order for the vital information in this book to reach the largest number of people, *Free to Fly* is available by mail-order directly from the publisher. This will enable those of you who do not have access to book stores or health food stores to purchase copies at competitive prices. In addition, discounts are being offered to individuals or groups who wish to purchase multiple copies. These discounts also apply to educational institutions, libraries, health, environmental, self-help groups, or professional associations. This book makes a wonderful gift for friends or relatives who may suffer from one or more of the symptoms discussed in this book. Or, you may know of parents with chronically unwell children or children with behavioral difficulties at home or in school. This book may provide them with answers to many of their health problems.

## How to Order

### In Canada

| Prices **per** book sent to a single location **on the same order:** | | | |
|---|---|---|---|
| Number of books | 1 | 2 - 4 | 5 - 9 | 10 or more |
| Cover price | $23.95 | $23.95 | $23.95 | $23.95 |
| Discount | 0% | 10% | 20% | 25% |
| Price per book | $23.95 | $21.55 | $19.15 | $17.95 |
| + S & H + GST | | | | |
| Total price **per** book | **$28.00** | **$24.00** | **$22.00** | **$20.00** |

### In the USA

| Prices **per** book sent to a single location **on the same order:** | | | |
|---|---|---|---|
| Number of books | 1 | 2- 4 | 5 - 9 | 10 or more |
| Cover price | $19.95 | $19.95 | $19.95 | $19.95 |
| Discount | 0% | 10% | 20% | 25% |
| Price per book | $19.95 | $17.95 | $15.95 | $14.95 |
| + S & H | | | | |
| Total price **per** book | **$24.00** | **$21.00** | **$18.00** | **$16.00** |

Send cheque or money order or call with VISA or MC to:

**New World Publishing**
P.O. Box 36075, Halifax, Nova Scotia, Canada B3J 3S9
Tel:  (902) 466-0000 or 466-5000  Fax: (902) 466-0005
Toll free orders: 1-877-211-3334    E-mail: sales@newworldpublishing.com
Website: www.newworldpublishing.com

# Publications to Improve Your Health and Your Life

## Judit Rajhathy Live! (audio) ISBN 1-895814-07-3 $17.97CAD/$14.95 USD

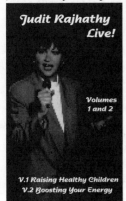

Double boxed set of audio cassettes on family health and wellness, recorded live by health educator and practitioner Judit Rajhathy, author of the Canadian best-seller *Free to Fly: a journey toward wellness*. It is the perfect learning tool as you drive to and from work or while running errands. Based on issues similar to those found in *Free to Fly*, these tapes are often used as a focal point for discussions with colleagues in the staff room or office; as a personal *aide memoire*; or with family members and friends who do not have time to read or attend workshops, but who need to hear this important information. This double set contains Volumes 1 and 2 described immediately below. The total running time for both volumes is 3 1/4 hours.

## Raising Healthy Children (audio)ISBN 1-895814-06-5 $11.95CAD/$9.95 USD

The focus of Volume1 is on children's health, including allergies, food sensitivities, chronic ear infections, colic, asthma, eczema, attention and behavioral problems, including ADD/ADHD and more! Run time: 90 minutes.

## Boosting Your Energy (audio) ISBN 1-895814-08-1 $11.95CAD/$9.95 USD

The focus of Volume 2 is on adult health including allergies, food sensitivities, chronic fatigue, headaches, depression, digestive and bowel disorders, yeast infections, PMS, sinusitis, asthma and lots more! Run time: 105 minutes.

## AEHA Guide to less toxic products (paper, 134 pp.) ISBN 0-9681359-0-0

Save money and time! The research has been done for you by theAllegy and Environmental Health Association (N.S. Branch) They have produced an inexpensive and invaluable guide for locating unscented personal care products, safer cleaning products, information on pest control and indoor air quality devices, low toxic building materials and school supplies. The final section lists sources for products in the Guide which strongly supports those sold in healthfood stores, wholefood markets and selected food outlets.   **Price: $6.95 CAD/$5.95USD**

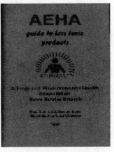

## George, the friendy dragon (E.T.Matthews) (40 pages; perfect/laminated)
### ISBN 1-895814-02-2 $15.95 CAD/$12.95 USD

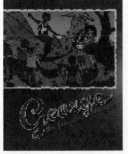

A heart warming tale by story-teller E.T. Matthews about tolerance and self-esteem for children. It's about being different and the struggle to be yourself. Bright, colorful characters dance from page to page, speaking and singing in rhyme - a guaranteed hit with both young and old. It is also a high quality production in three parts which can be read over several nights to younger children. Read to thousands of school children in the Maritimes, it contains bold and enchanting illustrations by Halifax artist Gizelle Erdei.

# More Books from New World Publishing

**An Unfortunate Likeness**...(Anna Careless)(140 pp., 6x9, illust., perfect, lam.)
©1998   ISBN 1-895814-05-7    $12.95 CAD/ $9.95 USD

A novel of romance and the supernatural where a vengeful act of the past plays itself out in the present - one that spans over a century in time and a thousand kilometers in distance. The crucial link is the incredible physical similarity between a young woman and her great-great-grandmother. Set in a small coastal town, this second novel by Anna Careless combines romance, intimacy and suspense in an intriguing struggle between the powers of darkness and unconditional love. Cover by well known maritime artist Laurie Mireau.

**Where the Fishermen Sing** ...... (Anna Careless) (198 pp., 6x9, perfect, laminated)
©1992   ISBN 0-921165-21-8    $14.95 CAD/ $10.95 USD

Anna's first novel of romance. A rather grim upbringing, convent school, several changes of location and time, and a cruel twist of fate combine to keep you in suspense until the conclusion of the story - one in which the heroine must discover something within herself to be complete. Contains original poems written and published by Anna in the 1980s. Cover by Michaela Ford.

**Leslie Braes** ...........(Murray Shoolbraid)(54 pp., 8 1/2 x 11, coil, annotated)
ISBN1-895814-03-0        $15.95 CAD/$12.95 USD

Sixty original compositions by the Scottish-born Canadian composer, writer and musician, Murray Shoolbraid. These are the best of over 400 works written and revised by Murray over 30 years and spanning two continents. It contains more than a dozen each of traditional Scottish-style jigs and reels, eight strathspeys, plus several airs and laments, schottische, two-steps and waltzes; as well as 17 other tunes arranged in five Scottish Country Dance Sets. For dance groups, as well as for those who play the violin, mandolin or accordion. Cover photo and sketch by Kirstie Shoolbraid.

## Mail-Order Option

Many of these books are stocked by bookstores and healthfood stores. If you cannot find the books you want, please ask you local bookseller to order them from the publisher for you. If there are no local bookstores in your area, you may purchase copies directly from the publisher at competitive prices. Please contact the publisher in writing or **call our toll free number, or fax or e-mail us at the addresses and numbers listed on the preceeding pages (pp. 326-8). Payment by cheque, VISA or MasterCard available.** Mail-order prices are listed in Canadian and USA dollars. Shipping rates are in Canadian dollars for Canada; US dollars for the United States. For rates for other countries, contact the publisher.

### Mail-Order Shipping Costs (GST included, if applicable):

The mailing address is listed on both pages 326 and 328. Please add shipping costs from the chart below to obtain your total cost:

```
... on an order of  $5.95 or less .............. $2.00
        - from $6.00 to $15.95 .............. $3.00
        - from $16.00 to $47.90 ............. $4.00
        - on orders of $48.00 or more ....... FREE
```

## Schools, Libraries, Professional Associations:

In addition, discounts are offered to selected groups who wish to purchase multiple copies of the books listed on these pages. These discounts apply to libraries, schools, health, self-help and environmental groups, or professional associations. Contact the publisher for current rates and shipping costs. Our publications are shipped world-wide.